Contemporary Approaches to Urinary Diversion and Reconstruction

Editor

MICHAEL S. COOKSON

UROLOGIC CLINICS
OF NORTH AMERICA

www.urologic.theclinics.com

Consulting Editor
SAMIR S. TANEJA

February 2018 • Volume 45 • Number 1

ELSEVIER

1600 John F. Kennedy Boulevard • Suite 1800 • Philadelphia, Pennsylvania, 19103-2899

http://www.theclinics.com

UROLOGIC CLINICS OF NORTH AMERICA Volume 45, Number 1
February 2018 ISSN 0094-0143, ISBN-13: 978-0-323-57006-0

Editor: Kerry Holland
Developmental Editor: Sara Watkins

Urologic Clinics of North America (ISSN 0094-0143) is published quarterly by Elsevier Inc., 360 Park Avenue South, New York, NY 10010-1710. Months of issue are February, May, August, and November. Business and Editorial Offices: 1600 John F. Kennedy Blvd., Suite 1800, Philadelphia, PA 19103-2899. Periodicals postage paid at New York, NY and additional mailing offices. Subscription prices are $374.00 per year (US individuals), $721.00 per year (US institutions), $100.00 per year (US students and residents), $431.00 per year (Canadian individuals), $901.00 per year (Canadian institutions), $515.00 per year (foreign individuals), $901.00 per year (foreign institutions), and $240.00 per year (Canadian and foreign students/residents). Foreign air speed delivery is included in all *Clinics* subscription prices. All prices are subject to change without notice. **POSTMASTER:** Send address changes to *Urologic Clinics of North America*, Elsevier Health Sciences Division, Subscription Customer Service, 3251 Riverport Lane, Maryland Heights, MO 63043. **Customer Service: 1-800-654-2452 (US). From outside the United States, call 1-314-447-8871. Fax: 1-314-447-8029. E-mail: JournalsCustomerServiceusa@elsevier.com (for print support) and JournalsOnlineSupport-usa@elsevier.com (for online support).**

Reprints. For copies of 100 or more, of articles in this publication, please contact the Commercial Reprints Department, Elsevier Inc., 360 Park Avenue South, New York, New York 10010-1710. Tel.: 212-633-3874; Fax: 212-633-3820; E-mail: reprints@elsevier.com.

Urologic Clinics of North America is covered in MEDLINE/PubMed (*Index Medicus*), *Excerpta Medica, Current Contents/Clinical Medicine, Science Citation Index,* and *ISI/BIOMED.*

PROGRAM OBJECTIVE

The goal of *Urologic Clinics of North America* is to keep practicing urologists and urology residents up to date with current clinical practice in urology by providing timely articles reviewing the state of the art in patient care.

TARGET AUDIENCE

Practicing urologists, urology residents and other healthcare professionals practicing in the discipline of urology.

LEARNING OBJECTIVES

Upon completion of this activity, participants will be able to:
1. Review preoperative considerations in urinary diversion and reconstruction.
2. Discuss urinary diversion procedures in adult and pediatric populations.
3. Recognize potential metabolic, nutritional, and other secondary consequences to urinary diversion and reconstruction.

ACCREDITATION

The Elsevier Office of Continuing Medical Education (EOCME) is accredited by the Accreditation Council for Continuing Medical Education (ACCME) to provide continuing medical education for physicians.

The EOCME designates this enduring material for a maximum of 15 *AMA PRA Category 1 Credit*(s)™. Physicians should claim only the credit commensurate with the extent of their participation in the activity.

All other healthcare professionals requesting continuing education credit for this enduring material will be issued a certificate of participation.

DISCLOSURE OF CONFLICTS OF INTEREST

The EOCME assesses conflict of interest with its instructors, faculty, planners, and other individuals who are in a position to control the content of CME activities. All relevant conflicts of interest that are identified are thoroughly vetted by EOCME for fair balance, scientific objectivity, and patient care recommendations. EOCME is committed to providing its learners with CME activities that promote improvements or quality in healthcare and not a specific proprietary business or a commercial interest.

The planning committee, staff, authors and editors listed below have identified no financial relationships or relationships to products or devices they or their spouse/life partner have with commercial interest related to the content of this CME activity:

Christopher B. Anderson, MD, MPH; Janet E. Bacck Kukreja, MD, MPH; Bernard H. Bochner, MD; Jeffrey D. Browning, MD; Sam S. Chang, MD, MBA; Alice Crane, MD, PhD; Siamak Daneshmand, MD; Timothy F. Donahue, MD; Mohamed Eltemamy, MD; Anjali Fortna; Scott M. Gilbert, MD, MS, FACS; Jessie R. Gills, MD; David A. Goldfarb, MD; Kerry Holland; Jeffrey M. Holzbeierlein, MD, FACS; Scott C. Johnson, MD; Ashish M. Kamat, MD, MBBS, FACS; Michael O. Koch, MD; Daniel J. Lee, MD; Roger Li, MD; Leah Logan; Matthew D. Lyons, MD; James M. McKiernan, MD; Sanjay Patel, MD; Shane M. Pearce, MD; Eugene J. Pietzak, MD; Raj S. Pruthi, MD; Joshua D. Roth, MD; Bryan S. Sak, MD; Eila C. Skinner, MD; Zachary L. Smith, MD; Elysia Sophie Spencer, MD; Gary D. Steinberg, MD; Heidi A. Stephany, MD; Tyler M. Thress, MD; Mark D. Tyson, MD; Vignesh Viswanathan; Dimitar V. Zlatev, MD.

The planning committee, staff, authors and editors listed below have identified financial relationships or relationships to products or devices they or their spouse/life partner have with commercial interest related to the content of this CME activity:

Michael S. Cookson, MD, MMHC, FACS is a is a consultant/advisor for Astellas Pharma US, Inc.; Myovant Sciences; TesoRx LLC; MDx Health; Janssen Global Services, LLC; and Pacific Edge.

UNAPPROVED/OFF-LABEL USE DISCLOSURE

The EOCME requires CME faculty to disclose to the participants:
1. When products or procedures being discussed are off-label, unlabelled, experimental, and/or investigational (not US Food and Drug Administration [FDA] approved); and
2. Any limitations on the information presented, such as data that are preliminary or that represent ongoing research, interim analyses, and/or unsupported opinions. Faculty may discuss information about pharmaceutical agents that is outside of FDA-approved labelling. This information is intended solely for CME and is not intended to promote off-label use of these medications. If you have any questions, contact the medical affairs department of the manufacturer for the most recent prescribing information.

TO ENROLL

To enroll in the *Urologic Clinics of North America* Continuing Medical Education program, call customer service at 1-800-654-2452 or sign up online at http://www.theclinics.com/home/cme. The CME program is available to subscribers for an additional annual fee of USD $270.

METHOD OF PARTICIPATION

In order to claim credit, participants must complete the following:

1. Complete enrolment as indicated above.
2. Read the activity.
3. Complete the CME Test and Evaluation. Participants must achieve a score of 70% on the test. All CME Tests and Evaluations must be completed online.

CME INQUIRIES/SPECIAL NEEDS

For all CME inquiries or special needs, please contact elsevierCME@elsevier.com.

Contributors

CONSULTING EDITOR

SAMIR S. TANEJA, MD
The James M. Neissa and Janet Riha Neissa
Professor of Urologic Oncology, Professor of
Urology and Radiology, Director, Division of
Urologic Oncology, Co-Director, Department
of Urology, Smilow Comprehensive Prostate
Cancer Center, NYU Langone Medical Center,
New York, New York

EDITOR

MICHAEL S. COOKSON, MD, MMHC, FACS
Professor and Chairman, Department
of Urology, The University of Oklahoma
Health Sciences Center, Oklahoma City,
Oklahoma

AUTHORS

CHRISTOPHER B. ANDERSON, MD, MPH
Assistant Professor, Department of Urology,
Columbia University Medical Center, New
York, New York

JANET E. BAACK KUKREJA, MD, MPH
Fellow, Department of Urology, The University
of Texas MD Anderson Cancer Center,
Houston, Texas

BERNARD H. BOCHNER, MD
Urology Service, Department of Surgery,
Memorial Sloan Kettering Cancer Center, New
York, New York

JEFFREY D. BROWNING, MD
Resident, Department of Urology, University of
Pittsburgh Medical Center, Pittsburgh,
Pennsylvania

SAM S. CHANG, MD, MBA
Department of Urologic Surgery, Vanderbilt
University Medical Center, Nashville,
Tennessee

MICHAEL S. COOKSON, MD, MMHC, FACS
Professor and Chairman, Department of
Urology, The University of Oklahoma Health
Sciences Center, Oklahoma City, Oklahoma

ALICE CRANE, MD, PhD
Glickman Urological & Kidney Institute,
Cleveland Clinic, Cleveland, Ohio

SIAMAK DANESHMAND, MD
Associate Professor of Urology (Clinical
Scholar), Director of Urologic Oncology,
Director of Clinical Research, Urologic
Oncology Fellowship Director, USC Norris
Comprehensive Cancer Center, Institute of
Urology, Los Angeles, California

TIMOTHY F. DONAHUE, MD
Urology Service, Department of Surgery,
Memorial Sloan Kettering Cancer Center, New
York, New York

MOHAMED ELTEMAMY, MD
Glickman Urological & Kidney Institute,
Cleveland Clinic, Cleveland, Ohio

SCOTT M. GILBERT, MD, MS, FACS
Associate Member, Departments of
Genitourinary Oncology and Health Outcomes
and Behavior, Moffitt Cancer Center and
Research Institute, Tampa, Florida

JESSIE R. GILLS, MD
University of Kansas Medical Center, Kansas
City, Kansas

DAVID A. GOLDFARB, MD
Professor of Surgery, Cleveland Clinic Lerner
College of Medicine, Glickman Urological &
Kidney Institute, Cleveland Clinic, Cleveland,
Ohio

JEFFREY M. HOLZBEIERLEIN, MD, FACS
Department of Urology, University of Kansas
Medical Center, Kansas City, Kansas

SCOTT C. JOHNSON, MD
Urologic Oncology Fellow, Department of
Surgery, Section of Urology, The University of
Chicago, Chicago, Illinois

ASHISH M. KAMAT, MD, MBBS, FACS
Professor, Department of Urology, The
University of Texas MD Anderson Cancer
Center, Houston, Texas

MICHAEL O. KOCH, MD
Chairman and Professor of Urology, Indiana
University School of Medicine, Indianapolis,
Indiana

DANIEL J. LEE, MD
Department of Urologic Surgery, Vanderbilt
University Medical Center, Nashville,
Tennessee

ROGER LI, MD
Fellow, Department of Urology, The University
of Texas MD Anderson Cancer Center,
Houston, Texas

MATTHEW D. LYONS, MD
Resident Physician, Department of Urology,
The University of North Carolina at Chapel Hill,
Chapel Hill, North Carolina

JAMES M. McKIERNAN, MD
John K. Lattimer Professor and
Chairman, Department of Urology, Columbia
University Medical Center, New York,
New York

SANJAY PATEL, MD
Assistant Professor, Department of Urology,
The University of Oklahoma Health Sciences
Center, Oklahoma City, Oklahoma

SHANE M. PEARCE, MD
Urologic Oncology Fellow, Clinical
Instructor, USC Norris Comprehensive Cancer
Center, Institute of Urology, Los Angeles,
California

EUGENE J. PIETZAK, MD
Urology Service, Department of Surgery,
Memorial Sloan Kettering Cancer Center, New
York, New York

RAJ S. PRUTHI, MD
Department of Urology, John Rhodes
Distinguished Professor of Urology,
Department of Urology, The University of North
Carolina at Chapel Hill, Chapel Hill, North
Carolina

JOSHUA D. ROTH, MD
Department of Urology, Indiana University
School of Medicine, Indianapolis, Indiana

BRYAN S. SACK, MD
Research Fellow in Surgery, Department of
Urology, Boston Children's Hospital, Boston,
Massachusetts

EILA C. SKINNER, MD
Professor and Chair, Department of Urology,
Stanford School of Medicine, Stanford
University Hospital and Clinics, Stanford,
California

ZACHARY L. SMITH, MD
Urologic Oncology Fellow, Department of
Surgery, Section of Urology, The University of
Chicago, Chicago, Illinois

ELYSIA SOPHIA SPENCER, MD
Resident Physician, Department of Urology,
The University of North Carolina at Chapel Hill,
Chapel Hill, North Carolina

GARY D. STEINBERG, MD
Professor of Surgery, Director of Urologic
Oncology, Department of Surgery, Section of
Urology, The University of Chicago, Chicago,
Illinois

HEIDI A. STEPHANY, MD
Assistant Professor of Urology, University of California, Irvine and Children's Hospital of Orange County, Orange, California

TYLER M. THRESS, MD
Resident Physician, PGY-5, Department of Urology, The University of Oklahoma Health Sciences Center, Oklahoma City, Oklahoma

MARK D. TYSON, MD
Department of Urologic Surgery, Vanderbilt University Medical Center, Nashville, Tennessee

DIMITAR V. ZLATEV, MD
Department of Urology, Stanford School of Medicine, Stanford University Hospital and Clinics, Stanford, California

Contents

Patient selection and preoperative counseling are critical aspects of determining which urinary diversion to perform and should be emphasized at each stage of preoperative planning. The surgeon must have a thorough understanding of the patient's disease process, functional and psycho-emotional status, and social support network so that they can set appropriate expectations. It is also crucial to have a multidisciplinary team of individuals who are experienced with all aspects of urinary diversion care, including ostomy nurses, nurse navigators, and urologic surgeons skilled at teaching and trouble-shooting self-catheterization for continent cutaneous diversion and orthotopic diversion in the setting of hypercontinence.

Patients undergoing urinary diversion are at high risk for complications in the perioperative period. The exact cause of these complications remains poorly defined but is likely multifactorial. Current efforts to optimize patients in the perioperative period, including prehabilitation, smoking cessation, recognition and treatment of comorbid conditions and malnutrition, immunonutrition supplementation, carbohydrate loading, and prevention of known complications and implementation of enhanced recovery after surgery pathways, seem beneficial in helping to improve outcomes in this at-risk population. Further studies (some of which are ongoing) are necessary to help optimize these strategies and identify which modifiable factors have the greatest impact.

Intestinal segments in various forms have been used to reconstruct the urinary tract since the mid-1800s. Currently, many different forms of continent and incontinent diversion options exist. Incorporating bowel mucosa within the urinary tract leads to predictable metabolic and nutritional consequences. The use of ileum or colon can cause a hyperchloremic metabolic acidosis, vitamin B12 deficiency, osteoporosis, fat malabsorption, urinary calculi, and ammoniagenic encephalopathy. Due to metabolic and nutritional consequences associated with the use of jejunum and gastric segments, the use of these bowel segments is not recommended.

Surgical Complications of Urinary Diversion

Christopher B. Anderson and James M. McKiernan

Urinary diversion (UD) with an intestinal segment has significant risks of short-term and long-term complications. With modern reporting criteria, understanding of the true prevalence and spectrum of these complications has improved. Methods to minimize early postoperative complications include enhanced recovery pathways, restricted intraoperative fluid protocols, and referral to high-volume centers. With long-term follow-up after UD, the risk of complications steadily rises. Late surgical complications include ureterointestinal anastomotic strictures, urolithiasis, and stomal issues. Patients with UDs require close surveillance to monitor for anatomic, infectious, and metabolic complications, and surgeons who perform UD should be aware of the risk and timing of postoperative complications.

Secondary Tumors After Urinary Diversion

Roger Li, Janet E. Baack Kukreja, and Ashish M. Kamat

It has been known that urinary diversions juxtaposing the urinary and intestinal tracts lead to increased incidence of secondary malignancies. Although tumorigenesis in ureterosigmoidostomies follows the typical course from adenomas to adenocarcinomas, secondary malignancies arising from isolated intestinal diversions are much more heterogeneous. Research over the past half century has unveiled patterns of incidence and progression, while also uncovering possible mechanisms driving the neoplastic changes. In this review, we summarize the current understanding of these unique tumors, with the hope that the knowledge gained may shed light on the etiologies of other cancers arising from the urinary and intestinal tracts.

Quality of Life and Urinary Diversion

Scott M. Gilbert

Health-related quality-of-life outcomes after urinary diversion vary significantly. Preserving and even improving health-related quality of life are highly relevant to urinary diversion. Life after urinary diversion is fundamentally different from before.

Urinary Diversion in Renal Transplantation

Mohamed Eltemamy, Alice Crane, and David A. Goldfarb

Renal transplantation involving anatomically or functionally altered recipient urinary reservoirs is a challenging procedure. Initial reports discouraged kidney transplantation in patients with urinary diversion due to inferior outcomes. However, more recent studies have shown that although there are more infectious complications, patients with urinary diversions have comparable long-term graft survival with those with native anatomy. Careful preoperative assessment of these candidates is mandatory. Unique technical and surgical concepts must be considered before embarking on transplanting this specific cohort of kidney transplantation candidates.

Advances in Pediatric Urinary Diversion

Jeffrey D. Browning and Heidi A. Stephany

Pediatric urinary diversion is performed for a unique set of indications with many options to consider. Although surgical intervention has decreased in necessity overall

UROLOGIC CLINICS OF NORTH AMERICA

THE CLINICS ARE AVAILABLE ONLINE!
Access your subscription at:
www.theclinics.com

Foreword

Re-Creating the Urinary Tract: An Art Derived from Science

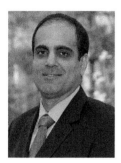

Samir S. Taneja, MD
Consulting Editor

The evolution of urinary diversion following radical cystectomy, or in bypass of a dysfunctional lower tract, has followed the lines of other surgical innovation: first a recognition of the need and desire to provide alternate options to conduit diversion; then an understanding of physiology and the functional storage limitations of tubularized bowel as well as other autologous or heterologous substitutes; then implementation of novel surgical techniques for re-creating the bladder; then recognition of the metabolic limitations of urinary storage in bowel; and finally, refined techniques to maximize function, minimize metabolic and functional derangement, and preserve quality of life. Along the way, surgeons learned from trial, error, complications, and oversights, and from this emerged the contemporary state-of-the-art.

As time goes on, efforts toward further innovation are underway, including the identification of alternate materials for bladder substitution, devising minimally invasive methods for urinary diversion, and understanding the relationship of urinary reconstruction and quality of life. The art of urinary reconstruction has evolved into a rigorous science, with preoperative assessment, patient optimization, and methodical repetition of process serving to improve outcomes for the individual patient. In this issue of *Urologic Clinics*, edited by Dr Michael Cookson, the contemporary science and art of urinary diversion are presented in comprehensive fashion. Dr Cookson has compiled an integrated spectrum of articles, authored by the top experts in the field, covering all the essential considerations in managing patients at the time of urinary reconstruction following bladder removal. For the practicing urologist, and even those not performing urinary diversion, this is a fantastic update on the topic that will serve as an essential tool in counseling patients. I am deeply indebted to Dr Cookson and all of the contributing authors for their generosity of time and their diligence in creating such a high-level resource.

Samir S. Taneja, MD
Division of Urologic Oncology
Smilow Comprehensive Prostate Cancer Center
Department of Urology
NYU Langone Medical Center
150 East 32nd Street, Suite 200
New York, NY 10016, USA

E-mail address:
samir.taneja@nyumc.org

Urol Clin N Am 45 (2018) xv
https://doi.org/10.1016/j.ucl.2017.11.001
0094-0143/17/© 2017 Published by Elsevier Inc.

Preface

Urinary Diversion: Nutritional Evolution and Surgical Revolution

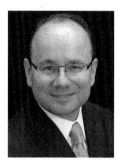

Michael S. Cookson, MD, MMHC, FACS
Editor

The field of urinary diversion continues to evolve. We as a specialty are pushing the envelope in terms of technical expertise with laparoscopic and robotic-assisted surgery, and we are in constant search of the holy grail of bowel replacement through research endeavors and tissue engineering. We are now faced with not only the technical challenges of often complex surgical reconstruction but also the burden of counseling patients on the known complications of these diversions and their impact on a patient's health-related quality of life (HRQOL).

In this issue of *Urology Clinics*, we review the field of urinary diversion from a very broad and comprehensive standpoint. Leaders in the field share both their clinical and their translational research, attempting to help surgeons in the clinical management of patients undergoing urinary diversion in a rapidly evolving field.

To accomplish our goal, we review not only patient selection and the types of urinary diversion but also the metabolic and surgical complications that may accompany these reconstructive procedures. Taking it back one step, we also review the evolving concept of perioperative preparation and immunonutrition and its importance in reducing complications and improving clinical outcomes prior to radical cystectomy and urinary diversion.

All aspects of urinary diversion were covered, including orthotopic urinary diversion in men and women. In addition, continent cutaneous diversion and conduit urinary diversion were reviewed. In addition to choice of bowel segments, the surgical approach, including the current status of laparoscopic robotic-assisted or intracorporeal diversion, is covered. Special circumstances, including urinary diversion in transplant patients and in children, are also discussed in this issue.

The impact of urinary diversion on HRQOL is better understood. Improvements in methodology and improved instruments to measure HRQOL are now being applied at baseline and in subsequent long-term follow-up. And, the impact of long-term oncologic concerns on the risk of secondary tumors that arise in the setting of urinary diversion is discussed.

I would like to thank the authors for their outstanding contributions to this issue and hope that this will serve as a reference for surgeons who evaluate, treat, and follow patients with urinary diversions. I would also like to thank my wife, Kimberly, and my children, Caroline, Connor, and Cooper, for their support and understanding of these academic endeavors.

Michael S. Cookson, MD, MMHC, FACS
Department of Urology
University of Oklahoma Health Sciences Center
920 Stanton L. Young Boulevard
WP 3150
Oklahoma City, OK 73104, USA

E-mail address:
michael-cookson@ouhsc.edu

Urol Clin N Am 45 (2018) xvii
https://doi.org/10.1016/j.ucl.2017.10.001
0094-0143/18/© 2017 Published by Elsevier Inc.

Patient Selection and Counseling for Urinary Diversion

Elysia Sophia Spencer, MD, Matthew D. Lyons, MD,
Raj S. Pruthi, MD*

KEYWORDS

- Urinary diversion • Ileal conduit • Continent urinary diversion • Orthotopic neobladder
- Continent cutaneous diversion • Patient selection • Preop counseling

KEY POINTS

- Incontinent diversions should be offered to all patients and recommended for those with comorbidities precluding a continent diversion and inability or unwillingness to perform self-catheterization.
- Patients should be counseled regarding the impact of a urostomy and should have access to a skilled ostomy care team.
- Orthotopic neobladder should be offered to all patients without an absolute contraindication due to preserved body image and potential for volitional voiding.
- Continent cutaneous diversion is a good option for patients who are not candidates for orthotopic diversions but desire a continent diversion and preservation of body image.
- Patient selection for continent cutaneous diversion is critical because failure to perform regular self-catheterization may result in life-threatening complications.

INTRODUCTION

Modern urinary diversions (UD) are globally categorized as either "incontinent" or "continent." The most commonly performed incontinent diversions use the distal ileum or the colon for the conduit. Cutaneous ureterostomies and pyelocutaneous stomas are less commonly used and are typically reserved for the pediatric and young adult population or for rare clinical scenarios in adults. Advantages of conduits include the relative ease of surgical technique, shorter operative times, and the elimination of the need for self-catheterization because of the passive nature of drainage.[1] However, the presence of a stoma and external appliance can be cosmetically unappealing and negatively affect body image.[1,2]

Continent diversions (CDs) can be further subdivided into orthotopic and nonorthotopic reservoirs. Orthotopic diversions (OD) use detubularized bowel to construct a reservoir, which is attached to the proximal urethral stump. Le Duc and colleagues[3] described the first OD in a male patient in 1979; however, the first female OD was not performed until the 1990s.[4] The advantage of the orthotopic neobladder (ONB) is its cosmetic, anatomic, and functional resemblance to the native bladder. Some experts advocate OD as the gold-standard therapy for all appropriately selected patients.[4]

Nonorthotopic reservoirs are continent cutaneous urinary diversions that were developed in the early twentieth century and initially varied greatly in terms of technique and bowel segment

Disclosure: The authors have nothing they wish to disclose.
Department of Urology, University of North Carolina at Chapel Hill, Chapel Hill, NC, USA
* Corresponding author. Department of Urology, University of North Carolina at Chapel Hill, 170 Manning Drive, 2115 Physicians Office Building, CB#7235, Chapel Hill, NC 27599-7235.
E-mail address: rpruthi@med.unc.edu

Urol Clin N Am 45 (2018) 1–9
https://doi.org/10.1016/j.ucl.2017.09.001
0094-0143/18/© 2017 Elsevier Inc. All rights reserved.

urologic.theclinics.com

used.[4,5] Most were associated with high complication rates, preventing widespread adoption.[4] Over time, several reliable techniques were developed making continent cutaneous diversion (CCD) more common.[4,6–10] CCD precludes the need for an external appliance, making it more cosmetically acceptable. However, CCD remains technically challenging and requires a mastery of several different surgical techniques and comfort with bowel anatomy.[4] Also, despite recent improvements, CCDs remain associated with the highest complication rates of all UDs and are therefore not widely used.

Given the diversity of available options for UD, the surgeon must decide which to perform based on the clinical scenario, patient-related factors, and impact on patient quality of life (QoL). As such, patient selection and preoperative counseling are critical aspects of diversion selection.

INDICATIONS FOR URINARY DIVERSION

Indications for diversion involve clinical scenarios in which the native bladder poses a serious threat to a patient's long-term survival or QoL. Most broadly, these indications can be categorized as malignant or benign. Overall, the most common indication for undergoing UD is high-grade muscle-invasive bladder cancer requiring radical cystectomy.

Malignant

Cystectomy with UD is the gold-standard treatment for patients with muscle invasive urothelial cell carcinoma of the bladder or nonmuscle invasive cancer with poor prognostic features. Less commonly, urothelial cell carcinoma of the urethra may be an indication for cystectomy with urethrectomy and UD. Other nongenitourinary malignancies such as locally invasive colorectal or gynecologic cancers may necessitate pelvic exenteration and also require diversion of the urine following cystectomy.

Benign

Benign indications for UD encompass a more diverse set of conditions in which first-line treatments typically involve conservative nonsurgical management. Surgical diversion is reserved for situations in which less invasive medical management has failed. Indications for surgical intervention include preservation of renal function, intractable gross hematuria, recurrent severe infections, medically refractory urinary incontinence, elimination of the need for a permanent indwelling catheter, and rarely, chronic pelvic pain.

INCONTINENT URINARY DIVERSIONS
Conduit Diversion

Procedure
Conduit diversions are constructed using a short segment of bowel that passively diverts urine from the upper urinary tract through the abdominal wall where the urine drains into an external urostomy appliance. Conduits are most often made from the distal ileum and less commonly from colon. Historically, jejunum and stomach were used for creation of a conduit; however, these were found to be associated with unacceptable metabolic derangement, risk of secondary malignancies, and other complications, and their utilization was largely abandoned. Typically, the terminal 10 to 15 cm of ileum are spared to prevent malabsorption of vitamin B12, fat-soluble vitamins, and bile salts.

Patient selection
Ileal conduit (IC) is the gold standard of incontinent diversions and is the default for patients who are not candidates for a continent diversion (CD).[2,4] ICs are the most commonly performed UD because of the familiar anatomy and relatively straightforward surgical technique.[1,2] These advantages translate into lower complication rates and operative times.[1,2,4] Conduits demand less rigorous, long-term care than CDs and are associated with lower rates of metabolic derangements.[11]

Patients who are not candidates for a CD typically default to an IC. ICs eliminate the need for self-catheterization, which make them the preferred option for patients with physical or mental impairment, poor dexterity, advanced age, or poor motivation, or those who are unwilling to perform clean intermittent self-catheterization (CISC).[2] In addition, it is the preferred diversion in the setting of severe renal or hepatic dysfunction. There are multiple relative contraindications to CDs that do not preclude construction of an IC (**Table 1**).

Table 1 Absolute and relative contraindications to continent urinary diversions	
Absolute Contraindications	**Relative Contraindications**
Renal insufficiency	Advanced age
Hepatic insufficiency	Multiple comorbidities
Inability to independently perform CISC	Prior pelvic radiation
	Inflammatory or malignant bowel disease
Unwillingness to perform CISC	Need for adjuvant chemotherapy

Accordingly, it is a good option for patients with a positive urethral margin, urethral abnormality, prior pelvic radiation, or bowel disease, and those at high risk for local recurrence, regional metastases, or need for adjuvant chemotherapy.[2]

Use of the ileum for formation of a conduit is not recommended in patients with short bowel syndrome, inflammatory small bowel disease, or extensive prior radiation to the ileum, most commonly as a result of prior pelvic malignancy.[12] Use of colon for diversion formation is often preferable in these clinical scenarios. The main disadvantage of IC is the presence of a stoma and need for an external appliance that can negatively affect a patient's body image and cause functional constraints.[1,2] Each type of diversion is associated with its own lifestyle adjustments and learning curve. Patients with an IC must adapt to wearing and changing a urostomy appliance, manage skin irritation, troubleshoot sleeping with a bag, and often deal with stomal retraction and parastomal hernias.[13]

Preoperative counseling

The principal goal in selecting a UD type is to attain the highest QoL while maintaining the lowest complication rate and balancing therapeutic targets.[2] Urinary diversion selection is a complex decision process, which must take into account a patient's comorbidities and functional status, cancer stage and future treatments, and patient preference with regards to QoL.[2] It is important to remember that what the physician perceives as the right UD for the patient may not be what the patient desires.[13] It is critical to elicit and clarify the patient's expectations of undergoing a UD and thoroughly counsel the patient preoperatively on the risks, side effects, postoperative rehabilitation, and long-term maintenance associated with each type of diversion.[4]

Although patient desire is important, this is only one factor in a complex clinical decision-making pathway. There are contraindications to CDs and utilization of bowel segments that may supersede patient preferences. It is important to counsel patients preoperatively that anatomic variance and other intraoperative findings can necessitate creation of a different type of diversion than planned.[2] An enterostomal nurse specialist can assist in the decision-making process by further educating the patient and their family on long-term functional outcomes after UD and provide preoperative stomal marking in the event that a conduit is required.[2]

Functional outcomes

Most studies that have evaluated QoL outcomes following IC formation versus CDs fail to demonstrate a difference in overall QoL.[2] One recent meta-analysis of 18 nonrandomized studies evaluating the pooled effect sizes of combined QoL following cystectomy with IC versus ONB found a trend toward slightly improved QoL for patients who underwent ONB; however, this did not reach significance.[14] However, subgroup analysis found significantly better QoL in those with ONB.[14] These results are limited by the retrospective nature, lack of randomization, and the fact that, in general, patients undergoing ONB were younger and healthier, which may confound QoL findings.[2] Prospective and randomized controlled trials using validated UD-specific QoL are needed in the future to further clarify differences in QoL.[2]

Complications

There is significant variability among the published rates of short- and long-term morbidity following UD. Morbidities within the first 30 days range from 20% to 56%, whereas long-term morbidity beyond 30 days varies between 28% and 94%.[15–17] Complications associated with diversions are typically unique to the diversion type and can be broadly categorized as related to bowel, conduit or reservoir type, stoma, or ureteroenteric anastomosis.[18]

Although ICs are generally perceived to be associated with comparatively low complication rates, there are still relatively high rates of short- and long-term complications. Sicker patients with more comorbidities are more likely to be offered IC in order to decrease operative time and surgical risks. As a result, the reported surgical complication rates associated with conduits approach that of CDs used in a healthier patient population.[2]

The most frequent complications associated with conduits are renal insufficiency, stomal and bowel problems, urinary tract infections (UTIs), ureteroenteric anastomotic or ureteral obstruction, and urinary calculi.[15,19] Stomal issues are the most common complications specific to conduits. Parastomal hernias, stomal retraction, and stenosis are often encountered, whereas stomal obstruction, necrosis, and prolapse occur less frequently.[18] Bowel complications can occur early or late in the postoperative period and typically result from issues with the bowel resection or anastomosis, such as prolonged ileus, bowel obstruction, anastomotic leak or breakdown, and enteric fistula.[18] Conduit complications may include retraction, elongation, ischemia, and necrosis. Ureteroenteric anastomotic stricture or breakdown can be one of the most challenging complications of ICs to manage.[20] The introduction and routine use of modern double J ureteral stents have significantly reduced the incidence of ureteroenteric anastomotic leaks to approximately 2% and strictures to 4%.[18]

Special considerations

Colon can be used to construct a conduit. Overall complication rates are similar to conduits constructed of ileum within properly selected patients.[15,21–23] However, the thicker bowel and larger circumference may result in higher rates of ureterocolonic obstruction and urinary retention.[4] Transverse colon can be used for a conduit in patients who have extensive prior pelvic radiation with exposure of the ileum. In the case of a pelvic exenteration with diverting colostomy, sigmoid colon conduit is often desirable as it obviates a bowel anastomosis. In addition, a sigmoid conduit is ideal for scenarios in which a left-sided stoma is preferable. Ileocecal conduit with a long segment of ileum can be used to make up distance when extended segments of ureter require replacement.[12] Contraindications to the use of colon conduits include inflammatory disease of the large bowel and severe chronic diarrhea.[12]

Cutaneous ureterostomy may be employed when use of a bowel segment is absolutely contraindicated and is most often used in the pediatric population. A stenosis rate greater than 50% and difficulty with pouching limit the applicability of this procedure.[4,24]

Summary

Incontinent diversions should be implemented in patients with significant medical comorbidities precluding them from CD, as well as those unable or unwilling to self-catheterize. Patients should be counseled extensively regarding the long-term physical and psychosocial impact of a urostomy and should have access to a skilled ostomy care team to help them transition to life with a stoma.

CONTINENT URINARY DIVERSIONS
Orthotopic Diversion

Procedure

ODs are constructed of detubularized bowel, formed into a spherical pouch and anastomosed to the native urethral stump. The internal reservoir allows for preserved body image by precluding the need for a stoma and more natural volitional voiding that relies on the external striated sphincter as the continence mechanism.[1] ODs can be constructed from small or large bowel; however, detubularized small bowel allows for greater compliance.[25] The ileal ONB is the most frequently used OD and is typically constructed from 40 to 50 cm of terminal ileum.

Patient selection

A patient's desire for a neobladder is one of the most important factors influencing the choice of UD.[4,26] Despite risks of incontinence or, rarely, retention with the need to perform CISC, many patients with adequate social support choose to undertake these potential side effects in order to avoid an external stoma.[4] As mentioned previously, it is critical to elicit and clarify the patient's expectations of undergoing a UD and thoroughly counsel the patient preoperatively on the risks and side effects associated with each type of diversion.[4]

Several recent studies have demonstrated the broad applicability of ODs, with as many as 90% of patients receiving neobladder after cystectomy at some institutions,[27] and others suggesting that 80% of men and 65% of women requiring cystectomy for bladder cancer are appropriate candidates for neobladder.[28] Despite this, several studies show that only 15% to 37% of patients undergoing cystectomy receive a CD.[1,29,30] Although these rates of CDs represent a wide array of hospitals, including nonacademic centers, the underlying reasons for lower adoption rates of ODs are not clear and may include patient- and provider-driven factors.

ONBs are ideal for young, healthy patients with good dexterity and an interest in maintaining a "natural" physical appearance (wanting to avoid a stoma or ostomy appliance). In addition, ODs allow for relatively normal and volitional voiding patterns after a period of postoperative recovery and intensive rehabilitation.[11] Daytime continence is another potential advantage of neobladder, with experienced centers reporting daytime continence rates as high as 90% to 95%.[31–33] Although this is likely an overestimate and not broadly applicable, it does demonstrate that experienced surgeons can attain excellent functional results in appropriately selected groups of patients. Several studies have found that urine leakage was of greater concern among patients with ICs compared with those with CDs.[34–36] Interestingly, another potential advantage of ODs is reduced risk of urethral recurrence. Two series found evidence of decreased urethral recurrence rates associated with ODs compared with heterotopic diversions after controlling for other pathologic variables.[37,38]

These advantages must be weighed against increased technical difficulty and surgical complexity, longer operative time, higher complication rates, and prolonged postoperative catheterization.[1] Advanced age has been associated with higher complication rates, and as a result, ICs are generally recommended for the elderly, whereas neobladders are more often used in younger, healthier patients.[39,40] However, physiologic age appears to be more closely associated with patient outcome when compared with chronologic age. For this reason, many centers advocate that no age limit should apply and that patient selection should instead be determined by surgical fitness, functional status, and motivation.[41,42]

There are several important contraindications to CDs in general, as well as those unique to ODs. It is important to distinguish absolute from relative contraindications. Crucially, these contraindications may vary between institutions based on surgeon experience and principles.[4] Absolute contraindications to CDs include impaired renal function (serum creatinine values of >2.0–2.5 mg/dL), hepatic insufficiency, and inability or unwillingness to independently perform CISC in the long term (see **Table 1**).[2] Positive intraoperative urethral margin in male and female patients is also an absolute contraindication to ONB (**Table 2**).[2]

Relative contraindications to CDs include advanced age (chronologic or physiologic), multiple comorbidities, prior pelvic radiation, chronic inflammatory or malignant bowel disease, and need for adjuvant chemotherapy (see **Table 2**).[2,4] Severe male urethral strictures, neurologic conditions impairing continence, extensive local disease with soft tissue or pubic bone extension, and planned postoperative pelvic radiation are relative contraindications to ODs (see **Table 2**).[4] ICs should be offered to patients with absolute contraindications or more than one relative contraindication to CD. Patients with absolute contraindications to ODs can be offered an IC or CCD if they desire a CD. In the setting of relative contraindications to CDs, a conduit should be strongly considered and patients should be counseled regarding possible adverse outcomes associated with CD. Likewise, patients with relative contraindications to neobladders should be primarily offered conduits or CCDs and informed of the potential risks of neobladder construction.

Table 2 Absolute and relative contraindications to orthotopic urinary diversions	
Absolute Contraindications	**Relative Contraindications**
Positive urethral margin	Male urethral stricture Preexisting incontinence Neurologic disease with impaired continence Extensive local disease Need for adjuvant radiation

Preoperative counseling

It is critical to clarify patient's expectations of undergoing an OD and adequately explain the short- and long-term risks and side effects of each type of diversion. The potential to void volitionally and avoid frequent self-catheterization or an external stoma make ONBs appealing. For these reasons, many patients with adequate social support opt for an OD despite the risk of possible daytime and nighttime incontinence, or more rarely, hypercontinence. However, patients should be counseled preoperatively that intraoperative findings, such as a positive urethral margin, may necessitate a change from the planned diversion type. As such, all patients slated to undergo OD should have a stoma site marked preoperatively by a stomal nurse in the event of urethral involvement precluding OD.[2]

It is also important to discuss the typical postoperative course and recovery with regard to the different diversion types. Components of recovery unique to ODs include prolonged need for indwelling urethral catheter and at least one cystogram before removal. Patients must be fully educated and committed to the labor-intensive rehabilitation process and pelvic floor retraining with physical therapy.[2] In addition, patients need to be informed of the necessity of postoperative bladder cycling or the slow and active process of progressively increasing duration between timed voids to allow for gentle expansion of the neobladder.

Functional outcomes

Urinary incontinence following continent OD can be very upsetting and difficult for patients to manage. Incontinence may present immediately postoperatively or have a delayed onset and can be temporary or permanent. Incontinence can affect patients during the day or, more commonly, at night because of lack of a guarding reflex with a neobladder. Typically, daytime continence is recovered more quickly than nighttime continence. A large meta-analysis found that 13% of patients with neobladders experienced daytime incontinence and that rates of nocturnal incontinence ranged from 15% to 40%.[43] It is important to counsel patients that overall continence rates decrease with advancing age and recovery in continence is often delayed in the elderly or the "physiologic elderly."[19,44]

Conversely, hypercontinence may also occur following OD. A meta-analysis of greater than 2000 patients found that 4% to 25% of neobladder patients performed CISC for incomplete emptying.[43] Important to patient selection is the fact that hypercontinence and urinary retention is more common in female patients following a neobladder with 16% to 25% eventually developing urinary retention.[45–48] Thus, patients must be willing and able to independently self-catheterize in the short and long term if they are to be considered candidates for an OD. Self-catheterization can be particularly difficult for obese, female, or disabled patients or those that have poor dexterity, mental incapacity, or neurologic or degenerative disorders.[2,25]

Complications

Many early complications of CDs are related to cystectomy and are not distinct to the diversion type. Bowel and ureteral complications can occur as a result of cystectomy and may also be contributed to by the UD. CDs use multiple suture lines, tapered limbs, and anti-incontinence mechanisms, which result in increased operative time when compared with ICs.[2] As a result, urine leaks are more common with CDs in the early postoperative period. In addition, pouch rupture may occur in the short or long term. Although both of these complications are often successfully managed conservatively with catheter drainage and maintenance of ureteral stents, some require additional diversion of the urine with percutaneous nephrostomy tubes or drain placement.[25]

The most common late complications associated with ODs include incontinence, hypercontinence, UTIs, ureteroenteric anastomotic stricture, afferent limb obstruction, urethral stricture, pouch and upper tract calculi, pouch rupture, and vaginal fistula.[25] With the exception of incontinence, these complications are less commonly encountered with OD compared with CCD. The vast majority of the time these complications can be managed endoscopically; however, infrequently they require open, laparoscopic, or robotic surgical revision.[25,49,50]

Summary

ONB should be offered to all patients without an absolute contraindication because many patients view the preservation of body image and the potential for volitional voiding highly desirable. Patients should be extensively counseled regarding the potential side effects of incontinence or hypercontinence with the need for short-term and possibly long-term catheterization. In addition, patients must be prepared for a longer and more rigorous postoperative recovery compared with incontinent diversions.

Continent Cutaneous Diversion

Procedure

CCDs consist of a pouch constructed from detubularized bowel, similar to a neoblabder, which is instead attached to anterior abdominal wall and skin via a nonrefluxing catheterizable channel. The reservoir is emptied by periodic CISC through a small cutaneous stoma within the umbilicus or either lower abdominal quadrant. The catheterizable channel can be constructed from various bowel segments, most commonly the appendix or small bowel. Multiple technical variations exist with regard to the type of valve mechanism, catheterizable channel, and bowel segment used, which has resulted in multiple surgical approaches, such as the Indiana, Kock, Miami, and right colon pouches.

Patient selection

In recent years, continent cutaneous pouches have largely been replaced by the ONBs. However, they remain an option for patients who desire a CD but are not a candidate for an OD. This form of diversion requires long-term active participation, and patients must demonstrate intact dexterity and the motivation to perform CISC multiple times daily. Continent cutaneous and ODs share all the same absolute and relative contraindications to CDs previously discussed (see **Table 1**). The contraindications specific to OD (see **Table 2**) do not, however, apply to CCDs. For this reason, continent cutaneous reservoirs are an excellent option for patients who do not qualify for ONBs, because of a positive urethral margin, nonfunctional urethra, or mesentery that will not reach the urethral stump during construction of an ONB, but still desire a CD.[51]

The major advantage of a continent cutaneous reservoir is daytime and nighttime continence precluding the need for an external appliance. Continent catheterizable diversions are associated with the highest continence rates of any diversion type, whereas the absence of a urostomy appliance and small and relatively subtle stoma help to preserve body image. However, these advantages must be balanced against the increased technical difficulty, operative time, and short- and long-term complication rates.

The critical importance of the patient's ability to independently self-catheterize and irrigate the pouch over a lifetime cannot be overemphasized.[2] Unlike a conduit or, in most circumstances, a neobladder, continent catheterizable diversions require continuous attention and active participation, which can be very difficult for caregivers to manage.[51] For this reason, patients with quadriplegia or multiple sclerosis, or those who are very frail, mentally impaired, or of advanced chronologic or physiologic age, are considered poor candidates for any form of CD, and particularly, cutaneous reservoirs.[51] Although these patient populations may require assistance with care of an external appliance as well, this is less burdensome because it requires less frequent care and expertise.[51]

Preoperative counseling

It is important to set realistic expectations for patients undergoing CCDs regarding the continuous and active role they will need to take in daily maintenance of their pouch for the remainder of their lifetime. Evaluation by an ostomy nurse can be very helpful in this regard. Patients must understand and be willing to catheterize and empty their pouch a minimum of 4 to 6 times daily as well as regularly irrigate excess mucous from the pouch. Equally importantly, they should understand the potential consequences of failure to do so: life-threatening pouch rupture, recurrent infections, stomal stenosis, upper tract deterioration, and pouch calculi requiring endoscopic or open surgical management. In the event that the patient is no longer able to self-catheterize their diversion because of impaired dexterity or cognitive decline, patients may become heavily dependent on their family or caregivers for round-the-clock care of their CCD. Also, importantly, this may limit long-term care and placement options for these patients in the future.[51]

Patients must also be made aware of the need for a prolonged indwelling catheter postoperatively and need for at least one cystogram before catheter removal. Similar to ONBs, pouch cycling is performed following indwelling catheter removal. Cycling initially requires frequent round-the-clock catheterization, which is progressively decreased over time as the reservoir volume increases. Finally, all patients opting for a CCD must also be adequately prepared for the potential, albeit rare, need for intraoperative conversion to IC. Preparation for this should include counseling as well as a preoperative visit with ileal stoma nurses for marking of the continent cutaneous stoma as well as a back-up IC stoma.

Functional outcomes

Continent cutaneous reservoirs remain a viable option for patients who are not candidates for ODs but are concerned with body image and functional concerns. Continence rates following CCD range from 90% to 98%.[52,53] Although still imperfect, this represents the highest continence rates of any CD. Incontinence typically results from uninhibited pouch contractions, inadequate continence mechanism, and poor reservoir compliance.[52,53] Reservoir urodynamics may be helpful in determining the cause of incontinence.

Anticholinergics may be trialed in the setting of a poorly compliant pouch; however, some more severe cases may require reservoir augmentation.[54–56] Incontinence as a result of failure of the continence mechanism typically necessitates surgical revision.[2]

Complications

CCDs are generally the most technically challenging and are associated with the highest short- and long-term complications. As with OD, long suture lines place patients at increased risk of urine leaks and even catastrophic pouch rupture. One large institutional series found an 18% to 36% risk of having a significant complication over the lifetime of the patient.[2,16,18,21,32] The rates of major complications are not necessarily higher when compared with ONBs; however, minor complications like stomal stenosis are relatively common (25%–50%).[10] The most common complications specific to CCD are difficulty with catheterization with the efferent limb, urine leaks, and development of reservoir calculi.[18] Other complications include recurrent UTIs, upper tract deterioration, pouchitis, ureteroenteric anastomotic strictures, small bowel obstruction, or bowel leak. Most complications can be managed conservatively with stomal dilation or leaving an indwelling catheter for a period of time and surgical revision or intervention is rarely required.[4]

Summary

CCD remains an available option for patients who do not meet criteria for OD but still desire a CD and preservation of body image. Patients must be counseled that although this diversion method has many advantages, it also is associated with the longest operative times and the highest rates of short- and long-term complications. Patient selection is especially critical, because it is essential that candidates be able to perform regimented intermittent catheterization reliably, because failure to do so can be life threatening.

OTHER CONTINENT DIVERSIONS

More rarely used diversions, including ureterosigmoidostomy or other variations that use the rectosigmoid for a reservoir such as the Mainz II pouch, rely on the anal sphincter for continence.[57] Ureterosigmoidostomy was one of the first UDs to use bowel and is constructed by anastomosing the ureters to the sigmoid colon. Ureterosigmoidostomy is most commonly used for patients who are not candidates for an orthotopic or CCD but insist on a CD.[4] Ureterosigmoidostomy is not preferred because of significant side effects, including chronic diarrhea, fecal incontinence, metabolic abnormalities, deterioration of the upper tracts, recurrent pyelonephritis, and higher risk of secondary colorectal malignancy.

SUMMARY

Patient selection and preoperative counseling are critical aspects of UD surgery. The surgeon must have an intimate knowledge of not only the patient's disease process but also their functional and psychoemotional status as well as their social support network so that he or she may be able to set appropriate expectations. Furthermore, the surgical care team must provide resources, in both the preoperative and postoperative period, to help optimize expectations, relieve anxiety, and help the patients adapt to their new diversion once they begin the recovery process. At the authors' institution, patients are introduced to ostomy nurses, nurse navigators, and nutritionists at their initial visit and continue to see these care team members during the immediate postoperative setting as well as at subsequent follow-up visits. This strategy enables them to set and manage expectations, while alleviating anxiety and optimizing outcomes.

REFERENCES

1. Gore JL, Saigal CS, Hanley JM, et al, Project Urologic Diseases in America Project. Variations in reconstruction after radical cystectomy. Cancer 2006;107(4):729–37.
2. Lee RK, Abol-Enein H, Artibani W, et al. Urinary diversion after radical cystectomy for bladder cancer: options, patient selection, and outcomes. BJU Int 2014;113(1):11–23.
3. Le Duc A, Camey M, Teillac P. Antireflux uretero-ileal implantation via a mucosal sulcus. Ann d'urologie 1987;21(1):33–4 [in French].
4. Daneshmand S, Bartsch G. Improving selection of appropriate urinary diversion following radical cystectomy for bladder cancer. Expert Rev Anticancer Ther 2011;11(6):941–8.
5. Fisch M, Thüroff JW. Continent cutaneous diversion. BJU Int 2008;102(9 Pt B):1314–9.
6. Skinner DG, Boyd SD, Lieskovsky G. Clinical experience with the Kock continent ileal reservoir for urinary diversion. J Urol 1984;132(6):1101–7.
7. Thüroff JW, Alken P, Riedmiller H, et al. The Mainz pouch (mixed augmentation ileum and cecum) for bladder augmentation and continent diversion. J Urol 1986;136(1):17–26.
8. Riedmiller H, Bürger R, Müller S, et al. Continent appendix stoma: a modification of the Mainz pouch technique. J Urol 1990;143(6):1115–7.
9. Rowland RG, Mitchell ME, Bihrle R, et al. Indiana continent urinary reservoir. J Urol 1987;137(6):1136–9.
10. Stein JP, Dunn MD, Quek ML, et al. The orthotopic T pouch ileal neobladder: experience with 209 patients. J Urol 2004;172(2):584–7.
11. Evans B, Montie JE, Gilbert SM. Incontinent or continent urinary diversion: how to make the right choice. Curr Opin Urol 2010;20(5):421–5.
12. Dahl DM. Use of intestinal segments in urinary diversion. In: Wein AJ, Kavoussi LR, Partin AW, et al, editors. Campbell-walsh urology, Vol. 3, 11th edition. Philadelphia: Elsevier; 2016. p. 2281–316.e2285.
13. Daneshmand S. Orthotopic urinary diversion. Curr Opin Urol 2015;25(6):545–9.
14. Cerruto MA, D'Elia C, Siracusano S, et al. Systematic review and meta-analysis of non RCT's on health related quality of life after radical cystectomy using validated questionnaires: better results with orthotopic neobladder versus ileal conduit. Eur J Surg Oncol 2016;42(3):343–60.
15. Madersbacher S, Schmidt J, Eberle JM, et al. Long-term outcome of ileal conduit diversion. J Urol 2003;169(3):985–90.
16. Killeen KP, Libertino JA. Management of bowel and urinary tract complications after urinary diversion. Urol Clin North Am 1988;15(2):183–94.
17. Perimenis P, Burkhard FC, Kessler TM, et al. Ileal orthotopic bladder substitute combined with an afferent tubular segment: long-term upper urinary tract changes and voiding pattern. Eur Urol 2004;46(5):604–9.
18. Farnham SB, Cookson MS. Surgical complications of urinary diversion. World J Urol 2004;22(3):157–67.
19. Madersbacher S, Möhrle K, Burkhard F, et al. Long-term voiding pattern of patients with ileal orthotopic bladder substitutes. J Urol 2002;167(5):2052–7.
20. Regan JB, Barrett DM. Stented versus nonstented ureteroileal anastomoses: is there a difference with regard to leak and stricture? J Urol 1985;134(6):1101–3.
21. Jahnson S, Pedersen J. Cystectomy and urinary diversion during twenty years–complications and metabolic implications. Eur Urol 1993;24(3):343–9.
22. Morales P, Golimbu M. Colonic urinary diversion: 10 years of experience. J Urol 1975;113(3):302–7.
23. Singh G, Wilkinson JM, Thomas DG. Supravesical diversion for incontinence: a long-term follow-up. Br J Urol 1997;79(3):348–53.
24. MacGregor PS, Montie JE, Straffon RA. Cutaneous ureterostomy as palliative diversion in adults with malignancy. Urology 1987;30(1):31–4.
25. Skinner E, Daneshmand S. Orthotopic urinary diversion. In: Wein AJ, Kavoussi LR, Partin AW, et al, editors. Campbell-Walsh urology, Vol. 3, 11th edition. Philadelphia: Elsevier; 2016. p. 2344–86.e2345.

26. Hautmann RE, Abol-Enein H, Hafez K, et al. Urinary diversion. Urology 2007;69(1 Suppl):17–49.

27. Hautmann RE. Urinary diversion: ileal conduit to neobladder. J Urol 2003;169(3):834–42.

28. Hautmann RE. Which patients with transitional cell carcinoma of the bladder or prostatic urethra are candidates for an orthotopic neobladder? Curr Urol Rep 2000;1(3):173–9.

29. Gore JL, Litwin MS. Project UDiA. Quality of care in bladder cancer: trends in urinary diversion following radical cystectomy. World J Urol 2009;27(1):45–50.

30. Lowrance WT, Rumohr JA, Clark PE, et al. Urinary diversion trends at a high volume, single American tertiary care center. J Urol 2009;182(5):2369–74.

31. Kessler TM, Burkhard FC, Perimenis P, et al. Attempted nerve sparing surgery and age have a significant effect on urinary continence and erectile function after radical cystoprostatectomy and ileal orthotopic bladder substitution. J Urol 2004;172(4 Pt 1):1323–7.

32. Hautmann RE, de Petriconi R, Gottfried HW, et al. The ileal neobladder: complications and functional results in 363 patients after 11 years of followup. J Urol 1999;161(2):422–7 [discussion: 427–8].

33. Hautmann RE, Volkmer BG, Schumacher MC, et al. Long-term results of standard procedures in urology: the ileal neobladder. World J Urol 2006;24(3):305–14.

34. Bjerre BD, Johansen C, Steven K. Health-related quality of life after cystectomy: bladder substitution compared with ileal conduit diversion. A questionnaire survey. Br J Urol 1995;75(2):200–5.

35. Conde Redondo C, Estebanez Zarranz J, Rodriguez Tovez A, et al. Quality of life in patients treated with orthotopic bladder substitution versus cutaneous ileostomy. Actas Urol Esp 2001;25(6):435–44 [in Spanish].

36. Månsson A, Johnson G, Månsson W. Quality of life after cystectomy. Comparison between patients with conduit and those with continent caecal reservoir urinary diversion. Br J Urol 1988;62(3):240–5.

37. Stein JP, Clark P, Miranda G, et al. Urethral tumor recurrence following cystectomy and urinary diversion: clinical and pathological characteristics in 768 male patients. J Urol 2005;173(4):1163–8.

38. Boorjian SA, Kim SP, Weight CJ, et al. Risk factors and outcomes of urethral recurrence following radical cystectomy. Eur Urol 2011;60(6):1266–72.

39. Stein JP, Lieskovsky G, Cote R, et al. Radical cystectomy in the treatment of invasive bladder cancer: long-term results in 1,054 patients. J Clin Oncol 2001;19(3):666–75.

40. Madersbacher S, Hochreiter W, Burkhard F, et al. Radical cystectomy for bladder cancer today–a homogeneous series without neoadjuvant therapy. J Clin Oncol 2003;21(4):690–6.

41. Sogni F, Brausi M, Frea B, et al. Morbidity and quality of life in elderly patients receiving ileal conduit or orthotopic neobladder after radical cystectomy for invasive bladder cancer. Urology 2008;71(5):919–23.

42. Clark PE, Stein JP, Groshen SG, et al. Radical cystectomy in the elderly: comparison of clincal outcomes between younger and older patients. Cancer 2005;104(1):36–43.

43. Steers WD. Voiding dysfunction in the orthotopic neobladder. World J Urol 2000;18(5):330–7.

44. Hautmann RE, Miller K, Steiner U, et al. The ileal neobladder: 6 years of experience with more than 200 patients. J Urol 1993;150(1):40–5.

45. Stenzl A, Holtl L. Orthotopic bladder reconstruction in women–what we have learned over the last decade. Crit Rev Oncol Hematol 2003;47(2):147–54.

46. Ali-El-Dein B, Gomha M, Ghoneim MA. Critical evaluation of the problem of chronic urinary retention after orthotopic bladder substitution in women. J Urol 2002;168(2):587–92.

47. Lee CT, Dunn RL, Chen BT, et al. Impact of body mass index on radical cystectomy. J Urol 2004; 172(4 Pt 1):1281–5.

48. Stein JP, Grossfeld GD, Freeman JA, et al. Orthotopic lower urinary tract reconstruction in women using the Kock ileal neobladder: updated experience in 34 patients. J Urol 1997;158(2):400–5.

49. Rowland RG. Complications of continent cutaneous reservoirs and neobladders: series using contemporary techniques. AUA Update Ser 1995;14(201).

50. Hautmann RE, de Petriconi RC, Volkmer BG. 25 years of experience with 1,000 neobladders: long-term complications. J Urol 2011;185(6):2207–12.

51. DeCastro GJ, McKiernan JM, Benson MC. Cutaneous continent urinary diversion. In: Wein AJ, Kavoussi LR, Partin AW, et al, editors. Campbellwalsh urology, Vol. 3, 11th edition. Philadelphia: Saunders/Elsevier; 2016. p. 2317–43.e2313.

52. Sumfest JM, Burns MW, Mitchell ME. The Mitrofanoff principle in urinary reconstruction. J Urol 1993; 150(6):1875–7 [discussion: 1877–8].

53. Bihrle R. The Indiana pouch continent urinary reservoir. Urol Clin North Am 1997;24(4):773–9.

54. Sheldon CA, Reeves D, Lewis AG. Oxybutynin administration diminishes the high gastric muscular tone associated with bladder reconstruction. J Urol 1995;153(2):461–2.

55. El-Bahnasawy MS, Shaaban H, Gomha MA, et al. Clinical and urodynamic efficacy of oxybutynin and verapamil in the treatment of nocturnal enuresis after formation of orthotopic ileal neobladders. A prospective, randomized, crossover study. Scand J Urol Nephrol 2008;42(4):344–51.

56. Christmas TJ, Smith GL, Rickards D. Diagnosis and management of high-pressure peristaltic contractions in cystoplasties. Br J Urol 1997;79(6):879–82.

57. Pajor L, Romics I. Modified ureterosigmoidostomy (Mainz II): technique and early results. BJU Int 1999;83(1):157–8.

Perioperative Preparation and Nutritional Considerations for Patients Undergoing Urinary Diversion

Jessie R. Gills, MD, Jeffrey M. Holzbeierlein, MD*

KEYWORDS

- Urinary diversion • Bladder cancer • Optimization • Cystectomy

KEY POINTS

- Patients undergoing urinary diversion are at high risk for complications in the perioperative period.
- The exact cause of these complications remains poorly defined but is likely multifactorial.
- Improvements in perioperative care may decrease complications.

Urinary diversions (UDs) carry significant morbidity regardless of indication. (1–5) When used in combination with extirpative surgery for nonmalignant urologic disease, 35% to 73%[1–3] of patients experience complications postoperatively. When UD alone (without bladder removal) is performed, 30.6% of patients still experience postoperative complications.[3] UD in the setting of urologic malignancy carries an attributable complication rate of 11% to 29%, specifically related to the diversion, whereas patients who undergo UD after pelvic exenteration experience the highest rate of complications, affecting up to 59% of patients.[3–5] Thus, factors influencing perioperative outcomes are of great interest to practitioners attempting to decrease perioperative complications in patients undergoing UD for any indication.

A majority of UDs are performed in the setting of a primary urologic malignancy, specifically muscle-invasive bladder cancer (MIBC), with UD after radical cystectomy (RC) the most common indication. Unfortunately this patient cohort is extremely vulnerable to the complications associated with UD because they are often affected by numerous comorbid conditions.[4,5] This review describes the perioperative assessment and preparation as well as any nutritional considerations that may be used to minimize the known associated complications in patients undergoing UD. Ideally, perioperative preparation and optimization should be patient specific, addressing patient-specific factors, such as frailty, malnutrition, and comorbid disease states that may or may not be readily evident. Thus a systematic approach to patient preparation for patients undergoing UD should be undertaken.

PERIOPERATIVE IMAGING

Perioperative imaging is essential for operative planning whether the indication for UD is benign or malignant. In the setting of benign disease, perioperative imaging can provide valuable information regarding the upper tracts, including presence of urolithiasis or obstruction, absence or malposition of a kidney, duplicated systems, or other anatomic variants. In addition, imaging may provide information regarding prior surgical interventions, abdominal/pelvic radiation, inflammatory bowel disease, or vascular graft placement.

Disclosures: The authors have nothing they wish to disclose.
University of Kansas Medical Center, Mail Stop 3016, 3901 Rainbow Boulevard, Kansas City, KS 66160, USA
* Corresponding author.
E-mail address: jholzbeierlein@kumc.edu

Urol Clin N Am 45 (2018) 11–17
https://doi.org/10.1016/j.ucl.2017.09.002
0094-0143/18/© 2017 Elsevier Inc. All rights reserved.

For MIBC, the European Association of Urology, National Comprehensive Cancer Network, and soon to be released American Urological Association guidelines incorporate clinical and radiologic staging as a common theme in their recommendations. Perioperative imaging plays a critical role in determining the most accurate clinical stage: extent of local tumor, lymph node involvement, concomitant upper tract, or distant organ disease, which ultimately determines treatment and prognosis. CT with excretory urography is the most widely available and used imaging modality, although not without limitation. Up to 42% of patients are up-staged at time of cystectomy using current imaging modalities,[6] with CT accuracy in predicting extravesical disease historically 35% to 55%.[7] Given the limitations of CT to accurately predict primary tumor stages, newer image modalities have been explored. MRI has been compared with CT and demonstrated no significant improvement in the detection of microscopic perivesical fat invasion,[8] although the sensitivity of detecting macroscopic perivesical tumor invasion was improved, with 73% to 96% for MRI[9] and 55% to 92% for CT.[10] When looking at the sensitivity of detecting lymph node metastases, MRI has shown the ability to accurately detect pelvic lymph node involvement in 80% of cases; however, specificity has not been as accurate. Looking to expand the accuracy of radiographic staging, the use of fluorodeoxyglucose–PET/CT has been studied in MIBC and found to accurately identify nodal metastatic disease in 48% of patients,[11] detecting up-staging in 20% of patients and changing treatment intent from curative to palliative in 8.5% of patients.[12] Currently the role of PET/CT in staging has been relegated to adjudicating equivocal findings on CT or MRI and is not recommended for routine staging of patients with MIBC. To date CT scans remain the recommended imaging modality due to their relatively low cost, their availability, and lack of proved superiority of other imaging modalities.

PERIOPERATIVE LABORATORY TESTING

Preoperative laboratory testing is one of the critical components of determining candidacy for specific types of UDs.[13] In particular, the assessment of renal function is paramount to decisions regarding UD, because more than 70% of patients undergoing UD have greater than expected renal function deterioration after UD.[14] Renal function deterioration occurs with both continent and incontinent UDs alike, with 74% and 71% of patients, respectively, experiencing significant declines in renal function over time.[15] The significant factors in determining the

risk of renal function declines include preoperative estimated glomerular filtration rate, hypertension, diabetes, postoperative hydronephrosis, presence of proteinuria, pyelonephritis, and the development of postoperative ureteroenteric strictures.[14,15] Classically, patients with an estimated glomerular filtration rate greater than 40 mL/min are candidates for continent diversions whereas patients with renal function less that this are recommended for incontinent diversions. In some cases, there is an expected improvement in renal function after diversion due to relief of obstruction. In these cases, additional evaluation and/or testing by nephrology is useful to determine if renal reserve is adequate for a continent diversion.

Other than renal function, hepatic function should also be evaluated because of the increased risk of hyperammonemic encephalopathy in patients with hepatic dysfunction who undergo continent UD.[13] This disturbance occurs due to the increase in ammonium chloride absorption across the luminal surface of the diversion. The treatment involves drainage of the continent UD with a catheter, administration of neomycin, and protein restriction along with treatment of any liver dysfunction.

Finally, all patients undergoing UD in the setting of bladder cancer should have complete blood cell counts and a comprehensive metabolic panel for staging, to identify any other underlying metabolic issues that may become exacerbated with UD.

MUSCLE INVASIVE BLADDER CANCER

Additional considerations must be given to MIBC perioperative preparation. Along with clinical staging with radiographic imaging, the roles of examination under anesthesia for clinical staging and administration of neoadjuvant chemotherapy are 2 crucial steps to perform prior to undergoing RC/UD. Although neither EUA nor CT alone is optimal for clinical staging of bladder cancer, the combination of EUA and cross-sectional imaging has a specificity of 89% and a negative predictive value of 74% for pathologic extravesical disease.[16,17] The role of prostatic urethral biopsy prior to orthotopic neobladder reconstruction remains controversial. Although several studies suggest an increased risk for patients with carcinoma in situ of the prostatic urethra, others support frozen section analysis of the urethral margin as the only predictive factor.[18]

Based on 2 well-performed randomized controlled trials, neoadjuvant multiagent cisplatin based chemotherapy should be offered to patients preparing to undergo RC/UD for MIBC,[19,20] which correlates with a long-term survival benefit of 5%

to 6% with a relative risk reduction of death at 10 years of 16%.[19] Although the receipt of neoadjuvant chemotherapy has not been shown to increase complications related to cystectomy and UD, there may be declines in renal function or general deconditioning that may effect the choice of UD.

COMPETING COMORBIDITIES

Competing comorbidities influence postoperative morbidity and mortality to the point that worse pathologic and clinical outcomes have been seen proportional to comorbid states,[5,21–24] making identification of comorbid conditions an area of great potential impact. This led to the EAU guideline for MIBC to recommend incorporating a validated comorbidity score, such as the Charlson Comorbidity Index into the Initial evaluation of patients with MIBC. In addition to age, comorbid conditions can predict risks of prolonged hospitalization (>10 days), likelihood of readmission, or discharge to somewhere other than home.[25] Increased mortality has been associated with 3 or greater comorbidities and age greater than 70.[25] Comorbid conditions seem more influential than chronologic age,[23] making modifications of comorbid conditions an area where alterations can show the greatest returns. Although there are no specific exclusionary criteria for patients with significant comorbidities (other than those discussed previously) in selecting the type of diversion, the general consensus is that patients with significant comorbidities should undergo ileal conduit UD.

PREHABILITATION

Frailty has been described as decreased functional reserve and resistance to stressors affecting multiple systems leaving patients vulnerable to adverse outcomes.[26] The Fried frailty phenotype was one of the first described metrics to identify this patient population and included at least 3 of the following: unintentional weight loss, self-reported exhaustion, weak grip strength, slow walking speed, and low physical activity.[26] Frailty in surgical patients has been associated with increased postoperative complications, adverse outcomes, and greater morbidity and mortality in patients undergoing UD.[27,28] This phenotype in conjunction with comorbid conditions, signs, and symptoms of deteriorating health is often found in patients who are undergoing UD and lead to a higher rate of adverse outcomes.

Prehabilitation has been proposed as a countermeasure to hopefully reduce the known increased risk within this population. The largest prospective randomized controlled trial of patients undergoing UD with or without prehabilitation using preoperative and postoperative strength and endurance exercise programs showed poor compliance, with only 59% of patients completing at least 75% of the prescribed exercise. Those in the treatment arm did show improved postoperative mobilization, endurance, and ability to perform activities of daily living but did not show a decrease in hospital length of stay or rate of postoperative complications.[29] Although promising, this demonstrates that multiple factors play a role in determining outcomes in patients undergoing UD, and currently designed programs have not addressed all issues adequately. It also brings to light patient compliance in this cohort and the need for better engagement tools and platforms.

ENHANCED RECOVERY AFTER SURGERY

To reduce complications associated with cystectomy and UD, multimodal multiphase approaches are clearly needed. Enhanced recovery after surgery (ERAS) pathways have been studied in RC/UD patients with promising results, and evidence-based ERAS Society guidelines for RC/UD patients exist. Of the 22 ERAS components considered by the ERAS Society as crucial for improving patient outcomes, the highest evidence was for early nasogastric tube removal, prevention of ileus, and minimally invasive surgery. At the time of publication of the Society's original guidelines in 2013, all the guidelines were extrapolations from colorectal literature.[30] Fortunately, since that time several ERAS prospective trials have been performed on RC/UD cohorts. None, however, has captured all 22 components that the ERAS Society hopes to incorporate. Interpreting the evidence-based data for patients undergoing UD is challenging due to the prospective but not randomized design and small number of trials with differing protocols and endpoints, leading to the inability to determine which component most influenced outcomes. Even with these limitations and variability, one constant remains in the literature: ERAS pathways positively effect patient recovery.[31]

Early enteral feeding is one common component of most RC/UD ERAS protocols, and although sufficient evidence exists within the colorectal surgery literature to support its use, the only randomized control trial in RC/UD patients recently closed prematurely due to poor accrual.[32] In the trial, the investigators found no statistical difference in complication rate, length of hospitalization, rate of ileus, or return of bowel function between early and traditional enteral feeding,[33] again stressing that the importance of the pathway as a whole is more important than its individual components.

Alvimopan (Entereg) is one ERAS component that has been shown in randomized trials to improve outcomes.[34] The addition of alvimopan, a μ-opioid receptor antagonist, in patients undergoing cystectomy and diversion has resulted in early return of feeding, decreased length of stay, and decreased costs. It was recently incorporated into the American Urological Association MIBC guidelines as a "Strong Recommendation."

VENOUS THROMBOEMBOLISM

Venous thromboembolism (VTE) has been reported to be 70-fold higher in bladder cancer patients than matched cohorts on large population-based studies,[35] with 6% to 8% of RC/UD patients experiencing a symptomatic VTE within 30 days of their procedure.[32,35,36] VTE prevention is part of all ERAS pathways, with prevention including early ambulation, compressive stocking, and chemoprophylaxis. At this time, the optimal duration of extended prophylaxis is unknown, although most protocols have recommended administration prior to induction of anesthesia and extending to 4 weeks postoperatively. In addition, it is unclear what the optimal agent is for VTE chemoprophylaxis, with low-molecular-weight heparin the most commonly used option. The risks of bleeding must be balanced against the use of VTE prophylaxis, leading to a patient-specific risk assessment being used in most protocols.

Another component of ERAS for an RC/UD patient that has been examined and shown to independently effect outcomes is the maintenance of euvolemia. The importance of this is specifically related to the maintenance of intraoperative euvolemia.

In regard to intraoperative euvolemia, 2 strategies have proved efficacious in preventing hypervolemia: image-guided goal-directed therapy[37] and fluid restriction with norepinephrine infusion.[37] Maintaining intraoperative euvolemia has been shown to decrease postoperative ileus, blood transfusions, wound infections, and quicker return of bowel functions.[38] Specific to fluid restriction using preemptive norepinephrine infusion, the overall complication rate was 52% in the norepinephrine group versus 73% in the control arm. Gastrointestinal and cardiac complications were 6% versus 31%, respectively, in the study, which also demonstrated an improvement in median length of hospitalization of 15 days versus 17 days, respectively, and a 90-day mortality rate of 0% versus 4.8%, respectively.[39]

BEHAVIORAL MODIFICATIONS
Tobacco Use

Tobacco use is the most established risk factor for bladder cancer,[40] causing up to 65% of cases.[41] Although studies examining the effects of smoking/smoking cessation have mixed results in predicting recurrence of bladder cancer and overall complication rate after RC/UD, the general principle of smoking cessation should be a core component of the perioperative period.[42–44] Smoking cessation has been shown in a randomized controlled trial to decrease the prevalence of overall complications (52% vs 18%), wound complications (31% vs 5%), cardiovascular complications (10% vs 0%), need for a secondary surgery (15% vs 4%), and median length of stay (13 days vs 11 days) for continued smokers versus perioperative smoking cessation, respectively, in patients undergoing hip or knee replacement.[45] This study has been reproduced in general surgery, plastic surgery, orthodontic surgery, and vascular and cardiovascular surgery populations, with all showing improvement in patient outcomes in the smoking cessation group. Despite currently published retrospective studies reviewing smoking cessation with mixed results on patient outcomes for patients undergoing UD, prospective randomized trials in every surgical population studied has shown a significant benefit to smoking cessation, supporting the importance of this measure.

Nutritional Considerations

Malnutrition is defined as the nutritional imbalance where calories, protein, or other nutrients are inadequate for tissue maintenance and repair.[46] The presence of significant malnutrition has been reported to be as high as 71% in cancer patients[47] and present in up to 55% of patients who undergo RC/UD.[48] Despite the fact that malnutrition is very prevalent in the UD population, it is likely under-recognized, under-reported, and undertreated.

Nutritional deficiency has been shown to be a predictor of poor overall survival and increased 90-day mortality in patients undergoing RC/UD.[49] Previous studies have looked at markers of nutritional status in efforts to predict poor outcomes and found that preoperative serum albumin less than 3.5 g/dL, body mass index less than 18.5 kg/m^2, and weight loss of 5% or greater of total body weight carried a hazard ratio of 2.9 for 90-day mortality for nutritionally deficit patients compared with patients without risk factors for malnutrition. This remained true even after controlling for comorbid conditions, pathologic stage, transfusion rate, and complications.[49] The identification of adverse markers of nutritional deficits highlights a potentially modifiable patient factor that has a known increased risk of death after RC/UD.

Total Parenteral Nutrition Versus Early Enteral Feeding

Postoperative total parenteral nutrition (TPN) has been explored to correct malnutrition seen in RC/UD patients. The best literature within the RC/UD population is a single-center, randomized trial of 157 consecutive patients undergoing RC/UD. In this study, 74 patients received TPN during the first 5 postoperative days with additional oral intake as desired compared with 83 patients who received oral nutrition alone.[50] Within the 2 groups, time to gastrointestinal recovery and length of hospital stay did not differ. Overall complications were higher (69% vs 49%) and, most significantly, infectious complications were higher (32% vs 11%; $P = .001$), in the TPN arm than in the oral enteral feeding arm, respectively. In addition serum prealbumin and total protein levels were significantly lower in the oral nutrition group on postoperative day 7 but not on day 12. TPN was also associated with a significantly higher cost per patient, leading the investigators to recommend against routine postoperative TPN in the setting of RC/UD.[50]

Immunonutrition

Immunonutrition is a nutritionally targeted therapeutic intervention using oral replacement therapies with supplements, to replace factors lost during surgery or in the malnourished immune system.[51] Primarily derived from the colorectal literature, a systematic review of 35 studies with implementation of perioperative immunonutrition with arginine supplementation decreased hospital length of stay and postoperative infections.[52] Immunonutrition has been studied in the RC/UD populations as well, although to a much smaller extent. A multicenter, case-controlled pilot study comparing arginine, fish oil, vitamin A, and nucleotides taken prior to surgery with historic controls found a significant reduction in postoperative complications (40% vs 77%) and infection rates (23% vs 60%), respectively.[53]

The only randomized controlled trial with immunonutrition intervention in the RC/UD population compared 29 patients with calorie-matched oral nutritional supplementation pre-RC/UD and post-RC/UD with or without arginine-enriched immunonutrition. Within the immunonutrition support group, the overall postoperative complication rate was decreased by 33% and the rate of postoperative infections was decreased by 39%.[54] Additional multicenter trials are currently under

way to further define the benefit of immunonutrition for patients undergoing RC/UD; however, early results show promise in mitigating the immune stressors of surgery in the often malnourished RC/UD patient.

Carbohydrate Loading

Insulin resistance and hyperglycemia are common in the fasting elective surgical patient.[55] In efforts to determine the effects of preoperative oral carbohydrate replacement, a meta-analysis of 21 randomized control trials, including surgical patients receiving greater than 50 g of carbohydrate prior to surgery, reviewed the safety and effectiveness of carbohydrate replacement. The investigators concluded based on the best available data that carbohydrate replacement up to 2 hours before surgery was safe, reduced postoperative insulin resistance, and decreased hospital length of stay in patients undergoing major abdominal surgery.[55] Although carbohydrate loading has been not been specifically studied in RC/UD, results from other organ systems suggest a benefit and thus is a component of many ERAS pathways.

SUMMARY

Patients undergoing UD are certainly at high risk for complications in the perioperative period. The exact cause of these complications remains poorly defined but is likely multifactorial. Current efforts to optimize patients in the perioperative period, including prehabilitation, smoking cessation, recognition and treatment of malnutrition, immunonutrition supplementation, carbohydrate loading, and implementation of ERAS pathways, seem beneficial in helping to improve outcomes in this at-risk population. Further studies (some of which are ongoing) are necessary to help optimize these strategies and identify which modifiable factors have the greatest impact.

REFERENCES

1. Osborn DJ, Dmochowski RR, Kaufman MR, et al. Cystectomy with urinary diversion for benign disease: indications and outcomes. Urology 2014; 83(6):1433–7.
2. Cohn JA, Large MC, Richards KA, et al. Cystectomy and urinary diversion as management of treatment-refractory benign disease: the impact of preoperative urological conditions on perioperative outcomes. Int J Urol 2014;21(4):382–6.
3. Brown KG, Solomon MJ, Latif ER, et al. Urological complications after cystectomy as part of pelvic exenteration are higher than that after cystectomy

for primary bladder malignancy. J Surg Oncol 2017; 115(3):307–11.

4. Shabsigh A, Korets R, Vora KC, et al. Defining early morbidity of radical cystectomy for patients with bladder cancer using a standardized reporting methodology. Eur Urol 2009;55(1):164–74.

5. Miller DC, Taub DA, Dunn RL, et al. The impact of co-morbid disease on cancer control and survival following radical cystectomy. J Urol 2003;169(1): 105–9.

6. Gray PJ, Lin CC, Jemal A, et al. Clinical-pathologic stage discrepancy in bladder cancer patients treated with radical cystectomy: results from the national cancer data base. Int J Radiat Oncol Biol Phys 2014;88(5):1048–56.

7. Lawrentschuk N, Lee ST, Scott AM. Current role of PET, CT, MR for invasive bladder cancer. Curr Urol Rep 2013;14(2):84–9.

8. Paik ML, Scolieri MJ, Brown SL, et al. Limitations of computerized tomography in staging invasive bladder cancer before radical cystectomy. J Urol 2000;163(6):1693–6.

9. Barentsz JO, Jager GJ, Witjes JA, et al. Primary staging of urinary bladder carcinoma: the role of MRI and a comparison with CT. Eur Radiol 1996; 6(2):129–33.

10. Kundra V, Silverman PM. Imaging in oncology from the University of Texas M. D. Anderson Cancer Center. Imaging in the diagnosis, staging, and follow-up of cancer of the urinary bladder. AJR Am J Roentgenol 2003;180(4):1045–54.

11. Goodfellow H, Viney Z, Hughes P, et al. Role of fluorodeoxyglucose positron emission tomography (FDG PET)-computed tomography (CT) in the staging of bladder cancer. BJU Int 2014;114(3):389–95.

12. Mertens LS, Fioole-Bruining A, Vegt E, et al. Impact of (18) F-fluorodeoxyglucose (FDG)-positron-emission tomography/computed tomography (PET/CT) on management of patients with carcinoma invading bladder muscle. BJU Int 2013;112(6):729–34.

13. Kassouf W, Hautmann RE, Bochner BH, et al. A critical analysis of orthotopic bladder substitutes in adult patients with bladder cancer: is there a perfect solution? Eur Urol 2010;58(3):374–83.

14. Robinson R, Tait CD, Somov P, et al. Estimated glomerular filtration rate is unreliable in detecting renal function loss during follow-up after cystectomy and urinary diversion. Int Urol Nephrol 2016;48(4):511–5.

15. Eisenberg MS, Thompson RH, Frank I, et al. Long-term renal function outcomes after radical cystectomy. J Urol 2014;191(3):619–25.

16. Rozanski A. Is exam under anesthesia still necessary for the staging of bladder cancer in t era of modern imaging? Bladder Cancer 2015;1(1):91–6.

17. von Rundstedt FC, Mata DA, Kryvenko ON, et al. Utility of clinical risk stratification in the selection of muscle-invasive bladder cancer patients for neoadjuvant chemotherapy: a retrospective cohort study. Bladder Cancer 2017;3(1):35–44.

18. Lebret T, Hervé JM, Barré P, et al. Urethral recurrence of transitional cell carcinoma of the bladder. Predictive value of preoperative latero-montanal biopsies and urethral frozen sections during prostato-cystectomy. Eur Urol 1998;33(2):170–4.

19. International Collaboration of Trialists, Medical Research Council advanced Bladder Cancer Working Party (now the National Cancer Research Institute Bladder Cancer Clinical Studies Group), European Organisation for Research and Treatment of Cancer Genito-Urinary Tract Cancer Group, et al. International phase III trial assessing neoadjuvant cisplatin, methotrexate, and vinblastine chemotherapy for muscle-invasive bladder cancer: long-term results of the BA06 30894 trial. J Clin Oncol 2011;29(16):2171–7.

20. Grossman HB, Natale RB, Tangen CM, et al. Neoadjuvant chemotherapy plus cystectomy compared with cystectomy alone for locally advanced bladder cancer. N Engl J Med 2003;349(9):859–66.

21. Dybowski B, Ossoliński K, Ossolińska A, et al. Impact of stage and comorbidities on five-year survival after radical cystectomy in Poland: single centre experience. Cent European J Urol 2015; 68(3):278–83.

22. Prout GR, Wesley MN, Yancik R, et al. Age and comorbidity impact surgical therapy in older bladder carcinoma patients: a population-based study. Cancer 2005;104(8):1638–47.

23. Rochon PA, Katz JN, Morrow LA, et al. Comorbid illness is associated with survival and length of hospital stay in patients with chronic disability. A prospective comparison of three comorbidity indices. Med Care 1996;34(11):1093–101.

24. Zietman AL, Shipley WU, Kaufman DS. Organ-conserving approaches to muscle-invasive bladder cancer: future alternatives to radical cystectomy. Ann Med 2000;32(1):34–42.

25. Nayak JG, Gore JL, Holt SK, et al. Patient-centered risk stratification of disposition outcomes following radical cystectomy. Urol Oncol 2016;34(5):235.e17-23.

26. Fried LP, Tangen CM, Walston J, et al. Frailty in older adults: evidence for a phenotype. J Gerontol A Biol Sci Med Sci 2001;56(3):M146–56.

27. Chappidi MR, Kates M, Patel HD, et al. Frailty as a marker of adverse outcomes in patients with bladder cancer undergoing radical cystectomy. Urol Oncol 2016;34(6):256.e1-6.

28. Lascano D, Pak JS, Kates M, et al. Validation of a frailty index in patients undergoing curative surgery for urologic malignancy and comparison with other risk stratification tools. Urol Oncol 2015;33(10):426.e1-12.

29. Jensen BT, Laustsen S, Jensen JB, et al. Exercise-based pre-habilitation is feasible and effective in radical cystectomy pathways-secondary results

from a randomized controlled trial. Support Care Cancer 2016;24(8):3325–31.

30. Cerantola Y, Valerio M, Persson B, et al. Guidelines for perioperative care after radical cystectomy for bladder cancer: Enhanced Recovery After Surgery (ERAS(®)) society recommendations. Clin Nutr 2013;32(6):879–87.

31. Danna BJ, Wood EL, Baack Kukreja JE, et al. The future of enhanced recovery for radical cystectomy: current evidence, barriers to adoption, and the next steps. Urology 2016;96:62–8.

32. Doiron RC, Booth CM, Wei X, et al. Risk factors and timing of venous thromboembolism after radical cystectomy in routine clinical practice: a population-based study. BJU Int 2016;118(5):714–22.

33. Deibert CM, Silva MV, RoyChoudhury A, et al. A prospective randomized trial of the effects of early enteral feeding after radical cystectomy. Urology 2016;96:69–73.

34. Lee CT, Chang SS, Kamat AM, et al. Alvimopan accelerates gastrointestinal recovery after radical cystectomy: a multicenter randomized placebo-controlled trial. Eur Urol 2014;66(2):265–72.

35. Ording AG, Nielsen ME, Smith AB, et al. Venous thromboembolism and effect of comorbidity in bladder cancer: a danish nationwide cohort study of 13,809 patients diagnosed between 1995 and 2011. Urol Oncol 2016;34(7):292.e1-8.

36. Stimson CJ, Chang SS, Barocas DA, et al. Early and late perioperative outcomes following radical cystectomy: 90-day readmissions, morbidity and mortality in a contemporary series. J Urol 2010;184(4):1296–300.

37. Wuethrich PY, Burkhard FC. Improved perioperative outcome with norepinephrine and a restrictive fluid administration during open radical cystectomy and urinary diversion. Urol Oncol 2015;33(2):66.e21-4.

38. Pillai P, McEleavy I, Gaughan M, et al. A double-blind randomized controlled clinical trial to assess the effect of Doppler optimized intraoperative fluid management on outcome following radical cystectomy. J Urol 2011;186(6):2201–6.

39. Wuethrich PY, Burkhard FC, Thalmann GN, et al. Restrictive deferred hydration combined with pre-emptive norepinephrine infusion during radical cystectomy reduces postoperative complications and hospitalization time: a randomized clinical trial. Anesthesiology 2014;120(2):365–77.

40. IARC Working Group on the Evaluation of Carcinogenic Risks to Humans. Tobacco smoke and involuntary smoking. IARC Monogr Eval Carcinog Risks Hum 2004;83:1437–8.

41. Freedman ND, Silverman DT, Hollenbeck AR, et al. Association between smoking and risk of bladder cancer among men and women. JAMA 2011; 306(7):737–45.

42. Johar RS, Hayn MH, Stegemann AP, et al. Complications after robot-assisted radical cystectomy: results from the international robotic cystectomy consortium. Eur Urol 2013;64(1):52–7.

43. Chang SS, Cookson MS, Baumgartner RG, et al. Analysis of early complications after radical cystectomy: results of a collaborative care pathway. J Urol 2002;167(5):2012–6.

44. Aveyard P, Adab P, Cheng KK, et al. Does smoking status influence the prognosis of bladder cancer? a systematic review. BJU Int 2002;90(3):228–39.

45. Møller AM, Villebro N, Pedersen T, et al. Effect of preoperative smoking intervention on postoperative complications: a randomised clinical trial. Lancet 2002;359(9301):114–7.

46. White JV, Guenter P, Jensen G, et al. Consensus statement: Academy of Nutrition and Dietetics and American Society for Parenteral and Enteral Nutrition: characteristics recommended for the identification and documentation of adult malnutrition (undernutrition). JPEN J Parenter Enteral Nutr 2012;36(3):275–83.

47. Lim SL, Ong KCB, Chan YH, et al. Malnutrition and its impact on cost of hospitalization, length of stay, readmission and 3-year mortality. Clin Nutr Edinb Scotl 2012;31(3):345–50.

48. Cerantola Y, Valerio M, Hubner M, et al. Are patients at nutritional risk more prone to complications after major urological surgery? J Urol 2013;190(6):2126–32.

49. Gregg JR, Cookson MS, Phillips S, et al. Effect of preoperative nutritional deficiency on mortality after radical cystectomy for bladder cancer. J Urol 2011;185(1):90–6.

50. Roth B, Birkhäuser FD, Zehnder P, et al. Parenteral nutrition does not improve postoperative recovery from radical cystectomy: results of a prospective randomised trial. Eur Urol 2013;63(3):475–82.

51. Tobert CM, Hamilton-Reeves JM, Norian LA, et al. The emerging impact of malnutrition on surgical patients: literature review and potential implications on cystectomy for bladder cancer. J Urol 2017;198(3):511–9.

52. Drover JW, Dhaliwal R, Weitzel L, et al. Perioperative use of arginine-supplemented diets: a systematic review of the evidence. J Am Coll Surg 2011;212(3):385–99, 399.e1.

53. Bertrand J, Siegler N, Murez T, et al. Impact of preoperative immunonutrition on morbidity following cystectomy for bladder cancer: a case-control pilot study. World J Urol 2014;32(1):233–7.

54. Hamilton-Reeves JM, Bechtel MD, Hand LK, et al. Effects of immunonutrition for cystectomy on immune response and infection rates: a pilot randomized controlled clinical trial. Eur Urol 2016;69(3):389–92.

55. Awad S, Varadhan KK, Ljungqvist O, et al. A meta-analysis of randomised controlled trials on preoperative oral carbohydrate treatment in elective surgery. Clin Nutr Edinb Scotl 2013;32(1):34–44.

Metabolic and Nutritional Consequences of Urinary Diversion Using Intestinal Segments to Reconstruct the Urinary Tract

Joshua D. Roth, MD[a], Michael O. Koch, MD[b],*

KEYWORDS

- Urinary diversion • Urinary reservoirs • Metabolic acidosis • Ileum • Colon
- Metabolic complications • Nutritional complications

KEY POINTS

- The bowel has been used in the urinary tract for many years.
- Urinary diversion with ileum or colon can lead to concentration defects or metabolic acidosis.
- Urinary diversion with jejunum or gastric segments is not recommended for use in urinary tract reconstruction due to metabolic consequences associated with their use.
- Nutritional consequences of urinary diversion with ileum or colon include vitamin B_{12} deficiency, osteoporosis, fat malabsorption, urinary calculi, and ammoniagenic encephalopathy.

INTRODUCTION

Intestinal segments in various forms have been used to reconstruct the urinary tract since the mid-1800s, with most initial reports focusing on the technical aspects of these procedures.[1] In the early twentieth century before 1950, the primary means of urinary diversion (UD) after cystectomy for any indication was bilateral ureterosigmoidostomy. Of all the past and present forms of UD, this particular technique created a conduit where the greatest amount of intestine was exposed to the excreted urine and, to some degree, where it was exposed to the urine for the greatest amount of time.[1,2] Because the metabolic conditions created by UD are directly and proportionally related to these factors, metabolic conditions are seen most commonly in ureterosigmoidostomy patients. In 1950, 2 physicians from the Mayo Clinic, Ferris and Odel,[3] were the first to recognize and publish on the condition of hyperchloremic metabolic acidosis.[3,4]

In the 1950s, there was a great interest in the etiologic factors of this metabolic acidosis and multiple theories were espoused by many of the leaders in urology of that generation. These theories included a renal acidifying defect from ureteral obstruction or pyelonephritis, secretion of bicarbonate (HCO_3^-) by the bowel into the urine, and the generation of ammonia (NH_3) from urea by the action of urease producing organisms in the urine, which was then reabsorbed.[3–5] All 3 of these theories were at least in part accurate and partially explain the abnormalities seen. It was at

Disclosure Statement: The authors have nothing they wish to disclose.
[a] Department of Urology, Indiana University School of Medicine, Suite 150 Indiana Cancer Pavilion, 535 North Barnhill Drive, Indianapolis, IN 46202, USA; [b] Indiana University School of Medicine, Suite 150 Indiana Cancer Pavilion, 535 North Barnhill Drive, Indianapolis, IN 46202, USA
* Corresponding author.
E-mail address: mkoch2@iuhealth.org

approximately the same time that Eugene Bricker first reported on the ileal conduit[6]. With a lower incidence of surgical and metabolic complications with the ileal conduit, UD via ureterosigmoidostomy was largely abandoned so that the issue of the hyperchloremic metabolic acidosis became a moot point.[7]

In the 1980s, there was a general recognition that patients with ileal conduit UD had significant issues over the long term. With the general acceptance of clean intermittent catheterization techniques, in many children who had neuropathic bladders that had been diverted with conduits, these were undiverted to an augmented bladder with bowel.[8] In addition, driven primarily by body image concerns after cystectomy, both continent cutaneous diversions (eg, Indiana Pouch, Kock pouch) and techniques for continent orthotopic bladder replacements were developed.[9–11] The continent orthotopic replacement was at least in part enabled by the refinement of radical prostatectomy and the ability of urologists to create a urethral-vesical anastomosis.[11] These new continent diversions created systems in which, once again, urine was exposed to large amounts of bowel surface area for protracted periods of time sufficient for the movement of urinary solutes across the intestinal mucosa, thereby leading to electrolyte abnormalities. In addition, the utilization of relatively large segments of ileum to create these diversions resulted in predictable nutritional complications.[12–14]

METABOLIC DERANGEMENTS

Normal urothelium is a highly impermeable barrier to urinary solutes. This property of urothelium allows the kidneys to excrete urinary waste products in concentrations vastly different than that seen in the serum. Specifically, urine is highly concentrated, has a low sodium (Na) content, high potassium content, and it is generally acidic with negligible bicarbonate levels. Whereas normal urine is acidic, normal feces are alkaline. The results seen with various forms of UD are a predictable result of the known physiology of various intestinal segments and the known concentrations of the solutes of urine.[13–16]

Concentration Defect

All forms of UD result in a concentrating defect that is generally well compensated but universally noticeable.[17] Normal urine generally has an osmolality of 500 to 850 mOsm per liter, whereas normal serum and tissue osmolality is around 290 mOsm per liter.[18] Generally, intestinal mucosa is highly permeable to water. As such, when concentrated urine is exposed to a bowel segment, there is movement of water into the intestinal lumen, which negates, in part, the body's ability to preserve volume status. Clinically, this partly accounts for the nocturia seen in these patients and it also results in a chronic prerenal state with an elevated blood urea nitrogen (BUN) to creatinine ratio. Ileum and colon are quite similar in this regard, with jejunum being more severe because of its more loose intra-epithelial junctions. Jejunal conduits also create a salt wasting condition, which further exacerbates the volume depletion.[16]

Ileum and Colon: Hyperchloremic Metabolic Acidosis

The apical membrane surface of both ileum and colon contains antiports, which are specific to certain electrolytes and exchange anions or cations in equimolar amounts. Normal ileum and colon absorb urinary chloride and excrete bicarbonate into the intestinal lumen. In the setting in which the urine has no bicarbonate but moderate amounts of chloride, bicarbonate moves into the lumen of the UD while chloride(Cl) is absorbed, thus initiating the observed acidosis.[19]

When an acidosis initially develops, the kidneys respond by excreting acid as free hydrogen (H) ions, which are buffered with phosphate (O_4P^{3-}) or, to a lesser degree, sulfate ($SO_4(2-)$) in the urine. This cannot continue indefinitely or the body would become deplete in phosphate (O_4P^{3-}), which is an essential part of bone mineralization.[17] The body adapts by creating another buffer in the distal tubule, ammonia, which is very avid for free hydrogen ions. This is readily generated in the kidney by converting glutamine to glutamate, and by deaminating glutamate to 2-oxo-glutarate^{2-} by gamma-glutamyl transferase in the proximal tubule. As abundant amounts of ammonia is generated, it passes through the loop of Henle and distal tubule, where some is reabsorbed and some of it binds to free hydrogen ions to become ammonium (NH_4^+).[20,21]

However, this leads to a second cause of acidosis. The ileum and colon also possess sodium-potassium (Na^+/K^+) antiports, which in normal circumstances allow for the absorption of sodium. In a patient with a UD, ammonium is reabsorbed in equimolar amounts to the amount of sodium excreted. The net effect of these 2 antiports in the patient with UD is the reabsorption of ammonium and chloride and a resulting hyperchloremic metabolic acidosis.[21,22] Ammonia reabsorption has been found to contribute more to the development of systemic acidosis than either the secretion of bicarbonate or the reabsorption of organic acids.[23–25]

These patients are generally depleted in potassium as well. In most circumstances, renal functional reserve can overcome the reabsorbed acid load and patients can maintain an appropriate acid-base balance within clinically acceptable parameters, although most will demonstrate serum bicarbonate and chloride levels that are at or slightly beyond the lower and upper rages of the reference ranges, respectively. The magnitude of these abnormalities will also become more severe with the development of renal insufficiency, as is often seen in these patients due to recurrent infections or obstruction.[26]

Jejunum: Hypochloremic, Hyponatremic, Hyperkalemic Metabolic Acidosis

Jejunum is unique with respect to electrolyte abnormalities after UD. Jejunum has a highly porous epithelium, which causes a large amount of water to be drawn into the bowel lumen, thus creating a significant state of chronic dehydration. In addition, the jejunum lacks the sodium-potassium antiports seen in ileum and colon but has chloride-bicarbonate antiports. With the excretion of normal urine into the jejunal lumen, sodium, chloride, and water rapidly pass down the concentration or osmolar gradients into the lumen. The sodium-hydrogen antiport then secretes further sodium in exchange for hydrogen, which is absorbed. The severe sodium and water loss creates a severe prerenal state that can initially create a contraction alkalosis but, once severe enough, can lead to severe acidosis. This leads to a jejunal conduit syndrome manifested by hyponatremia, hypochloremia, hyperkalemia, azotemia, and usually presents with metabolic acidosis and symptoms of nausea, vomiting, dehydration, muscular weakness, lethargy, and sometimes seizures.[27–30] Because the metabolic derangements in jejunal conduits are so severe, they should never be used for urinary reconstruction.

Gastric Segments: Hypochloremic, Hypokalemic Metabolic Alkalosis

Gastric segments came into prominence following experiments by Sinaiko[31] in 1956 that used gastric segments for lower urinary tract reconstruction in dogs. It was believed that the using gastric segments conferred many benefits, including compensation for preexisting metabolic acidosis in patients with impaired renal function, less mucus production, and conservation of gastrointestinal absorptive surface in patients with foreshortened or compromised bowel.[32] It briefly became an acceptable and favorable alterative to small and large bowel for use in bladder augmentation in children with renal insufficiency.[33] However, due to the severe metabolic side effects found in patients with gastric segment augments, its use is not recommended. The physiologic secretion of hydrogen and chloride ions in gastric mucosa via potassium-hydrogen antiports, as well as considerable amounts of water secretion across the gastric mucosa, lead to a hypokalemic, hypochloremic metabolic alkalosis, hematuria-dysuria syndrome, and hypergastrinemia.[34] This results in lethargy, mental status changes, and intractable seizures, and can lead to respiratory insufficiency related to a compensatory respiratory acidosis. Further, this can result acutely from dehydration from a gastrointestinal illness or, more insidiously, can be chronic in nature.[35]

NUTRITIONAL COMPLICATIONS

The nutritional complications of UD with large segments of ileum or colon are generally predictable and result from the loss of the normal function of these segments in the normal intestinal tract. The latter half of the ileum is largely responsible for the absorption of vitamin B_{12}, fatty acids, bile salts, and multiple other nutrients.[13–16]

Vitamin B_{12}

B_{12} receptors are located in the distal three-fifths of ileum, but are most densely located in the terminal 3 to 5 feet of this segment of the intestinal tract. UD with segments of terminal ileum 60 cm or more diminishes the body's ability to absorb ingested vitamin B_{12}.[14,36] However, human vitamin B_{12} stores are quite large, with stores decreasing very slowly over time, usually taking 3 to 4 years in the absence of any absorption to deplete stores.[14] The consequences of severe B12 deficiency, when they occur, are significant. This presents with chronic macrocytic anemia and, more importantly, an irreversible peripheral neuropathy. Fortunately, vitamin B12 levels are easily monitored by checking serum B_{12} levels and are easy to replace by prescribing B_{12} supplementation.[37,38]

Osteoporosis or Osteopenia

The inability of the kidney to effectively excrete urinary acid as ammonium due to its reabsorption by the intestinal segment results in the excessive waste of phosphate from bone for use as a urinary buffer for the excreted acid. Animal models demonstrate that over the long term this results in bone demineralization.[39] In practice, and especially in adults, this issue seems to be minor and often does not require treatment.[40,41] In children, there remains a concern that this will have an adverse result on bone health over the long term.[42] Rather than resorting to agents that act at the bone level to prevent bone reabsorption, bone demineralization is best managed by correcting the acidosis with the administration of citrate or bicarbonate salts. If there is no clinical response to the correction of acidosis, calcium and vitamin D should be administered.[14,16]

Fatty Acid and Bile Salts

Fatty acids are absorbed in the small intestine after binding with bile salts excreted from the biliary system. These bile salts are reabsorbed in the distal ileum and reexcreted through the liver. If bile salts pass unabsorbed into the colon, they can damage the colonic mucosa, leading to a decreased absorption surface, and can also cause an active secretion of chloride and water, which contributes to secretory diarrhea. Loss of significant portions of small bowel for the UD and/or rapid intestinal transit from loss of the ileocecal valve can result in bile salt depletion over time with resultant abnormalities in fat malabsorption and chronic diarrhea.[43–47] Cholestyramine can be effective in managing these patients.

Urinary Calculi

There are many reasons that patients with intestinal diversions are more likely to have urinary tract calculi. First, patients can be chronically dehydrated due to water loss through the diversion, which is a risk factor for stone formation. Further, patients with long segments of ileum can develop enteric hyperoxaluria due to fat saponification of intestinal calcium, thus increasing unbound oxalate for absorption, which can lead to creation of calcium oxalate stones.[48] In addition, those in a state of chronic acidosis have impaired renal production of citrate, leading to hypocitraturia, and any type of malabsorption problem will often lead to reduced urinary excretion of citrate. Citrate is an inhibitor of stone crystallization and the decreased amount of urinary citrate helps further promote stone formation.[49,50] Finally, urinary reservoirs are frequently colonized with urea-splitting organisms, which can often predispose patients to form magnesium ammonium phosphate stones.[16]

Ammoniagenic Encephalopathy

Ammoniagenic encephalopathy occurs due to excess ammonia absorption. Urinary ammonium produced by the kidney to buffer the increased urinary acid is reabsorbed by the intestinal segment into the portal circulation. Via the ornithine cycle, the liver metabolizes ammonia to urea, which is

Table 1 Summary of metabolic disturbances of urinary diversion using intestinal segments				
Bowel	Sodium	Potassium	Chloride	pH
Stomach	—	↓	↓	↑
Jejunum	↓	↑	↓	↓
Ileum or Colon	—	↓	↑	↓

Abbreviations: —, electrolyte or pH should remain unchanged; ↑, increase; ↓, decrease.

excreted by the kidney. Although the liver can typically handle excess serum ammonia produced as a result of reabsorption of urinary ammonium, this becomes problematic in the setting of hepatic insufficiency or an increased ammonia load caused by the presence of urea-splitting organisms in the urinary tract. The excess ammonia load can overwhelm the detoxification abilities of the liver, resulting in a rare syndrome of an ammoniagenic encephalopathy, which is characterized by seizures, confusion, personality changes, and progressive periods of unresponsiveness that can result in an ammoniagenic coma.[51–55] This condition is very rare with only a few case reports in the literature.

SUMMARY

Overall, the metabolic and nutritional consequences of using intestinal segments to reconstruct the urinary tract are not severe enough to avoid their use. A summary of the expected metabolic disturbances seen with each intestinal segment can be seen in **Table 1**. These patients generally do quite well and the abnormalities seen generally require limited or no interventions. However, the complexities of mixing mucosa between the intestinal and urinary tracts are not well understood by nonurologists and thus it is the urologists who should bear the responsibility of monitoring these patients for potential abnormalities.

REFERENCES

1. Hendren WH. Historical perspective of the use of bowel in urology. Urol Clin North Am 1997;24(4): 703–13.
2. Boyd JD. Chronic acidosis secondary to ureteral transplantation. Arch Pediatr Adolesc Med 1931; 42(2):366–71.
3. Ferris DO, Odel HM. Electrolyte pattern of the blood after bilateral ureterosigmoidostomy. J Am Med Assoc 1950;142(9):634–41.

4. Odel HM, Ferris DO, Priestley JT. Further observations on the electrolyte pattern of the blood after bilateral ureterosigmoidostomy. J Urol 1951;65(6):1013–20.

5. Duckett JW, Gazak JM. Complications of ureterosigmoidostomy. Urol Clin North Am 1983;10(3):473–81.

6. Bricker EM. Bladder substitution after pelvic evisceration. Surg Clin North Am 1950;30(5):1511–21.

7. Butcher HR, Sugg WL, McAfee CA, et al. Ileal conduit method of ureteral urinary diversion. Ann Surg 1962;156(4):682–91.

8. Hendren WH. Reconstruction ("undiversion") of the diverted urinary tract. Hosp Pract 1976;11(1):70–9.

9. Rowland RG, Mitchell ME, Bihrle R, et al. Indiana continent urinary reservoir. J Urol 1987;137(6):1136–9.

10. Kock NG. Intra-abdominal "reservoir" in patients with permanent ileostomy. Preliminary observations on a procedure resulting in fecal "continence" in five ileostomy patients. Arch Surg 1969;99(2):223–31.

11. Studer UE, Ackermann D, Casanova GA, et al. A newer form of bladder substitute based on historical perspectives. Semin Urol 1988;6(1):57–65.

12. Boyd SD, Schiff WM, Skinner DG, et al. Prospective study of metabolic abnormalities in patient with continent Kock pouch urinary diversion. Urology 1989;33(2):85–8.

13. Cruz DN, Huot SJ. Metabolic complications of urinary diversions: an overview. Am J Med 1997;102(5):477–84.

14. Mills RD, Studer UE. Metabolic consequences of continent urinary diversion. J Urol 1999;161(4):1057–66.

15. Mundy AR. Metabolic complications of urinary diversion. Lancet 1999;353(9167):1813–4.

16. Chang SS, Koch MO. The metabolic complications of urinary diversion. Urol Oncol 2000;5(2):60–70.

17. Newman DJ, Price CP. Renal function and nitrogen metabolites. In: Burtis CA, Ashwood ER, editors. Tietz Textbook of Clinical Chemistry. 3rd edition. Philadelphia: Tietz textbook of clinical chemistry. 4th edition. Philadelphia, PA: WB Saunders Company; 1999. p. 1204–70.

18. Newman DJ, Price CP. Renal function and nitrogen metabolites. In: Burtis CA, Ashwood ER, editors. Tietz textbook of clinical chemistry. 4th edition. Philadelphia: WB Saunders Company; 2006. p. 1204–70.

19. Turnberg LA, Bieberdorf FA, Morawski SG, et al. Interrelationships of chloride, bicarbonate, sodium, and hydrogen transport in the human ileum. J Clin Invest 1970;49(3):557–67.

20. Silbernagl S, Scheller D. Formation and excretion of NH3—NH4+. New aspects of an old problem. Klin Wochenschr 1986;64(18):862–70.

21. Garvin JL, Burg MB, Knepper MA. Active NH4+ absorption by the thick ascending limb. Am J Physiol 1988;255(1 Pt 2):F57–65.

22. Stampfer DS, McDougal WS. Inhibition of the sodium/hydrogen antiport by ammonium ion. J Urol 1997;157(1):362–5.

23. Koch MO, McDougal WS. The pathophysiology of hyperchloremic metabolic acidosis after urinary diversion through intestinal segments. Surgery 1985;98(3):561–70.

24. Koch MO, Gurevitch E, Hill DE, et al. Urinary solute transport by intestinal segments: a comparative study of ileum and colon in rats. J Urol 1990;143(6):1275–9.

25. McDougal WS, Stampfer DS, Kirley S, et al. Intestinal ammonium transport by ammonium and hydrogen exchange. J Am Coll Surg 1995;181(3):241–8.

26. Hall MC, Koch MO, McDougal WS. Metabolic consequences of urinary diversion through intestinal segments. Urol Clin North Am 1991;18(4):725–35.

27. Clark SS. Electrolyte disturbance associated with jejunal conduit. J Urol 1974;112(1):42–7.

28. Golimbu M, Morales P. Electrolyte disturbances in jejunal urinary diversion. Urology 1973;1(5):432–8.

29. Golimbu M, Morales P. Jejunal conduits: technique and complications. J Urol 1975;113(6):787–95.

30. Klein EA, Montie JE, Montague DK, et al. Jejunal conduit urinary diversion. J Urol 1986;135(2):244–6.

31. Sinaiko E. Artificial bladder from segment of stomach and study of effect of urine on gastric secretion. Surg Gynecol Obstet 1956;102(4):433–8.

32. Kurzrock EA, Baskin LS, Kogan BA. Gastrocystoplasty: is there a consensus? World J Urol 1998;16(4):242–50.

33. Adams MC, Mitchell ME, Rink RC. Gastrocystoplasty: an alternative solution to the problem of urological reconstruction in the severely compromised patient. J Urol 1988;140(5 Pt 2):1152–6.

34. Peters CA. Bladder reconstruction in children. Curr Opin Pediatr 1994;6(2):183–93.

35. Gosalbez R, Woodard JR, Broecker BH, et al. Metabolic complications of the use of stomach for urinary reconstruction. J Urol 1993;150(2 Pt 2):710–2.

36. Thompson WG, Wrathell E. The relation between ileal resection and vitamin B12 absorption. Can J Surg 1977;20(5):461–4.

37. Steiner MS, Morton RA, Marshall FF. Vitamin B12 deficiency in patients with ileocolic neobladders. J Urol 1993;149(2):255–7.

38. Jahnson S, Pedersen J. Cystectomy and urinary diversion during twenty years–complications and metabolic implications. Eur Urol 1993;24(3):343–9.

39. Lemann J, Litzow JR, Lennon EJ. Studies of the mechanism by which chronic metabolic acidosis augments urinary calcium excretion in man. J Clin Invest 1967;46(8):1318–28.

40. Sevin G, Koşar A, Perk H, et al. Bone mineral content and related biochemical variables in patients with

ileal bladder substitution and colonic Indiana pouch. Eur Urol 2002;41(6):655–9.

41. Fujisawa M, Nakamura I, Yamanaka N, et al. Changes in calcium metabolism and bone demineralization after orthotopic intestinal neobladder creation. J Urol 2000;163(4):1108–11 [quiz: 1295].

42. Gros DA, Dodson JL, Lopatin UA, et al. Decreased linear growth associated with intestinal bladder augmentation in children with bladder exstrophy. J Urol 2000;164(3 Pt 2):917–20.

43. Mekjian HS, Phillips SF, Hofmann AF. Colonic secretion of water and electrolytes induced by bile acids: perfusion studies in man. J Clin Invest 1971;50(8):1569–77.

44. Binder HJ, Rawlins CL. Effect of conjugated dihydroxy bile salts on electrolyte transport in rat colon. J Clin Invest 1973;52(6):1460–6.

45. Hofmann AF, Poley JR. Role of bile acid malabsorption in pathogenesis of diarrhea and steatorrhea in patients with ileal resection. I. Response to cholestyramine or replacement of dietary long chain triglyceride by medium chain triglyceride. Gastroenterology 1972;62(5):918–34.

46. Durrans D, Wujanto R, Carroll RN, et al. Bile acid malabsorption: a complication of conduit surgery. Br J Urol 1989;64(5):485–8.

47. Chadwick VS, Gaginella TS, Carlson GL, et al. Effect of molecular structure on bile acid-induced alterations in absorptive function, permeability, and morphology in the perfused rabbit colon. J Lab Clin Med 1979;94(5):661–74.

48. Steiner MS, Morton RA. Nutritional and gastrointestinal complications of the use of bowel segments in the lower urinary tract. Urol Clin North Am 1991;18(4):743–54.

49. Rudman D, Dedonis JL, Fountain MT, et al. Hypocitraturia in patients with gastrointestinal malabsorption. N Engl J Med 1980;303(12):657–61.

50. Pak CY. Citrate and renal calculi: new insights and future directions. Am J Kidney Dis 1991;17(4):420–5.

51. Kaufman JJ. Ammoniagenic coma following ureterosigmoidostomy. J Urol 1984;131(4):743–5.

52. McDermott WV. Diversion of urine to the intestines as a factor in ammoniagenic coma. N Engl J Med 1957;256(10):460–2.

53. Donnard G, Dumotier J, Le Dantec P, et al. Hyperammonemia encephalopathy after ureterosigmoidostomy. Cah Anesthesiol 1996;44(2):149–51 [in French].

54. Edwards RH. Hyperammonemic encephalopathy related to ureterosigmoidostomy. Arch Neurol 1984;41(11):1211–2.

55. Silberman R. Ammonia intoxication following ureterosigmoidostomy in a patient with liver disease. Lancet 1958;2(7053):937–9.

Conduit Urinary Diversion

Daniel J. Lee, MD*, Mark D. Tyson, MD, Sam S. Chang, MD, MBA

KEYWORDS

- Cystectomy • Ileal conduit • Urinary diversion • Stomal hernia • Ureteroenteric anastomosis

KEY POINTS

- Urinary conduits are the most common urinary diversion performed.
- The surgical technique is reproducible, with acceptable levels of postoperative complications.
- Despite advances in technique, there remain areas of unmet needs in the care for patients with a urinary conduit.

INTRODUCTION

Radical cystectomy with urinary diversion has been the historical standard therapy for localized muscle-invasive bladder cancer.[1] Although multiple various intestinal segments have been described for urinary diversions, the most common urinary diversion has been the ileal conduit, accounting for anywhere from 33% to 84% of all types of urinary diversions.[2,3] Since the first published description of the ileal conduit by Verhoogen and de Graeuve in 1909,[4] there have been multiple refinements in surgical technique[5,6] and perioperative management that have helped to improve patient outcomes and quality of life.[7] Despite these innovations, radical cystectomy is still associated with potentially significant risks of postoperative complications,[1,8–11] mortality rates of up to 10%,[11–13] and can have a significant impact on patients' quality of life.[7,14]

Urinary conduits warrant special consideration in patient counseling and education, because a visible stoma can affect a patient's lifestyle, social relationships, dependence on others for care, and self-image.[3,15] In this review, we characterize the use of the urinary conduit in the contemporary era, focusing primarily on the ileal conduit; examine the evidence behind recent advances in surgical technique; and identify potential unmet needs for patients undergoing a cystectomy and urinary conduit to help improve health care services for patients. In this article, we review the salient aspects of the ileal conduit with 3 educational objectives for the reader: (1) to describe the surgical steps emphasizing important surgical principles, (2) to provide commentary on various preoperative and postoperative considerations, and (3) to summarize long-term complications and quality of life.

SURGICAL PRINCIPLES

The surgical technique varies somewhat according to patient characteristics, surgeon, and institution. The intent is not to present a single "best practice" for the ileal conduit, but rather to present our technique within the context of several surgical principles that require fastidious attention regardless of the technique used.

Isolating the Ileal Loop

In his original description, Bricker isolated a segment of ileum "6 to 8 inches in length about 4 to 5 inches from the ileocecal junction."[5] Similarly, a 15-cm segment of ileum is isolated about 15 cm

Disclosure: This work was in part supported by NIH/NCI Grant 5T32CA106183 (M.D. Tyson).
Department of Urologic Surgery, Vanderbilt University Medical Center, A1302 Medical Center North, Nashville, TN 37232, USA
* Corresponding author.
E-mail address: Daniel.Lee.1@Vanderbilt.edu

proximal to the ileocecal junction if there are no signs of inflammatory bowel disease or radiation changes involving this segment. Owing to variations in individual anatomy, it is best to ensure that 15 cm is enough ileum by juxtaposing the provisional loop of ileum to the site chosen for the urostomy before dividing the bowel. Once the segment has been identified, it is marked to aid in orientation during the ureteroenteric anastomosis.

Before dividing the bowel, the vascular arcade is identified using transillumination. The branches from the superior mesenteric artery are vertically oriented toward the mesenteric border of the bowel and are connected to each other by an arcade of vessels. The mesentery is then divided to an approximate depth of 5 cm, but the distal end of the conduit may need greater mobilization to reach the stoma site. After division of the proximal and distal ends of the conduit, a side-to-side ileo-ileostomy is performed. A hand-sewn or stapled anastomosis is performed; if stapling, a 60 to 80 mm GIA staple is used to approximate the antimesenteric border of the 2 cut ends of the ileum. A separate 60- to 80-mm load of the GIA stapler or a TA stapler is used to approximate the open end of the ileostomy. The staple line is oversewn with running 4-0 Vicryl sutures and staple line is buttressed along the antimesenteric border of the ileo-ileostomy using interrupted 4-0 Vicryl sutures. The mesenteric window (ie, "the trap door") of the ileo-ileostomy is then closed using 3-0 Vicryl sutures so as to prevent internal bowel herniation.

Complications

Nevertheless, there are a couple of worthy considerations regarding the isolation of the ileal segment. First, the terminal ileum is the predominant site of absorption of micronutrients such as cobalamin (vitamin B_{12}) and magnesium.[16] Cobalamin evades the digestive enzymes of the upper gastrointestinal tract by binding to intrinsic factor, a glycoprotein synthesized by gastric parietal cells.[17] The cobalamin-intrinsic factor complex is subsequently absorbed by the Cubam receptor located at the apical brush border membrane of polarized enterocytes of the terminal ileum.[18] Therefore, the classic teaching is to avoid using large distal segments of the terminal ileum in an effort to avert vitamin B_{12} deficiency syndromes, such as megaloblastic anemia, particularly in patients with extensive ileal disease such as Crohn's disease. However, for most patients without malabsorption syndromes, large resections of ileum (>100 cm) would be required before clinical manifestations of vitamin B_{12} deficiency would be evident.[19] Therefore, under most circumstances, the urologist can safely harvest larger segments of ileum should it be necessary for anatomic reasons, such as obesity or a short mesentery, because ileal conduits that are too short may not easily reach the stoma site, resulting in unnecessary tension on the ureteroenteric anastomosis.

Jejunal Conduit

Jejunal conduits are not commonly used, and are usually only used when there has been extensive radiation of the ileum, severe adhesions of the ileum, or unusable or absent sections of the large bowel. Use of the jejunum is contraindicated in patients with severe bowel-related nutritional disease and when another, more appropriate segment of bowel is available. The jejunum has the largest diameter of the small bowel and also has a relatively long mesentery. The surgical technique to isolate the jejunal segment is similar to that described for the ileal conduit. A 10- to 15-cm segment is isolated about 10 to 15 cm from the ligament of Treitz. In addition, the stoma is usually best situated in the left upper quadrant, but can be placed wherever it can reasonably reach without any tension. The complications in general are similar to those of an ileal conduit, except that the electrolyte abnormality is a hyperkalemic hyponatremic metabolic acidosis,[20] which can be treated with sodium bicarbonate and thiazide diuretics.[21] The routine use of this diversion has been discouraged for decades.

Colon Conduit

Three different segments of the colon can be used as a conduit, each with their own strengths and weaknesses. The transverse colon is normally used in patients with extensive pelvic radiation, or when a colopyelostomy needs to be done. The sigmoid colon can be used if the patient is undergoing a pelvic exenteration with a colostomy, so that no bowel reanastomosis is necessary and can allow a refluxing or a nonrefluxing submucosal ureteral implantation and a left-sided stoma when needed. However, the sigmoid colon should be avoided after pelvic radiation or when there is disease of that segment, such as inflammatory bowel disease. The ileocecal conduit can provide a long segment of ileum that can be helpful when the ureters need more proximal transection.

The blood supply for the transverse colon conduit should be based on either the right or middle colic arteries. The gastrocolic ligament is incised, the omentum is freed from the colon conduit, and splenic and hepatic flexures are mobilized. Usually about 15 cm of the transverse colon is measured out for the conduit, but the length should be sufficient to reach the retroperitoneum and ureters without any tension. The segment is isolated and the reanastomosis can be performed as described previously for the ileal conduit. The segment should be caudad to the bowel anastomosis, or placed cephalad to the anastomosis if a colopyelostomy needs to be performed. For a sigmoid colon conduit, the peritoneal attachments and the line of Toldt should be incised. The segment of the sigmoid conduit is then isolated on the vessels and placed lateral to the sigmoid colon anastomosis. The ileocecal conduit should be based on the ileocecal artery, with the segment placed caudad to the anastomosis.

Ureteroenteric Anastomosis

There are many different techniques for the ureteroenteric anastomosis, but this discussion is limited to the 2 most commonly used techniques: the Bricker and the Wallace techniques. The Bricker technique is a freely refluxing end-to-side anastomotic technique whereby the ureters are placed at 2 separate locations on the proximal end of the conduit. An enterotomy is first made followed by eversion of the mucosa using 4-0 chromic sutures. The ureter is then spatulated and a single layer full-thickness anastomosis is performed using 4-0 or 5-0 absorbable sutures in a running or interrupted fashion. Before completing the anastomosis, a stent is placed in the ureter and delivered through the conduit using a Yankeur suction tip or an instrument such as a Tonsil clamp. Before completing the anastomosis, the stent is secured to the conduit using 5-0 chromic suture. If feasible, some of the periureteral fat can be approximated over the top of the anastomosis before turning to the other side to help decrease ureteroenteric anastomotic leaks. Once this maneuver is complete, the other side is anastomosed in the same fashion, but usually not directly across from the other ureter so as not to compromise the blood supply of that portion of the conduit.

For the Wallace technique, the proximal end of the conduit is left open. The ureters are spatulated for a distance that is slightly greater than the diameter of the conduit. The inner walls of the ureters are joined to each other using a running 4-0 absorbable suture followed by joining of the outer walls to the proximal end of the conduit. Similar to the Bricker technique, stents can be placed before completion of the anastomosis. One potential downside to the Wallace technique is that a recurrence in 1 ureter may compromise the other ureter. No matter which technique is used, there are several surgical principles that apply to both techniques, including maintenance of an adequate distal ureteral blood supply, a tension-free anastomosis, and avoidance of ureteral kinking or twisting. Finally, after completing the ureteroenteric anastomosis, the proximal end of the conduit is retroperitonealized by approximating the cut edges of the peritoneum of the sigmoid colon.

Maturation of the Stoma

The standard rosebud technique begins by excising a circular piece of skin around the site marked by the enterostomal nurses. Dissection is carried down to the anterior rectus sheath in which a cruciate incision is made. The dissection is carried through the belly of the rectus muscle followed by digital dilation of the stomal site, usually with 2 fingers. The distal end of the conduit is then delivered through the stoma site using a Babcock, ensuring that it is 2 to 3 cm above the level of the skin. Although some surgeons may place facial sutures, the stoma can be matured by passing absorbable suture through the dermal tissue just deep to the skin, through the serosa of the conduit several centimeters proximal to the mucosa, and then through the mucosa in all 4 quadrants of the conduit. The skin is then reapproximated to the mucosa of the conduit to ensure proper eversion of the mucosa into a rosebud. A red rubber catheter or Foley can be placed into the conduit, although this measure is not necessary. It is critical to ensure that the conduit is not twisted on its mesentery, so after the stoma has been matured, it is prudent to inspect the conduit before maturing the stoma.

A Turnbull, or loop stoma, can also be performed with equivalent functional outcomes as end ileal stomas.[22] To construct a loop stoma, the distal end of the ileal segment is closed in the same manner as the proximal end, and a loop of the segment is brought up through the rectus muscle and onto the anterior abdominal wall. A piece of umbilical tape can be passed through a small opening of the mesentery at a location where the distal portion of the loop will remain in the abdomen when the rest of the loop is brought up to the skin. A slightly larger skin opening is made compared with the end ileal stoma, and the peritoneum is entered as described previously. The ileal loop can then be brought up by the umbilical tape that was placed previously, and positioned such that the closed distal portion of the loop is cephalad to the main portion of the loop conduit. A small rod then replaces the umbilical tape to hold the loop in position. The bowel wall is then opened by a transverse incision closer to the most cephalad and nonfunctioning portion of the loop. The cephalad portion is then sutured to the skin, and the caudal portion is then everted and sutured as in the rosebud technique. The loop stoma has been found to have lower rates of stomal stenosis, but can have a higher risk of parastomal hernias.[23] Loop stomas may be easier to place in obese patients where the abdominal wall is often thick and the ileal mesentery is often short and thick.[20]

PREOPERATIVE CONSIDERATIONS
Impact of Age in Radical Cystectomy and Urinary Conduit

Age is an important factor to consider in patients undergoing a radical cystectomy and urinary conduit. The median age at diagnosis of urothelial carcinoma of the bladder is 73 years,[24] and almost 90% of patients aged 65 to 74 years undergoing a radical cystectomy receive an ileal conduit urinary diversion.[2] Older patients tend to have more comorbidities and disabling illnesses; by the age of 65, more than 50% will have 2 or more chronic diseases,[25] and more than 60% report some major disability.[26] Most studies, especially those from population-based registries, have found that older patients have higher morbidity and mortality rates after cystectomy.[27,28] An analysis of the Surveillance, Epidemiology, and End Results registry data found that the 90-day mortality rate after cystectomy of patients 70 to 79 years of age and those 80 years of age and older was 10.4% and 14.3%, respectively.[13] However, other studies from centers of excellence have found that, with careful selection of elderly patients, a radical cystectomy can be safely done, even in those 80 years of age and older, without an increased risk of major complications.[29] radical cystectomy may be underused in elderly patients; approximately 20% of Medicare beneficiaries aged 66 years or older diagnosed with muscle-invasive bladder cancer underwent a radical cystectomy,[30] and the prognosis for patients with invasive bladder cancer is more highly correlated with the extent of the cancer than with patient age.[31–34] Moreover, radical cystectomy has previously demonstrated survival benefits even among the elderly,[33,35] and overall survival was found to be higher patients who underwent radical cystectomy compared with those who underwent alternative treatments such as chemotherapy and/or radiation therapy or no active treatment.[30] Although age is an important factor for those considering a radical cystectomy, elderly patients are a heterogeneous population with varying degrees of comorbidities and functional impairments, and chronologic age must be considered in the context of the whole patient and all other possible risk factors.

Psychosocial Considerations for a Urinary Conduit

Psychosocial factors are also an important consideration for patients undergoing a cystectomy with urinary diversion. Up to two-thirds of patient with an ileal conduit require help from their spouse or another caretaker to take care of their appliance and urostomy,[36] but almost one-third of the people age 65 and older live by themselves without anybody else to help take care of them.[37] For those who are discharged to a skilled nursing facility, it is imperative that the facility have experience with urostomy management to prevent complications and the decreases in quality of life associated with poor stomal management. Also, stomal care such as peristomal skin maintenance is particularly important because the skin is often sensitive to effects of exposure to urine. Going from diagnosis through treatment to survivorship may be an extremely difficult process that reveals a large unmet need for improved counseling and support; up to 50% of survivors after cystectomy experience depression.[36] Preoperative counseling and shared decision making may be difficult, especially in elderly patients, because one-third of people 65 years and older have a less than basic health literacy and would not be able to understand clearly written material from a pamphlet.[38] In addition, cognitive deficits have been found in up to 50% of patients in elderly patients with cancer.[39] In fact, low health literacy is related to increased postcystectomy complication rates,[40] and many of the cancer society websites on bladder cancer are written at an 11th- to 12th-grade reading level.[41] Each individual's social factors must therefore be evaluated to assess the availability of support in terms of long-term care and assistance with daily function, transportation, and living arrangements. These discussions and evaluations could drastically influence the individual's treatment plans, and affect the social network and family dynamics, warranting careful consideration in the decision making.

Choice of Urinary Diversion

There is large variation in the use of different urinary diversion techniques, with some centers of excellence performing 70% to 90% of all of their cystectomies with an orthotopic diversion,[1,42] whereas 80% to 90% of cystectomies in population-based datasets are performed with an ileal conduit.[43,44] The reasons behind this great variation are likely multifactorial, with multiple oncologic, functional, and quality-of-life considerations in choosing an appropriate urinary diversion, whether it is an incontinent conduit, continent cutaneous, or continent orthotopic diversion. There are several important oncologic and patient factors that are contraindications for an orthotopic or continent diversion where the patient should then receive a urinary conduit (**Table 1**).[45]

Prostatic urethral involvement has been associated with a higher risk of urethral recurrence. In pooled analyses, urethral recurrence occurs in up to 25% of men with prostatic urethral involvement[46] compared with about 5% without any involvement.[47] Interestingly, carcinoma in situ in the bladder and tumor multifocality have not been associated individually with anterior urethral recurrence.[47] Extensive disease detected at the time of surgery has been considered a relative contraindication, because patients with orthotopic diversions tolerate adjuvant chemotherapy as well as those with incontinent diversions, and local recurrence tends not to interfere with the urinary diversion itself.[48,49] One important consideration is in those patients with disease invading the pelvic sidewall with grossly positive margins, who are at very high risk of local pelvic recurrence and may require radiation treatment after surgery, which can damage an orthotopic diversion; these patients may benefit from a urinary conduit instead.

Other important patient factors that can preclude the possibility of an orthotopic or continent diversion include urethral strictures, and conditions that can affect the quality of the small bowel, including a history of enteric inflammatory diseases or pelvic radiation. Severe urethral stricture disease is a contraindication to orthotopic urinary diversion, because it can increase outflow resistance and hinder the possibility of catheterization if needed for complete bladder emptying. A history of pelvic radiation is not necessarily a contraindication to the use of an orthotopic diversion, because certain series in centers of excellence have found similar complication rates in those who did or did not receive pelvic radiation.[50] Instead, careful intraoperative assessment is recommended to determine the viability of the bowel and ureters to determine the safety and feasibility of performing an orthotopic diversion as opposed to a urinary conduit with an uninvolved segment of bowel such as the transverse colon.[51–53]

An important consideration is the degree of the patient's manual dexterity. For orthotopic diversions, about 10% of men and 50% of women will require self-catheterization to completely empty their orthotopic diversion.[54,55] For urinary conduits, manual dexterity is also important to assess the ability to change the urostomy appliance, and may determine future patient independence.

Renal Function

The patient's renal function is one of the most important patient factors to consider in choosing a urinary diversion. Urea, potassium, and chloride are reabsorbed by the small bowel mucosa, and sodium and bicarbonate are excreted normally, causing an increased acid load to the kidneys. The surface area and time that the urine is in contact with the gastrointestinal tract are directly related to the increase in acid load to the kidneys. In patients with renal failure, worsening hyperchloremic metabolic acidosis can develop with worsening uremia, bone loss, and dehydration. The ileal conduit is ideal for elderly patients and for those with impaired renal function, because the segment of bowel is short and there is minimal contact time with the urine. This is a particularly important consideration for those undergoing cisplatin-based chemotherapy,[56] because a

Table 1	
Contraindications to orthotopic or continent diversion	
Absolute Contraindications	**Relative Contraindications**
Positive intraoperative urethral margin	Extensive disease outside the bladder or pubic bone
Chronic renal failure (serum creatinine >1.7–2.2 mg/dL or estimated creatinine clearance of <35–40 mL/min)	Plan for postoperative pelvic radiation
	Neurologic diseases impairing the patient's continence
Physical, neurologic, or mental impairment to performing self-catheterization	Chronic enteric inflammatory diseases or malignant bowel diseases
Hepatic insufficiency	
Severe urethral strictures	

Data from Skinner EC, Daneshmand S. Orthotopic urinary diversion. 11th edition. Dallas (TX): Elsevier; 2016.

significant proportion will eventually develop renal impairment. Over time, there is a long-term decrease in renal function, regardless of the type of urinary diversion.[57,58] One important exception is the ureterosigmoidostomy, where the incidence of renal failure and sepsis is more common than in ileal conduits, with about 10% to 22% of these patients dying of renal failure or sepsis.[59] Although it is generally accepted that patients with renal failure, defined as a serum creatinine of greater than 1.7 to 2.2 mg/dL or an estimated creatinine clearance of less than 35 to 40 mL/min, should not receive continent or orthotopic diversions, the optimal limit for acceptable renal function has not been well-established.[45] If patients with a serum creatinine of greater than 2 mg/dL are being considered for an orthotopic diversion or continent cutaneous diversion, then a more detailed analysis of the renal function would be warranted. A patient with a higher creatinine can be considered for a continent diversion if the patient has urine with a pH of 5.8 or less after an ammonium chloride load, the glomerular filtration rate exceeds 35 mL/min, the urine has minimal protein, and has a urine osmolality of 600 mOsm/kg or higher after water deprivation.[20]

PERIOPERATIVE AND INTRAOPERATIVE CONSIDERATIONS
Preoperative Bowel Preparation

The routine use of mechanical bowel preparation before undergoing intestinal surgery was previously thought to reduce infectious and anastomotic complications.[60] However, a growing body of evidence is challenging these assertions in patients undergoing an ileal conduit. In several prospective studies and 2 randomized trials, there seems to be little decrease in complications, including abdominal abscess formation, sepsis, wound complications, bowel obstruction, fistulas, or leaks.[61–66] In fact, in 1 study, the rate of *Clostridium difficile* colitis seemed to be higher among patients treated with a bowel preparation, although the authors cautioned that this may have been due to a higher rate of hospital-wide *C difficile* in that particular year of the study.[67]

Stoma Marking and Preparation

Preoperative marking of the potential stoma site has been shown to decrease stoma-related complications and help to increase the likelihood of independent care.[68] The preoperative marking helps to determine the optimal location of the stoma by giving time to evaluate the abdomen from multiple positions. This allows for ideal placement of the stoma in an easy-to-reach location within the line of sight, which will help to improve the patient's ability to adapt to the urostomy and encourage independent self-care. The preoperative marking gives time for the trained clinicians and staff to educate and familiarize the patient with the urostomy care, hygiene, and the application of the appliance. Furthermore, use of preoperative marking by specially trained wound ostomy nurses and clinicians have been found to decrease stoma-related complications such as stomal hernias and peristomal dermatitis, enhance independent self-care, improve the reliability of stomal appliance functioning, and improve the likelihood of resuming normal activities.[69–73]

Ureteral Stent Placement

The need for ureteral stents across ureteroenteric anastomoses has been debated in the urologic literature. Ureteroenteric anastomoses are often stented out of concern for mechanical obstruction from postoperative tissue edema. Stents were not routinely used in the early experience with urinary diversions because of a lack of evidence that they prevented a urine leak.[74] In addition, there has been concern that indwelling stents could increase the risk for infections and eventually propagate the formation of strictures.[75] In a randomized trial of urinary diversions with or without ureteral stenting, Mattei and colleagues[76] found that, although stenting was not associated with the long-term stricture rate, patients with ureteral stents had lower urine leaks in the early postoperative period with lower measured fluid creatinine levels from the drains, decreased metabolic acidosis, and improved recovery of bowel function. Other studies have had similar findings that suggest that ureteral stent placement could help to decrease the urinary leak rate and improve return of bowel function,[77,78] although the evidence on the actual effect on long-term stricture rates is still inconsistent.[77–79]

Prophylactic Mesh Placement to Prevent Parastomal Hernias

Parastomal hernias are among the most frequent complications after a urinary conduit; however, the actual rates vary widely from 5% to 65% depending on the cohort studied, duration of follow-up, and means of diagnosis.[80–86] Parastomal hernias can have a significant effect on the quality of life and can occasionally cause life-threatening situations with bowel strangulation or obstruction.[87] About one-third of patients with a parastomal hernia require surgical repair,[87] and anywhere from 30% to 75% of those will recur.[83,88–91]

With the high rates of morbidity and recurrence with parastomal hernias, there have been significant efforts to identify risk factors for developing hernias and evaluate methods to prophylactically prevent hernias from recurring. Certain patient factors have been found to be associated independently with radiographically detected parastomal hernias, such as obesity, female gender, and poor nutrition.[80,81,92,93] In fact, 1 study found that severely obese patients with a body mass index of greater than 40 kg/m^2 had 4 times the risk of developing a parastomal hernia than those with a normal body mass index.[81] The size of the abdominal fascia opening for the stoma has been found to be a significant risk factor for the development of parastomal hernias.[92,93] The widely used criteria to determine the size of the stoma has been the width of 2 fingers, which correlates with about a 35-mm defect.[93,94] Some studies suggest that, for every millimeter increase in size of the abdominal fascia defect of greater than 35 mm, the risk of developing a parastomal hernia increases by about 10%.[95] Another commonly used technique is the use of anchoring sutures to secure the conduit to the fascia. However, in the urologic and colorectal literature, this maneuver has not been found to reduce parastomal hernia rates.[88,90,96]

There have been multiple prospective randomized trials in the colorectal literature of mesh placement at the time of stoma formation.[97–102] All of the studies have found significant reductions in parastomal hernia rates without any long-term morbidity or complications associated with the mesh placement. In the study with the longest follow-up, with an average of 6 years of follow-up, the clinically detected parastomal hernia rate was 13% with the mesh placement compared with 81% without the mesh, with no fistulas, strictures, mesh infections, or need for mesh removal in any of the patients.[99]

Prophylactic mesh placement at the time of a urinary conduit has not been well-studied. One study evaluated 33 patients, 16 men with a body mass index of greater than 30 kg/m^2 and 17 women of all body mass indexes, who underwent prophylactic partially absorbable mesh placement at the time of the urinary conduit.[103] The mesh was anchored to the posterior rectus sheath and placed circumferentially around the conduit. At 1 year, 12% of those patients developed a radiographically detected parastomal hernia compared with 27% of historic controls, with no complications, fistulas, or need to remove the mesh.[103] Another study of 114 patients who underwent a urinary conduit with prophylactic mesh placement with a median follow-up of almost 3 years found a similar parastomal hernia rate around 14% with the mesh, with no mesh-related complications.[104] These studies provide promising evidence that may be able to help decrease the rates of parastomal hernias. However, there is a need for long-term follow-up and randomized, controlled trials before the use of prophylactic mesh placement in urinary conduits can be recommended.

COMPLICATIONS AFTER A URINARY CONDUIT

Urinary conduits are often considered easier to perform compared with continent diversions. However, urinary conduits have not necessarily been associated with lower complication rates compared with other diversion techniques.[3,105] This finding may be due to a significant selection bias present in many studies, where those receiving an ileal conduit have more comorbidities, are higher surgical risk candidates, and have poorer tumor characteristics.[106,107] Most of the complications related to urinary conduits are grouped into early (<90 days) and late (>90 days) categories[54] (**Table 2**).

In general, the early complication rate in the literature ranges from 20% to 64%,[107,108] with the majority related to complications involving the gastrointestinal tract. Paralytic ileus can occur in up to about 20% of cases and is often one of the determining factors for the duration of stay after a cystectomy.[109] An anastomotic bowel leakage is a relatively uncommon but potentially devastating complication, with increased rates of related morbidity and mortality.[107] Although this outcome is often related to the surgical technique, there have been no associations between the risk of

Table 2	
Complications after urinary conduit	
Early Complications	**Late Complications**
Bowel related	Stoma related
Bowel anastomosis related	Abdominal wall related
Ureteroenteric anastomosis leakage	Conduit stenosis
Enteric fistula	Ureteroenteric anastomotic stricture
Bowel obstruction	Hydronephrosis
Prolonged ileus	Kidney failure
Conduit necrosis	Metabolic changes

Data from Hautmann RE. Urinary diversion: ileal conduit to neobladder. J Urol 2003;169(3):834–42.

an anastomotic leak and the use of a stapled or hand-sewn closure.[43] Urine leak from the ureteroenteric anastomosis can be a challenging early complication, accounting for up to about 7% of complications.[82] This complication is often related to the surgical technique, such as tension at the anastomosis or ureteral devascularization as opposed to the type of anastomosis used.[109]

In 1 long-term study of more than 1000 patients who underwent cystectomy with a urinary conduit and who were followed for a median of more than 15 years found that, overall, about 20% of the patients developed bowel complications, 20% developed renal complications, 17% had infectious complications, 15% had stomal complications, and 15% developed renal stones.[110] Bowel obstruction occurred in 16%, and 7% of the patients required a reoperation. Stomal stenosis has been described in about 2% to 8% of urinary conduits.[111,112] Stenosis at the skin can be managed with gentle dilation, but often requires surgical intervention to repair. Benign ureteral strictures occur in about 7% to 14% of cases and normally occur within the first 2 years.[107] Endourological techniques, such as stent placement, balloon dilatation, and endoureterotomy are being increasingly used with excellent results in select patients[113]; however, open revision remains the gold standard for repair. The type of ureteroenteric anastomosis used (Bricker vs Wallace technique) has not been consistently associated with long-term stricture rates in urinary conduits.[114,115] The reabsorption of acid by the urinary conduit increases the mobilization of calcium from the bones to act as a buffer, which weakens the bones and increases the risk of kidney stones.[116]

Quality of Life

There have been multiple studies assessing the health-related quality of life after different types of urinary diversions using different assessment tools. These tools have included general health related quality of life instruments, such as the 36-Item Short Form Health Survey, but have also included a few questionnaires specific to patients with muscle-invasive bladder cancer, such as the Functional Assessment of Cancer Therapy-Bladder, the European Organization for Research and Treatment of Cancer 30-item quality of life questionnaire for patients with muscle-invasive bladder cancer, the Bladder Cancer Index, and the Vanderbilt Cystectomy Index.[117,118] Despite multiple studies and systematic reviews of the primary data, there has been conflicting evidence and no clear advantage in the quality of life for orthotopic diversions over incontinent urinary

conduits.[119–121] Some of the main limitations of these studies have been the lack of prospective studies, lack of baseline data in a cross-sectional analysis, and the use of general health-related quality-of-life outcome instruments instead of validated, disease-specific tools.[119,120]

The main advantages for orthotopic diversions over a urinary conduit would potentially involve an improved body image, satisfaction with continence, and potentially improved lifestyle and social functioning.[122] Orthotopic diversions, especially in centers of excellence, have reported high daytime continence rates of 80% to 90%,[45,48] but this benefit needs to be balanced by the risks of nighttime incontinence and urinary retention, with about 20% of men and about 40% to 60% of women requiring self-catheterization.[55] Despite the lack of a consistent advantage for orthotopic diversions over urinary conduits, it is important to take into consideration the priorities of the patients and clearly depict the possible risks and complications for each process.

SUMMARY

Urinary conduits are the most commonly used urinary diversions after radical cystectomy, owing in large part to the relative simplicity of the technique and acceptable complication rates. These factors allow the urinary conduit to be widely used in elderly patients with comorbidities. Despite many advances in technique and care management that have improved outcomes, there remain many unmet needs that should be further studied and evaluated so that patient's outcomes and quality of life can continue to improve.

REFERENCES

1. Stein JP, Lieskovsky G, Cote R, et al. Radical cystectomy in the treatment of invasive bladder cancer: long-term results in 1,054 patients. J Clin Oncol 2001;19(3):666–75.
2. Gore JL, Yu HY, Setodji C, et al. Urinary diversion and morbidity after radical cystectomy for bladder cancer. Cancer 2010;116(2):331–9.
3. Hautmann RE, Abol-Enein H, Hafez K, et al. Urinary diversion. Urology 2007;69(1 Suppl):17–49.
4. Verhoogen J, de Graeuve A. La cystectomie totale. Folia Urol 1909;3:629.
5. Bricker EM. Bladder substitution after pelvic evisceration. Surg Clin North Am 1950;30(5):1511–21.
6. Wallace DM. Uretero-ileostomy. Br J Urol 1970; 42(5):529–34.
7. Tyson MD, Chang SS. Enhanced recovery pathways versus standard care after cystectomy: a

meta-analysis of the effect on perioperative outcomes. Eur Urol 2016;70(6):995–1003.

8. Sood A, Kachroo N, Abdollah F, et al. An evaluation of the timing of surgical complications following radical cystectomy: data from the American College of Surgeons National Surgical Quality Improvement Program. Urology 2017;103:91–8.

9. Kim SP, Boorjian SA, Shah ND, et al. Contemporary trends of in-hospital complications and mortality for radical cystectomy. BJU Int 2012;110(8):1163–8.

10. Cookson MS, Chang SS, Wells N, et al. Complications of radical cystectomy for nonmuscle invasive disease: comparison with muscle invasive disease. J Urol 2003;169(1):101–4.

11. Stimson CJ, Chang SS, Barocas DA, et al. Early and late perioperative outcomes following radical cystectomy: 90-day readmissions, morbidity and mortality in a contemporary series. J Urol 2010; 184(4):1296–300.

12. Dell'Oglio P, Tian Z, Leyh-Bannurah SR, et al. Short-form Charlson Comorbidity index for assessment of perioperative mortality after radical cystectomy. J Natl Compr Canc Netw 2017;15(3):327–33.

13. Schiffmann J, Gandaglia G, Larcher A, et al. Contemporary 90-day mortality rates after radical cystectomy in the elderly. Eur J Surg Oncol 2014; 40(12):1738–45.

14. Yang LS, Shan BL, Shan LL, et al. A systematic review and meta-analysis of quality of life outcomes after radical cystectomy for bladder cancer. Surg Oncol 2016;25(3):281–97.

15. Boyd SD, Feinberg SM, Skinner DG, et al. Quality of life survey of urinary diversion patients: comparison of ileal conduits versus continent Kock ileal reservoirs. J Urol 1987;138(6):1386–9.

16. Said H, Trebble T. Intestinal digestion and absorption of micronutrients. 10th edition. Philadelphia: Saunders; 2016.

17. Levine JS, Nakane PK, Allen RH. Immunocytochemical localization of human intrinsic factor: the nonstimulated stomach. Gastroenterology 1980; 79(3):493–502.

18. Fyfe JC, Madsen M, Højrup P, et al. The functional cobalamin (vitamin B12)-intrinsic factor receptor is a novel complex of cubilin and amnionless. Blood 2004;103(5):1573–9.

19. Mason JB. Mechanisms of nutrient absorption and malabsorption - UpToDate. 2016. Available at: https://www.uptodate.com/contents/mechanisms-of-nutrient-absorption-and-malabsorption?source=search_result&search=vitaminabsorption&selectedTitle=1~150#H5. Accessed January 25, 2017.

20. Dahl DM. Use of intestinal segments in urinary diversion. 11th edition. Dallas (TX): Elsevier; 2016.

21. Hasan ST, Coorsh J, Tapson JS. Use of bendrofluazide in the management of recurrent jejunal conduit syndrome. Br J Urol 1994;73(1):101–2.

22. Chechile G, Klein EA, Bauer L, et al. Functional equivalence of end and loop ileal conduit stomas. J Urol 1992;147(3):582–6.

23. Emmott D, Noble MJ, Mebust WK. A comparison of end versus loop stomas for ileal conduit urinary diversion. J Urol 1985;133(4):588–90.

24. "Cancer stat facts: bladder cancer." Surveillance, Epidemiology, and End Results Program. Available at: https://seer.cancer.gov/statfacts/html/urinb.html. Accessed March 1, 2017.

25. Wolff JL, Starfield B, Anderson G. Prevalence, expenditures, and complications of multiple chronic conditions in the elderly. Arch Intern Med 2002; 162(20):2269–76.

26. Aging SNMtNshTiHa. 2008. Available at: http://www.cdc.gov/nchs/agingact.thm. Accessed December 14, 2008.

27. Froehner M, Brausi MA, Herr HW, et al. Complications following radical cystectomy for bladder cancer in the elderly. Eur Urol 2009;56(3):443–54.

28. Lavallée LT, Schramm D, Witiuk K, et al. Peri-operative morbidity associated with radical cystectomy in a multicenter database of community and academic hospitals. PLoS One 2014;9(10):e111281.

29. Donat SM, Siegrist T, Cronin A, et al. Radical cystectomy in octogenarians–does morbidity outweigh the potential survival benefits? J Urol 2010;183(6): 2171–7.

30. Gore JL, Litwin MS, Lai J, et al. Use of radical cystectomy for patients with invasive bladder cancer. J Natl Cancer Inst 2010;102(11):802–11.

31. Konety BR, Joslyn SA. Factors influencing aggressive therapy for bladder cancer: an analysis of data from the SEER program. J Urol 2003;170(5):1765–71.

32. Clark PE, Stein JP, Groshen SG, et al. Radical cystectomy in the elderly: comparison of clincal outcomes between younger and older patients. Cancer 2005;104(1):36–43.

33. Nielsen ME, Shariat SF, Karakiewicz PI, et al. Advanced age is associated with poorer bladder cancer-specific survival in patients treated with radical cystectomy. Eur Urol 2007;51(3):699–706 [discussion: 706–8].

34. Prout GR, Marshall VF. The prognosis with untreated bladder tumors. Cancer 1956;9(3):551–8.

35. Hollenbeck BK, Miller DC, Taub D, et al. Aggressive treatment for bladder cancer is associated with improved overall survival among patients 80 years old or older. Urology 2004;64(2):292–7.

36. Mohamed NE, Pisipati S, Lee CT, et al. Unmet informational and supportive care needs of patients following cystectomy for bladder cancer based on age, sex, and treatment choices. Urol Oncol 2016;34(12):531.e7-14.

37. "Share of U.S. population living alone." Pew Research Center. Available at: http://www.pewsocialtrends.

org/2010/03/18/the-return-of-the-multi-generational-family-household/. Accessed March 1, 2017.

38. "The health literacy of America's adults." National Assessment of Adult Literacy. U.S. Department of Education. Available at: https://nces.ed.gov/pubs2006/2006483.pdf. Accessed March 15, 2017.

39. Extermann M, Hurria A. Comprehensive geriatric assessment for older patients with cancer. J Clin Oncol 2007;25(14):1824–31.

40. Scarpato KR, Kappa SF, Goggins KM, et al. The impact of health literacy on surgical outcomes following radical cystectomy. J Health Commun 2016;21(sup2):99–104.

41. Azer SA, Alghofaili MM, Alsultan RM, et al. Accuracy and readability of websites on kidney and bladder cancers. J Cancer Educ 2017. [Epub ahead of print].

42. Ghoneim MA, Abdel-Latif M, el-Mekresh M, et al. Radical cystectomy for carcinoma of the bladder: 2,720 consecutive cases 5 years later. J Urol 2008;180(1):121–7.

43. Gore JL, Saigal CS, Hanley JM, et al, Urologic Diseases in America Project. Variations in reconstruction after radical cystectomy. Cancer 2006;107(4):729–37.

44. Gore JL, Litwin MS, Urologic Diseases in America Project. Quality of care in bladder cancer: trends in urinary diversion following radical cystectomy. World J Urol 2009;27(1):45–50.

45. Skinner EC, Daneshmand S. Orthotopic urinary diversion. 11th edition. Dallas (TX): Elsevier; 2016.

46. Freeman JA, Tarter TA, Esrig D, et al. Urethral recurrence in patients with orthotopic ileal neobladders. J Urol 1996;156(5):1615–9.

47. Stein JP, Clark P, Miranda G, et al. Urethral tumor recurrence following cystectomy and urinary diversion: clinical and pathological characteristics in 768 male patients. J Urol 2005;173(4):1163–8.

48. Hautmann RE, de Petriconi R, Gottfried HW, et al. The ileal neobladder: complications and functional results in 363 patients after 11 years of followup. J Urol 1999;161(2):422–7 [discussion: 427–8].

49. Hautmann RE, Simon J. Ileal neobladder and local recurrence of bladder cancer: patterns of failure and impact on function in men. J Urol 1999;162(6):1963–6.

50. Bochner BH, Figueroa AJ, Skinner EC, et al. Salvage radical cystoprostatectomy and orthotopic urinary diversion following radiation failure. J Urol 1998;160(1):29–33.

51. Abbas F, Biyabani SR, Talati J. Orthotopic bladder replacement to the urethra following salvage radical cystoprostatectomy in men with failed radiation therapy. Tech Urol 2001;7(1):20–6.

52. Hautmann RE. Editorial comment. Urology 2009;74(5):1149 [author reply: 1149].

53. Hautmann RE, de Petriconi R, Volkmer BG. Neobladder formation after pelvic irradiation. World J Urol 2009;27(1):57–62.

54. Hautmann RE. Urinary diversion: ileal conduit to neobladder. J Urol 2003;169(3):834–42.

55. Stein JP, Dunn MD, Quek ML, et al. The orthotopic T pouch ileal neobladder: experience with 209 patients. J Urol 2004;172(2):584–7.

56. Grossman HB, Natale RB, Tangen CM, et al. Neoadjuvant chemotherapy plus cystectomy compared with cystectomy alone for locally advanced bladder cancer. N Engl J Med 2003;349(9):859–66.

57. Nishikawa M, Miyake H, Yamashita M, et al. Long-term changes in renal function outcomes following radical cystectomy and urinary diversion. Int J Clin Oncol 2014;19(6):1105–11.

58. Eisenberg MS, Thompson RH, Frank I, et al. Long-term renal function outcomes after radical cystectomy. J Urol 2014;191(3):619–25.

59. Zabbo A, Kay R. Ureterosigmoidostomy and bladder exstrophy: a long-term followup. J Urol 1986;136(2):396–8.

60. Nichols RL, Condon RE. Preoperative preparation of the colon. Surg Gynecol Obstet 1971;132(2):323–37.

61. Raynor MC, Lavien G, Nielsen M, et al. Elimination of preoperative mechanical bowel preparation in patients undergoing cystectomy and urinary diversion. Urol Oncol 2013;31(1):32–5.

62. Hashad MM, Atta M, Elabbady A, et al. Safety of no bowel preparation before ileal urinary diversion. BJU Int 2012;110(11 Pt C):E1109–13.

63. Arumainayagam N, McGrath J, Jefferson KP, et al. Introduction of an enhanced recovery protocol for radical cystectomy. BJU Int 2008;101(6):698–701.

64. Tabibi A, Simforoosh N, Basiri A, et al. Bowel preparation versus no preparation before ileal urinary diversion. Urology 2007;70(4):654–8.

65. Xu R, Zhao X, Zhong Z, et al. No advantage is gained by preoperative bowel preparation in radical cystectomy and ileal conduit: a randomized controlled trial of 86 patients. Int Urol Nephrol 2010;42(4):947–50.

66. Shafii M, Murphy DM, Donovan MG, et al. Is mechanical bowel preparation necessary in patients undergoing cystectomy and urinary diversion? BJU Int 2002;89(9):879–81.

67. Large MC, Kiriluk KJ, DeCastro GJ, et al. The impact of mechanical bowel preparation on postoperative complications for patients undergoing cystectomy and urinary diversion. J Urol 2012;188(5):1801–5.

68. Salvadalena G, Hendren S, McKenna L, et al. WOCN society and AUA position statement on preoperative stoma site marking for patients

undergoing urostomy surgery. J Wound Ostomy Continence Nurs 2015;42(3):253–6.

69. Millan M, Tegido M, Biondo S, et al. Preoperative stoma siting and education by stomatherapists of colorectal cancer patients: a descriptive study in twelve Spanish colorectal surgical units. Colorectal Dis 2010;12(7 Online):e88–92.

70. Gulbiniene J, Markelis R, Tamelis A, et al. The impact of preoperative stoma siting and stoma care education on patient's quality of life. Medicina (Kaunas) 2004;40(11):1045–53 [in Lithuanian].

71. Park JJ, Del Pino A, Orsay CP, et al. Stoma complications: the Cook County Hospital experience. Dis Colon Rectum 1999;42(12):1575–80.

72. Parmar KL, Zammit M, Smith A, et al, Greater Manchester and Cheshire Colorectal Cancer Network. A prospective audit of early stoma complications in colorectal cancer treatment throughout the Greater Manchester and Cheshire colorectal cancer network. Colorectal Dis 2011;13(8):935–8.

73. Pittman J, Rawl SM, Schmidt CM, et al. Demographic and clinical factors related to ostomy complications and quality of life in veterans with an ostomy. J Wound Ostomy Continence Nurs 2008; 35(5):493–503.

74. Richie J, Skinner D. Complications of urinary conduit diversion. Philadelphia: Saunders; 1976.

75. Keane PF, Bonner MC, Johnston SR, et al. Characterization of biofilm and encrustation on ureteric stents in vivo. Br J Urol 1994;73(6):687–91.

76. Mattei A, Birkhaeuser FD, Baermann C, et al. To stent or not to stent perioperatively the ureteroileal anastomosis of ileal orthotopic bladder substitutes and ileal conduits? Results of a prospective randomized trial. J Urol 2008;179(2):582–6.

77. Mullins JK, Guzzo TJ, Ball MW, et al. Ureteral stents placed at the time of urinary diversion decreases postoperative morbidity. Urol Int 2012;88(1):66–70.

78. Regan JB, Barrett DM. Stented versus nonstented ureteroileal anastomoses: is there a difference with regard to leak and stricture? J Urol 1985; 134(6):1101–3.

79. Beddoe AM, Boyce JG, Remy JC, et al. Stented versus nonstented transverse colon conduits: a comparative report. Gynecol Oncol 1987;27(3): 305–15.

80. Donahue TF, Bochner BH, Sfakianos JP, et al. Risk factors for the development of parastomal hernia after radical cystectomy. J Urol 2014;191(6): 1708–13.

81. Liu NW, Hackney JT, Gellhaus PT, et al. Incidence and risk factors of parastomal hernia in patients undergoing radical cystectomy and ileal conduit diversion. J Urol 2014;191(5):1313–8.

82. Farnham SB, Cookson MS. Surgical complications of urinary diversion. World J Urol 2004;22(3): 157–67.

83. Kouba E, Sands M, Lentz A, et al. Incidence and risk factors of stomal complications in patients undergoing cystectomy with ileal conduit urinary diversion for bladder cancer. J Urol 2007;178(3 Pt 1):950–4.

84. Wood DN, Allen SE, Hussain M, et al. Stomal complications of ileal conduits are significantly higher when formed in women with intractable urinary incontinence. J Urol 2004;172(6 Pt 1): 2300–3.

85. Bloom DA, Grossman HB, Konnak JW. Stomal construction and reconstruction. Urol Clin North Am 1986;13(2):275–83.

86. Fontaine E, Barthelemy Y, Houlgatte A, et al. Twenty-year experience with jejunal conduits. Urology 1997;50(2):207–13.

87. Marimuthu K, Vijayasekar C, Ghosh D, et al. Prevention of parastomal hernia using preperitoneal mesh: a prospective observational study. Colorectal Dis 2006;8(8):672–5.

88. Israelsson LA. Parastomal hernias. Surg Clin North Am 2008;88(1):113–25, ix.

89. Ripoche J, Basurko C, Fabbro-Perray P, et al. Parastomal hernia. A study of the French federation of ostomy patients. J Visc Surg 2011;148(6): e435–441.

90. Carne PW, Robertson GM, Frizelle FA. Parastomal hernia. Br J Surg 2003;90(7):784–93.

91. Horgan K, Hughes LE. Para-ileostomy hernia: failure of a local repair technique. Br J Surg 1986; 73(6):439–40.

92. Seo SH, Kim HJ, Oh SY, et al. Computed tomography classification for parastomal hernia. J Korean Surg Soc 2011;81(2):111–4.

93. Hotouras A, Murphy J, Power N, et al. Radiological incidence of parastomal herniation in cancer patients with permanent colostomy: what is the ideal size of the surgical aperture? Int J Surg 2013; 11(5):425–7.

94. Keeling NJ, Ataullah CM, Wastell C. A survey of glove preferences of general and orthopaedic surgeons in North West Thames Regional Health Authority. J Hosp Infect 1995;30(4):305–8.

95. Pilgrim CH, McIntyre R, Bailey M. Prospective audit of parastomal hernia: prevalence and associated comorbidities. Dis Colon Rectum 2010; 53(1):71–6.

96. Pisters AL, Kamat AM, Wei W, et al. Anterior fascial fixation does not reduce the parastomal hernia rate after radical cystectomy and ileal conduit. Urology 2014;83(6):1427–31.

97. Serra-Aracil X, Bombardo-Junca J, Moreno-Matias J, et al. Randomized, controlled, prospective trial of the use of a mesh to prevent parastomal hernia. Ann Surg 2009;249(4):583–7.

98. Jänes A, Cengiz Y, Israelsson LA. Randomized clinical trial of the use of a prosthetic mesh to

prevent parastomal hernia. Br J Surg 2004;91(3): 280–2.

99. Jänes A, Cengiz Y, Israelsson LA. Preventing parastomal hernia with a prosthetic mesh: a 5-year follow-up of a randomized study. World J Surg 2009;33(1):118–21 [discussion: 122–3].

100. Hammond TM, Huang A, Prosser K, et al. Parastomal hernia prevention using a novel collagen implant: a randomised controlled phase 1 study. Hernia 2008;12(5):475–81.

101. Lambrecht JR, Larsen SG, Reiertsen O, et al. Prophylactic mesh at end-colostomy construction reduces parastomal hernia rate: a randomized trial. Colorectal Dis 2015;17(10):O191–7.

102. Vierimaa M, Klintrup K, Biancari F, et al. Prospective, randomized study on the use of a prosthetic mesh for prevention of parastomal hernia of permanent colostomy. Dis Colon Rectum 2015;58(10): 943–9.

103. Donahue TF, Cha EK, Bochner BH. Rationale and early experience with prophylactic placement of mesh to prevent parastomal hernia formation after ileal conduit urinary diversion and cystectomy for bladder cancer. Curr Urol Rep 2016;17(2):9.

104. Styrke J, Johansson M, Granåsen G, et al. Parastomal hernia after ileal conduit with a prophylactic mesh: a 10 year consecutive case series. Scand J Urol 2015;49(4):308–12.

105. Madersbacher S, Schmidt J, Eberle JM, et al. Long-term outcome of ileal conduit diversion. J Urol 2003;169(3):985–90.

106. Gburek BM, Lieber MM, Blute ML. Comparison of Studer ileal neobladder and ileal conduit urinary diversion with respect to perioperative outcome and late complications. J Urol 1998;160(3 Pt 1): 721–3.

107. Gudjónsson S, Davidsson T, Månsson W. Incontinent urinary diversion. BJU Int 2008;102(9 Pt B): 1320–5.

108. Shabsigh A, Korets R, Vora KC, et al. Defining early morbidity of radical cystectomy for patients with bladder cancer using a standardized reporting methodology. Eur Urol 2009;55(1):164–74.

109. Lawrentschuk N, Colombo R, Hakenberg OW, et al. Prevention and management of complications following radical cystectomy for bladder cancer. Eur Urol 2010;57(6):983–1001.

110. Shimko MS, Tollefson MK, Umbreit EC, et al. Long-term complications of conduit urinary diversion. J Urol 2011;185(2):562–7.

111. Magnusson B, Carlén B, Bak-Jensen E, et al. Ileal conduit stenosis–an enigma. Scand J Urol Nephrol 1996;30(3):193–7.

112. Colwell JC, Goldberg M, Carmel J. The state of the standard diversion. J Wound Ostomy Continence Nurs 2001;28(1):6–17.

113. Lobo N, Dupré S, Sahai A, et al. Getting out of a tight spot: an overview of ureteroenteric anastomotic strictures. Nat Rev Urol 2016;13(8):447–55.

114. Kouba E, Sands M, Lentz A, et al. A comparison of the Bricker versus Wallace ureteroileal anastomosis in patients undergoing urinary diversion for bladder cancer. J Urol 2007;178(3 Pt 1):945–8 [discussion: 948–9].

115. Davis NF, Burke JP, McDermott T, et al. Bricker versus Wallace anastomosis: a meta-analysis of ureteroenteric stricture rates after ileal conduit urinary diversion. Can Urol Assoc J 2015;9(5–6): E284–90.

116. Terai A, Arai Y, Kawakita M, et al. Effect of urinary intestinal diversion on urinary risk factors for urolithiasis. J Urol 1995;153(1):37–41.

117. Cookson MS, Dutta SC, Chang SS, et al. Health related quality of life in patients treated with radical cystectomy and urinary diversion for urothelial carcinoma of the bladder: development and validation of a new disease specific questionnaire. J Urol 2003;170(5):1926–30.

118. Gilbert SM, Wood DP, Dunn RL, et al. Measuring health-related quality of life outcomes in bladder cancer patients using the Bladder Cancer Index (BCI). Cancer 2007;109(9):1756–62.

119. Porter MP, Penson DF. Health related quality of life after radical cystectomy and urinary diversion for bladder cancer: a systematic review and critical analysis of the literature. J Urol 2005;173(4): 1318–22.

120. Gerharz EW. Is there any evidence that one continent diversion is any better than any other or than ileal conduit? Curr Opin Urol 2007;17(6):402–7.

121. Crozier J, Hennessey D, Sengupta S, et al. A systematic review of ileal conduit and neobladder outcomes in primary bladder cancer. Urology 2016;96:74–9.

122. Kretschmer A, Grimm T, Buchner A, et al. Prospective evaluation of health-related quality of life after radical cystectomy: focus on peri- and postoperative complications. World J Urol 2017;35(8): 1223–31.

Male Neobladder

Eugene J. Pietzak, MD, Timothy F. Donahue, MD, Bernard H. Bochner, MD*

KEYWORDS

- Urinary diversion • Radical cystectomy • Neobladder • Bladder Cancer

KEY POINTS

- The goals for urinary diversion are to store urine at low pressure, protect renal function, allow for complete volitional emptying, and provide socially acceptable continence.
- The diversion should have minimal absorption of excreted urinary metabolites to avoid major metabolic abnormalities and also have acceptable rates of early and late complications.
- Finding a suitable replacement for the native bladder is one of the great challenges after radical cystectomy.

BACKGROUND

Finding a suitable replacement for the native bladder is one of the great challenges after radical cystectomy. The goals for urinary diversion are to store urine at low pressure, protect renal function, allow for complete volitional emptying, and provide socially acceptable continence. The diversion should have minimal absorption of excreted urinary metabolites to avoid major metabolic abnormalities and also have acceptable rates of early and late complications. Recapitulating many of the intrinsic properties of the native bladder and understanding the impact of the choice of bowel segments are paramount to successfully reconstructing the urinary tract. This article reviews the principles, surgical technique, perioperative management, and long-term issues associated with orthotopic continent urinary diversion in male patients.

SURGICAL PRINCIPLES
Development of a Low-Pressure System

The fundamental principle behind any form of continent urinary diversion is the creation of a low-pressure reservoir that protects the upper tracts, optimizes continence, and allows for volitional voiding. Low-pressure storage is achieved by detubularization of the bowel segment and cross-folding into a spheroid shape to maximize reservoir capacity. Detubularization disrupts rhythmic peristaltic bowel contractions, thereby protecting the upper and lower urinary tracts from intermittent increases in pressure.[1] The spherical configuration maximizes the radius of the reservoir, which according to Laplace's law (pressure = tension/radius), translates into lower filling and storage pressures. The spherical configuration also minimizes the surface area that is in contact with urine, thus reducing reabsorption and metabolic complications. Furthermore, continence is best with a low-pressure reservoir.

Because reconfiguration into a spheroid shape maximizes capacity, the overall length of bowel required for the diversion is not excessively long. Although capacity of the reservoir is limited immediately after surgery, it increases over time as the viscoelastic properties of bowel wall allows stretch.[2] The temptation to use too long an ileal segment for the neobladder must be avoided because this can result in an excessively large, flaccid reservoir with high postvoid residual urine volumes requiring intermittent self-catheterization to empty. Large reservoirs also place patients at higher risk for metabolic disorders and infections

Disclosure: E.J. Pietzak, T.F. Donahue, and B.H. Bochner have nothing they wish to disclose.
Urology Service, Department of Surgery, Memorial Sloan Kettering Cancer Center, New York, NY, USA
* Corresponding author. Urology Service, Department of Surgery, Kimmel Center for Prostate and Urologic Cancers, Memorial Sloan Kettering Cancer Center, 353 East 68th Street, New York, NY 10065.
E-mail address: bochnerb@mskcc.org

Urol Clin N Am 45 (2018) 37–48
https://doi.org/10.1016/j.ucl.2017.09.003
0094-0143/18/© 2017 Elsevier Inc. All rights reserved.

urologic.theclinics.com

from chronic colonization and bacteriuria. If this occurs, patients are usually managed with medical therapy and possible long-term intermittent or chronic catheterization.

Maintenance of Intrinsic Continence Mechanism

Central to the successful outcome after orthotopic reconstruction is the ability to maintain urinary continence. The continence of an orthotopic neobladder is dependent on an anatomically and neurologically intact native urethra and sphincter. The distal external sphincter is composed of an omega-shaped striated rhabdosphincter at the level of the membranous urethra in men and is under voluntary control by the somatic nervous system. Meticulous apical dissection during cystoprostatectomy is required to ensure the sphincter is not damaged and maximal functional urethral length is maintained. To help achieve these aims, complete control of the dorsal venous complex is paramount to obtain a bloodless field that allows the contours of the prostatic apex to be properly visualized, thus minimizing the risk of excessive distal dissection or damage to the muscular or neural components.

Additionally, nerve-sparing cystectomy can result in preserved sexual function and may improve continence outcomes in men. Attempted nerve sparing in men has been shown to improve nighttime continence rates compared with those whom nerve sparing was not attempted.[3] Nerving sparing is thought to preserve the somatic efferent innervation to the pelvic floor and external urethral sphincter as well as the autonomic innervation to the smooth muscle component of the sphincter complex.[4] Urethral sensation may also be preserved by nerve sparing, which may contribute to improved continence in orthotopic diversions.[5] Although nerve sparing can potentially improve continence rates and preserve sexual function, this should never be performed at the expense of the oncological objective.[3] Careful patient selection in nerve sparing is paramount to reduce the risk of positive surgical margins.

Some investigators advocate for sparing of the prostatic apex, prostatic capsule, and/or seminal vesicles during the extirpative part of radical cystectomy.[6] Although these efforts are intended to preserve sexual function and continence, these modifications have not been shown to improve continence rates and may have worse oncological outcomes.[6] Thus, the authors do not support these techniques in routine practice and advocate for a more radical resection, particularly in patients with invasive disease or high-risk histologic subtypes.

Refluxing Versus Antirefluxing Upper Tract Systems

A long-standing controversy in urinary diversions is whether the upper urinary tracts need protection against the effects of reflux to prevent long-term renal deterioration. Similar to the function of the vesicoureteral junction of the native bladder, the principle behind constructing antirefluxing ureteral anastomoses is to protect the kidneys and upper tracts from sustained increases in pressures during voiding and to prevent ascending bacteriuria. Although this was particularly relevant for patients undergoing ureterosigmoidostomy, which diverts the urine into a high-pressure chronically infected system, ureteral reflux may be less of a concern with the development of lower pressure, high-capacity orthotopic reservoirs. Yet, proponents of antireflux mechanisms in orthotopic diversions argue that there are high rates of bacteria colonization, and intraluminal pressures can substantially increase during voiding.[7] There are several different antireflux techniques described, including extramural and transmural tunneling, as well as creating nipple valve mechanisms with ileum or the ureter directly.[8-10] Randomized controlled trials comparing refluxing and nonrefluxing anastomoses have not demonstrated a benefit for nonrefluxing anastomosis but have found them associated with an increased risk of ureteral strictures and complications.[11,12] Not only are ureteral strictures seen, but the antireflux mechanism itself is at risk for stricture and can result in obstruction as demonstrated in the long term follow-up for the Kock valve, Ghoneim subserosal tunneling system, and T-pouch reconstructions.[8,10,12] A randomized trial demonstrated a reoperative rate for the T-pouch antireflux mechanism was 22% at 3 years compared with 13% for refluxing ureteral anastomoses.[12] There seems a greater risk of gradual renal deterioration from ureterointestinal anastomotic strictures than from reflux of urine into the upper tracts. Refluxing anastomosis into an isoperistaltic tubular afferent limb of the orthotopic reservoir has demonstrated excellent long-term protection against renal deterioration.[13] Hautmann and colleagues[14] reported a 20.6% ureteroileal stricture rate at 10 years with the Le Duc antirefluxing technique, which was reduced to 7.0% when they switched to refluxing Wallace anastomoses. Because refluxing anastomoses are technically simpler to complete and have not been associated with significant rates of upper tract deterioration in patients undergoing orthotopic reconstruction, they are a widely accepted design.[15-19]

INDICATIONS AND CLINICAL APPLICATIONS
Patient Selection Criteria

Patients considering orthotopic urinary diversion should be motivated, be carefully selected, and have realistic expectations regarding the functional outcomes after reconstruction. They must be willing to follow a prescribed voiding time regimen, have the ability to generate an adequate Valsalva pressure to empty the neobladder, and should also possess the ability to perform self-catheterization if needed. Although chronologic age is not a contraindication to neobladder reconstruction, patients at advanced ages must be carefully selected and counseled that they are at greater risk for a delayed recovery of daytime urinary control and that nocturnal incontinence is a greater long-term risk. Patients who have undergone prior pelvic surgery, in particular radical prostatectomy, or those having received extensive pelvic radiation therapy may also be at risk for continence issues postoperatively.

Patients with serum creatinine levels greater than 2.0 mg/dL or glomerular filtration rates less than 35 mL/min are also not optimal candidates for continent diversion. Reabsorption of urinary components by the urinary diversion bowel wall may lead to severe systemic electrolyte abnormalities in patients with limited renal function. Additionally free water loss occurs within continent reservoirs, which may lead to dehydration in those patients with impaired renal concentrating ability. Patients with severe hepatic dysfunction are at risk for hyperammonemia due to an impaired ability to process the ammonia absorbed by the reservoir.

Relative contraindications to orthotopic diversion are inflammatory bowel disease, an inability or unwillingness to self-catheterize, and mental impairment. Patients with a history of urethral stricture disease or external urethral sphincter dysfunction may not be candidates for orthotopic reconstruction.

All patients who undergo continent urinary diversion need to receive detailed preoperative counseling and teaching about the planned reconstructive procedure and postoperative recovery. Patients must be aware that although the goal of reconstruction is to provide an acceptable substitute for the native bladder, there are inherent differences with the voiding technique and voiding regimen that the patient must be willing to accept.

Oncological Considerations for Orthotopic Neobladder

Preoperative and intraoperative evaluation of the urethra is necessary to select patients most appropriate for orthotopic reconstruction. An orthotopic diversion is contraindicated when high-grade tumor is present within the pendulous or membranous urethra. Additionally patients with extensive involvement of the prostatic urethra, particularly with high-grade or invasive disease, are at a significantly higher risk for having a positive urethral margin at the time of frozen section during cystectomy and subsequent tumor formation within the remaining urethra. The risk of urethral recurrence is observed to be 2% to 5% after orthotopic diversion but can range from 0.5% to 13.7%.[20] The median time to urethral recurrence in most large series ranges from 8 months to 28 months.[20] Studer and colleagues[21] reported a 5% urethral recurrence rate in 482 neobladder patients, with a median time to recurrence of 14 months (range 3–158 months). The strongest risk factor associated with a subsequent urethral recurrence is prostatic urethral involvement, particularly if prostatic stroma invasion is found.[22,23] Bladder pathology, such as multifocal disease, diffuse carcinoma in situ, prior recurrent nonmuscle invasive tumors, and ureteric disease, have previously been associated with an increased urethral recurrence risk; however, large, long-term series of men undergoing orthotopic diversion have not verified these associations.[20] The rate of urethral recurrence is lower in orthotopic urinary diversions compared with defunctionalized urethras after heterotopic diversions.[20] This leads some investigators to suggest that a yet to be determined substance in the urine or produced by the ileum is protective against tumor recurrence.[20] Stricter selection criteria for orthotopic diversion, however, might be the main contributing factor.[20]

The optimal technique for assessing suitability of the urethra and future urethral recurrence risk is subject to debate. Some investigators advocate for routine precystectomy biopsies of the prostatic urethra regardless of cystoscopic findings, arguing that paraffin-embedded biopsies are more accurate than intraoperative frozen section.[20] Others have found that a frozen section at the time of radical cystectomy can accurately identify disease at the urethral margin.[20] A frozen section of the full circumferential distal urethral margin during cystectomy is an excellent technique to determine patient eligibility for orthotopic diversion and has repeatedly demonstrated reliability in selecting appropriate orthotopic neobladder candidates intraoperatively.[20]

Although most recurrences are reported within the first 2 years to 3 years, urethral recurrence is a time-dependent event that needs to be assessed long term. Urethral recurrence after orthotopic neobladder may present as hematuria (microscopic or gross) or as a change in voiding pattern, such as obstructive voiding symptoms. Detection of urethral recurrence while patients are asymptomatic is associated with significantly lower stage of disease and improved patient survival.[24] For this reason, the authors routinely obtain a voided urine cytology and perform a dedicated physical examination of the entire urethra, perineum, and rectal fossa.[24]

In the absence of overt disease at the prostatic apex, a thorough and complete radical oncological procedure can be performed in patients who are selected for orthotopic reconstruction. If sound oncological principles are followed during cystectomy, there should be no difference in disease recurrence rates in those undergoing orthotopic diversion compared with heterotopic diversions.[25] Furthermore, patients with pelvic nodal disease may be offered a neobladder reconstruction without compromising pelvic disease control and should still be able to achieve the same function results as node-negative patients.[25] It is rare for a subsequent pelvic recurrence to have a direct impact on the function of the neobladder and, if this does occur, it can typically be managed with catheter drainage.[25]

SELECTION OF BOWEL SEGMENT

Selection of the proper segment of bowel for reservoir construction should be based on a patient's renal function, history of prior abdominal surgery or radiation therapy, and the type of reconstruction planned. Each bowel segment has its own relative advantages and disadvantages, including metabolic sequelae, when used for urinary diversion.

Ileum and colon have similar characteristics and are associated with fewer electrolyte disturbances, greater redundancy, and ease of mobilization into the pelvis and have robust, anatomically consistent blood supplies. Both segments absorb ammonium chloride from the urine that can result in a hyperchloremic metabolic acidosis. Patients with impaired renal function are more susceptible to developing clinically detectable or severe metabolic abnormalities, which may manifest as lethargy, anorexia, and weight loss. Over the long term, patients are at risk for bone demineralization leading to osteopenia. Symptomatic metabolic acidosis can be treated with alkalinizing agents, maintaining good hydration, and minimizing dwell time of urine stored within the reservoir.

The terminal ileum handles absorption of bile salts, fat-soluble vitamins (A, D, E, and K), and the absorption of vitamin B_{12}. Some patients, in whom the ileum is used for diversion, can develop steatorrhea leading to fat-induced diarrhea, vitamin B_{12} deficiency, and dehydration. Drugs excreted unchanged in the urine and absorbed by the urinary reservoir can be problematic, especially in patients receiving adjuvant chemotherapy. Methotrexate toxicity has been described in patients with urinary diversions due to absorption of the agent and its active metabolites.[26,27] To minimize the reabsorption of excreted drugs and/or metabolites, patients undergoing chemotherapy should have the neobladder drained with a urethral catheter during treatment. Those patients taking phenytoin, theophylline, lithium, and certain antibiotics excreted in an active form into the urine should be monitored closely.[28–30]

BRIEF HISTORY OF ORTHOTOPIC ILEAL NEOBLADDERS

The modern concept of orthotopic urinary diversion begin in the 1880s with the works of Tizzoni and Poggi, who interposed an isolated ileal segment to connect the ureters and urethra of a dog in a 2-stage experimental procedure.[31] The evolution of this technique led to the eventual first-in-human report of a tubulized U-shaped ileal reservoir by Couvelaire in 1951.[31] Over time the importance of detubularization was better understood, thus making the development of low-pressure reservoirs possible.[31] The concept of orthotopic neobladder was later popularized by Le Duc and Camey, who reported on their extensive clinical experience in 1979 with the development of Camey I pouch and then the Camey II pouch.[32] The initial S configuration used by Camey evolved in the 1980s into a W-configuration as popularized by Hautmann and a U-configuration as popularized by Studer.[15,31,33] Simultaneously with these advancements, many of the techniques introduced by the continent ileostomy Kock pouch used after protocolectomy were adapted for urinary diversion.[31] This led to a further expansion of both continent catheterizable reservoirs and orthotopic urinary diversions for which ileal, ileoceceal, and colonic segments have all been described.[34–37]

Over the past 30 years, orthotopic neobladder reconstruction has become increasingly used in patients undergoing radical cystectomy. Some evidence suggests that orthotopic reservoirs are associated with improved quality of life and may provide improved body image, sexuality, sociability, and sense of well-being compared with other forms of urinary diversion.[38] Multiple descriptions and iterations have been described for the construction of orthotopic urinary diversions sharing the same goal to closely resemble the function of the native bladder by storing urine at low pressures and allowing patients to volitionally void per urethra with acceptable urinary control.

All modern orthotopic diversions regardless of whether they are constructed of small or large bowel follow the principles of detubularization and cross-folding according to Goodwin's principle of achieving these goals.[39,40] The authors prefer to construct a folded detubulized U-shaped ileal orothotopic neobladder with a isoperistaltic tubular afferent limb into which the ureters are anastomosed, discuss in detail later.[1] Another popular orthotopic construction is the W-ileal configuration, as popularized by Hautmann and colleauges.[15] This diversion uses 60 cm to 70 cm of distal ileum opened along its antimesenteric border except for short 2 cm to 3 cm chimneys on each end. The 4 limbs of the detubularized bowel are closed with a running suture to form an ileal plate. A small opening for the neourethra is made in the middle of the dependent U flap of the W-shaped ileal plate. The urethrointestinal anastomosis can be performed from inside the neobladder. Before the anterior wall is closed, the ureteral anastomosis can be performed in an end-to-side fashion directly to the top of the open chimneys or directly implanted to the chimney in a Nesbit/Bricker fashion. The larger capacity of the Hautmann pouch allows for shorter afferent limbs to be used and may allow for improved nighttime continence, albeit with a potentially higher risk of metabolic acidosis.[15]

SURGICAL TECHNIQUE OF ORTHOTOPIC ILEAL NEOBLADDER

Measures taken at the time of the extirpative portion of radical cystectomy can help optimize outcomes of the ileal neobladder. An infraumbilical skin incision is made with the fascial incision extended slightly left of the umbilicus to allow for greater exposure during the extended lymphadenectomy. The ureters are mobilized only as high as needed to complete the pelvic lymph node dissection being mindful to maintain the surrounding periureteral tissue, such as that provided by the adjacent gonadal vessels to prevent ischemia of the remaining ureter. Fully mobilizing the sigmoid colon off the sacral promontory not only facilitates the pelvic lymph node dissection but also assists in passing the left ureter under the sigmoid without extensive angulation.

Many of the lessons learned from the experience with retropubic prostatectomy can be applied to optimize cystectomy outcomes.

Preservation of the neurovascular bundle bilaterally for patients without invasive disease or on the non–tumor-bearing side may help with sexual function and continence by maintaining autonomic innervation. Meticulous apical dissection is required during the extirpation to ensure the sphincter is not damaged and that adequate functional urethral length is maintained. The authors prefer to place 6 to 8 anastomotic stitches with 2-0 monocryl sutures prior to transecting the posterior urethra. Only 2 mm to 4 mm of urethra are included to minimize ischemic insult to the anastomosis.

The authors routinely send a frozen section on the complete circumferential distal urethral margin. If cancer is present on frozen section, the neobladder is aborted and either a continent cutaneous diversion or ileal conduit proceeded with, depending on the patient's preoperative preference.

After completion of the extirpative portion and once hemostasis is achieved, attention is turned to the orthotopic neobladder. There are multiple designs of orthotopic diversions that can be constructed.[10,12,14,31,32,36,37,41,42] As previously discussed, the authors prefer to use ileum because it is abundant, has acceptable metabolic consequences when exposed to urine, and can be easily mobilized into the pelvis. To select the portion of the terminal ileum to construct the orthotopic ileal neobladder, identify the avascular line of Treves between terminal branches of the superior mesentery artery and ileocolic artery. This usually leads to a point along the small bowel approximately 15 cm to 20 cm from the ileocecal valve. This marks the distal division of the mesentery to be divided with Bovie cautery, staples, or LigaSure device. To facilitate adequate mobility of the neobladder reservoir mesentery, carry the division deep into the mesentery between the terminal inferior mesenteric artery and ileocolic vessels; this requires dividing the vascular arcade connecting these 2 vessels. Two 20-cm segments of more proximal bowel are then measured to serve as the eventual reservoir. Next approximately 12 cm to 15 cm of ileum destined to become the afferent chimney limb is identified. This serves as the most proximal part of the pouch and the length can be modified depending on the length of ureter that needs to be removed. The authors prefer to isolate and discard approximately 2 cm of more proximal small bowel to improve mobility of the neobladder and increase the distance between the neobladder and small bowel anastomosis.

A Parker-Kerr stitch is used to close the proximal end of afferent limb. The ileoileal anastomosis is created in standard side-to-side fashion, with the mesentery to the reservoir passed underneath the mesenteric trap, which is closed in a fashion that allows the mesentery to the reservoir to drop down and free of the terminal ileum mesenteric segment.

The back wall of the 2 adjacent 20-cm bowel limbs are approximated as close to the mesenteric border as possible to bring the segments into a U-shaped configuration. This initial suture line is not part of the closure of the reservoir but is used to bring the limbs of the U in close proximity to each other to facilitate detubularization and sewing of the back wall of the pouch. A small opening is made near the apex of the U shape approximately 4 mm from the suture line and mesenteric border. Using cautery the entire length of each 20-cm limb is detubularized up to the takeoff of the afferent limb. The afferent limb is left intact as a tube. Next, the posterior plate of the reservoir is created by approximating the inner bowel edges with running 3-0 Vicryl sutures. It is important to maintain constant tension on suture line with each throw of the suture to ensure a watertight closure. A second layer of 3-0 Vicryl is placed in a running fashion over the first suture line with each pass of the needle aimed between the sutures of the first layer.

To create a low-pressure, high-capacity spherical reservoir, the pouch is then folded in half in the opposite direction bringing the apex of the U toward the opposite side. The anterior wall is closed in 2 layers. The authors prefer to leave the distal end of the suture line open for the site of the urethral anastomosis in men. Other investigators prefer to close the reservoir and make a new opening in the dependent portion of the pouch for the urethral connection.[21]

With the reservoir fashioned, attention is turned to the ureterointestinal anastomoses. The left ureter is brought below the inferior mesenteric artery under the previously mobilized base of the sigmoid mesentery. Care is taken to minimize ureteral mobilization proximally to limit devascularization of the distal segment. If the distal ureter needs to be resected due to cancer or damage from prior therapy, the tubularized ileal limb can be brought underneath the sigmoid mesentery and the left ureteral anastomosis can be completed on the left side of the retroperitoneum.

The author prefer to make end-to-side Bricker-style ureterointestinal anastomoses as advocated by Leadbetter.[43] Only a small opening in the bowel serosa is made, because there is a tendency for this opening to increase in size. A holding stitch is placed on the lateral aspect of the ureter so a no-touch technique can be performed and the ureter is spatulated along its medial side. The authors prefer to use interrupted 4-0 polyglycolic acid sutures. In general, only 2 mm to 3 mm bites of ureteral wall are needed to avoid reducing the size of the lumen and the stitches on the bowel side are passed so generous amounts of serosa are included but minimal mucosa. The result is a watertight, tension-free mucosa-to-mucosa ureteroileal anastomosis. Eight French (F) infant feeding tubes or single J-stents are used to stent the anastomoses. These are threaded through the pouch and out the end of the open suture line to be connected to the urethral catheter once the neobladder-urethral anastomosis is formed.

With the ureters attached to the afferent limb, attention is turned to the neobladder-urethral anastomosis. The 4 posterior stitches are placed in an in-to-out fashion into the neobladder. Next, a 24F 30-mL Rusch hematuria catheter is passed through the urethra to the entrance of the neobladder. The 8F pediatric feeding tubes that serve as the ureteral stents are secured to end of Rusch catheter with a 3-0 nylon. This facilitates removal of the stents at time of urethral catheter removal 3 weeks postoperatively. The Rusch catheter is then inserted into the neobladder and anterior urethral sutures are then placed into the neobladder. A 2-0 polyglycolic acid suture is placed in a figure-of-8 fashion on the anterior aspect of the neobladder in its midline approximately 3 cm to 4 cm from the urethral connection site that will be used later to secure the neobladder to the pubic symphysis after the urethral anastomotic sutures are tied. After the neobladder urethral anastomotic stitches are tied, the previously placed 2-0 polyglycolic acid stitch is secured to the abdominal surface of the pubic symphysis to stabilize the neobladder, prevent rotation, and minimize tension on the anastomosis. The ureterointestinal anastomoses are retroperitonealized by bringing the sigmoid mesentery over the top of the afferent limb and securing this into position. The small bowel is inspected from the ligament of Treitz to the cecum, the ileoileal anastomosis is re-examined, and whenever possible omentum and small bowel is used to separate the intestinal anastomosis from the neobladder to prevent fistula formation.

PREOPERATIVE PREPARATION AND POSTOPERATIVE CARE

Optimizing postoperative outcomes should start in the preoperative period. Preoperative counseling and education provided by experienced nurses with specialty training are standard practice in the authors' clinics. Preoperative teaching and training allow patients to develop a better under-standing of expectations and what is required for long-term successful outcomes with their ortho-topic diversion. Patients must be educated preop-eratively and instructed about proper voiding technique with the neobladder, which occurs with a combination of abdominal pressure (Valsalva or Crede voiding), pelvic floor relaxation, and timed voiding to avoid overdistension and to facilitate complete emptying.[44–49] Counseling regarding alternative urinary diversion options is provided preoperatively to ensure patients have realistic expectations after surgery. Patients are marked prior to surgery for the possible stoma site in the event that intraoperative findings require conversion to an incontinent diversion. Preopera-tive cardiovascular risk assessments and medical optimization is routine.

The authors advocate for the use of standard-ized clinical pathways to reduce postoperative complications, decrease length of hospital stay, and provide cost-effective care for patients under-going radical cystectomy. In the authors' institu-tion, a standardized clinical pathway is used for all patients undergoing radical cystectomy and uri-nary diversion. The pathways delineate milestones anticipated on each postoperative day and order sets are available to standardize the care such that all members of the team caring for the patient know what to expect on subsequent days of admission. The order sets are used as guidelines and clinical judgment may dictate removing a patient from the prescribed pathway. The authors' pathway has undergone continuous reassessment and outcomes reviewed to optimize clinical outcome. Thus, the authors' pathway is in con-stant state of evolution aiming for continuous improvement.

Preoperative outpatient bowel preparation with an oral polyethylene glycol solution is only given when a colon-based reservoir is planned. Prepara-tion for an ileal neobladder does not require formal bowel preparation; the authors prefer to keep pa-tients on clear liquids only starting the day before surgery. On arrival to the preoperative area on the day of surgery, patients are routinely given oral gabapentin, diclofenac, and alvimopan, unless there is a contraindication. Although an orogastric tube is routinely used intraoperatively, it is typically removed prior to extubation. The authors' preference for pain control is with an epidural patient-controlled analgesic pump, intra-venous ketorolac, intravenous acetaminophen, and oral gabapentin to minimize exposure to sys-temic narcotics. All patients receive deep venous thrombosis prophylaxis with subcutaneous heparin prior to incision along with pneumatic compression devices. Low-molecular-weight heparin is initiated on postoperative day 1 as long as the hemoglobin remains stable. Incentive spirometry, aggressive pulmonary therapy regi-mens, and early and frequent ambulation are pre-scribed for all patients. On postoperative day 1, patients are advanced to a clear liquid diet. If toler-ated, patients are advanced to a regular diet on postoperative day 2 irrespective of flatus and bowel movements. In addition, oral docusate sodium stool softeners and bisacodyl supposi-tories are initiated as long as the rectal wall was not thinned during resection. Alvimopan is continued until a patient's first bowel movement. Since adopting this current clinical pathway, the authors have routinely noted an increase in pa-tients meeting the milestones for safe discharge to home on postoperative days 3 and 4.

The neobladder is irrigated every 4 hours daily beginning in the recovery room to clear any accu-mulated mucous. The patient and family are instructed on irrigations prior to discharge and at home continue regimented irrigations until the catheter is removed 3 weeks after surgery. Routine fluoroscopy to assess the integrity of the neoblad-der is not necessary if there is no evidence of uri-nary leakage perioperatively. In heavily radiated patients, a pouchogram to confirm complete reservoir healing is reasonable.[50]

Once the catheter is removed, patients are instructed to void every 2 hours to 3 hours during the day and every 3 hours to 4 hours at night. Patients can expect to gradually increase the void-ing interval as the capacity of the reservoir increases.[51] Strict adherence to timed voiding schedules is advised because the orthotopic neo-bladder lacks the sensation to reliably prompt voiding.

LONG-TERM OUTCOMES
Voiding and Continence

One of the main goals behind construction of an orthotopic neobladder is the resumption of normal, volitional emptying of urine. Patients void with a combination of abdominal pressure (Valsalva or Crede voiding) along with pelvic floor relaxation. The authors advise men sit to void because it is easier for them to learn to relax their pelvic floor in this position. Patients need to learn in the postoperative period the different sensation of filling evoked by the intestinal stretch receptors. Timed voiding to avoid overdistension of the neobladder and facilitate complete emptying is critical.

Continence after an orthotopic urinary diversion is dependent on an intact external urinary sphincter, intact pelvic floor, adequate functional urethral length, and the age of the patient. Generally, continence continues to improve over the first year after surgery as the capacity and compliance of the neobladder increase.[51,52] The initial volume of most neobladders is 100 mL to 150 mL with the viscoelastic properties of bowel allowing for rapid increases in capacity over the next several months. Typically a reservoir constructed from 40 cm to 45 cm of doubly cross-folded detubulized bowel reaches a maximal capacity of 500 mL. This volume is sufficient for excellent continence with long intervals between voiding while simultaneously minimizing the risk of metabolic acidosis and incomplete emptying.[21,33]

Daytime continence with orthotopic diversions is generally better and typically precedes nighttime urinary control by 6 months to 12 months. Daytime continence rates after orthotopic diversions generally exceed 85% to 90% at centers of excellence but have been reported to range from 47% to 100% depending on the definition used for continence and the time after surgery when it is measured.[15,42,53–58] Daytime pad-free rates range between 64% and 87%.[15,42,53–58] Surgical technique and anatomic constraints may also influence continence rates after orthotopic diversion, because a shorter urethral length is associated with an increased risk of urinary leakage, especially when walking.[51]

As with daytime control, nocturnal continence is achieved gradually over the first year once the capacity and compliance of the continent diversion increases. Satisfactory nighttime continence rates at 1 year range between 71% and 80% at high-volume centers.[15,21,42,59] Complete nighttime control without any pads is reported to be between 45% and 65% of patients.[55,56] Until the functional capacity of the bladder is greater than nocturnal urine production, patients should continue to awaken at night to empty their neobladder. Some patients may never gain adequate capacity to store a large volume of urine during sleeping hours, which may contribute to the high long-term rates of nocturnal enuresis in neobladders.[1]

Additionally, older age is associated with poorer continence rates due to weaker pelvic floors and external urinary sphincters.[2] Often daytime continence remain intact but nighttime continence rate slowly decline over time as external urethral sphincter tone decreases and patients are less willing or able to wake up to empty overnight.

Inability to adequately empty the neobladder is another potential concern after orthotopic reconstruction. The etiology of retention, or so-called hypercontinence, often remains unclear; however, strictures must always be excluded in any patient with an inability to empty the neobladder. In several large series, the rate of male patients who perform intermittent self-catheterization due to incomplete emptying of the neobladder approaches 4% to 5% but has been reported to be as high as 25% at some centers.[60] Hautmann and colleagues[61] reported failure to empty occurred in 11.5% of 655 men with orthotopic urinary diversions at median follow-up of 36.5 months. This included dysfunctional voiding in 3.5% and mechanical obstruction in 8.5% (benign anastomotic stricture, 3.5%; benign urethral stricture, 1.7%; tumor recurrence, 2.0%; nonurological malignancy, 0.2%; mucosal valves, 0.5%; and foreign body, 0.2%).[61] Studer and other investigators[62] argue against a funnel-shaped outlet for the neobladder, claiming that it leads to kinking and obstruction. This has not, however, been the authors' experience nor that of many other high-volume centers.[63] Daneshmand and colleagues[63] prospectively evaluated urinary continence in 188 men undergoing orthotropic ileal diversion using a validated questionnaire and reported intermittent self-catheterization rates in 10% of men at any point in time and 5.3% due to incomplete emptying. Suspected causes of inability to empty in men are urethral angulation, elongation of the neobladder neck, the neobladder neck being in nondependent portion of pouch, an oversized floppy neobladder, a preserved but dysfunctional native bladder neck, denervated proximal urethra, inadequate pelvic floor relaxation during voiding, and ineffective Valsalva straining.[61]

Ureterointestinal Strictures

Ureterointestinal stricture rates reported in the large orthotopic series approach less than 3% to 4% and serve as the benchmark. The rate of ureterointestinal strictures is dependent on the anastomotic technique used and the length of follow-up reported. Risk factors for strictures include ischemia, prior radiation, periureteral fibrosis from a urine leak, and infection. Most strictures are thought to occur due to ureteral ischemia and may occur within the first 1 year to 2 years after surgery irrespective of the type of anastomosis performed. These strictures may create symptoms, such as infection in the obstructed system, or they can remain asymptomatic and only be identified by changes in creatinine levels over time or on surveillance imaging studies.[51,64–66] Minimizing mobilization and devascularization of ureters is of paramount importance in reducing the risk of postoperative strictures. Care must be taken in routing the left ureter under the sigmoid colon. Adequate mobilization of the sigmoid off the sacral promontory creates a sufficient opening under the mesentery below the inferior mesenteric vessels to eliminate excessive angulation or tension on the left ureteroenteric anastomosis.

Urinary tract infections

It is important to distinguish between bacterial colonization and symptomatic urinary tract infections in patients with neobladders. Rates of asymptomatic bacteriuria in neobladders can be as high as 78% and may be even higher in patients who need to self-catheterize; thus, asymptomatic bacteriuria in neobladder patients more likely represents colonization rather than a clinical infection that mandates antibiotic therapy.[67] In the absence of symptoms, such as fever, flank pain, abdominal pain, purulent urine, leukocytosis, or high clinical suspicion, bacteriuria should usually not be treated to minimize the development of antibiotic resistance and potential medication side effects. Treatment should be considered in select cases involving colonization with pathologic bacteria, such as proteus, that can lead to stone formation.[68,69]

Vitamin deficiency

Vitamin B_{12} absorption occurs primarily in the terminal ileum so construction of an orthotopic ileal neobladder increases the risk for vitamin B_{12} deficiency that can result in irreversible neurologic and hematologic derangements. Vitamin B_{12} levels deplete slowly after surgery, often taking 3 years to 5 years to drop to a level sufficiently low enough to produce symptoms.[70–73] Of 314 evaluable patients in 482 patient series, Studer and colleagues[21] reported that 12% had low vitamin B_{12} levels at some point during follow-up with 32 months' median follow-up (0.4–208). Hautmann and colleagues[14] reported on 923 patients with a minimum of 3 months; follow-up (median of 72 months), all with ileal-based reservoirs. They found that only 2 of 923 were treated with vitamin B_{12} supplementation for values less than 200 pmol/L.[14] It is the authors' practice to monitor vitamin B_{12} levels and to replace on an as-needed basis after urinary diversion.

Metabolic complications

Acidosis after radical cystectomy and orthopotic reconstruction is a commonly observed event. Studer and colleagues[21] found that of 482 neobladder patients, metabolic acidosis noted in the majority in early postoperative period. Given the high frequency of this finding, their center gives routine prophylactic oral sodium bicarbonate for 3 months after catheter removal.[21] Overall 6.2%

of patients in their series were readmitted to the hospital for salt losing and acidotic states.[21] Similarly, Hautmann and colleagues[14] found that 70% of 923 neobladder patients developed acidosis in the early postoperative period, with 33% requiring sodium bicarbonate replacement beyond 1 year. They noted that treating underlying urinary tract infections and ensuring adequate emptying improved the ability to resolve the acidosis.[14]

Chronic acidosis after urinary diversion occurs in 5.5% to 13.3% of patients and can eventually result in bone demineralization and osteomalacia.[54] Bone minerals, such as calcium and carbonate, act as buffers against hydrogen ions, leading to decreased skeletal calcium content. Chronic acidosis can activate bone resorption by osteoclasts and induce vitamin D deficiency that can result in further bone demineralization.[74–77] Furthermore, decreased intestinal absorption of calcium can occur with resection of longer segments of ileum. It could take years to develop radiographic evidence of bone demineralization, but the optimal timing for bone mineral density measurement by dual energy x-ray absorptiometry scans after cystectomy is not known. Population-based studies suggest that fractures occur in approximately 21% of patients after cystectomy and urinary diversion.[78] To reduce the likelihood of developing bone sequelae from chronic acidosis, patients with a base deficit of -2.5 mmol/L should be considered for supplementation with oral sodium bicarbonate and potentially calcium and vitamin D.[79–81] The authors recommend that monitoring of metabolic complications should be a part of early and long-term follow-up of patients with orthotopic reconstruction. Maintenance of optimal renal function is necessary to minimize the risk for developing metabolic changes. All metabolic abnormalities should be corrected early. Future consideration should be aimed at investigating active intervention for long-term bone health in patients undergoing urinary diversion.

REFERENCES

1. Studer UE, Zingg EJ. Ileal orthotopic bladder substitutes. What we have learned from 12 years' experience with 200 patients. Urol Clin North Am 1997; 24(4):781–93.
2. Madersbacher S, Mohrle K, Burkhard F, et al. Long-term voiding pattern of patients with ileal orthotopic bladder substitutes. J Urol 2002;167(5):2052–7.
3. Kessler TM, Burkhard FC, Perimenis P, et al. Attempted nerve sparing surgery and age have a significant effect on urinary continence and erectile function after radical cystoprostatectomy and ileal

orthotopic bladder substitution. J Urol 2004; 172(4 Pt 1):1323–7.

4. Nelson CP, Montie JE, McGuire EJ, et al. Intraoperative nerve stimulation with measurement of urethral sphincter pressure changes during radical retropubic prostatectomy: a feasibility study. J Urol 2003; 169(6):2225–8.

5. Hugonnet CL, Danuser H, Springer JP, et al. Urethral sensitivity and the impact on urinary continence in patients with an ileal bladder substitute after cystectomy. J Urol 2001;165(5):1502–5.

6. Hernandez V, Espinos EL, Dunn J, et al. Oncological and functional outcomes of sexual function-preserving cystectomy compared with standard radical cystectomy in men: a systematic review. Urol Oncol 2017;35(9):539.e17-29.

7. Gotoh M, Yoshikawa Y, Sahashi M, et al. Urodynamic study of storage and evacuation of urine in patients with a urethral Kock pouch. J Urol 1995;154(5): 1850–3.

8. Ghoneim MA, Osman Y. Uretero-intestinal anastomosis in low-pressure reservoirs: refluxing or antirefluxing? BJU Int 2007;100(6):1229–33.

9. Stein JP, Skinner DG. T-mechanism applied to urinary diversion: the orthotopic T-pouch ileal neobladder and cutaneous double-T-pouch ileal reservoir. Tech Urol 2001;7(3):209–22.

10. Skinner DG, Lieskovsky G, Boyd SD. Continent urinary diversion. A 5 1/2 year experience. Ann Surg 1988;208(3):337–44.

11. Studer UE, Danuser H, Thalmann GN, et al. Antireflux nipples or afferent tubular segments in 70 patients with ileal low pressure bladder substitutes: long-term results of a prospective randomized trial. J Urol 1996;156(6):1913–7.

12. Skinner EC, Fairey AS, Groshen S, et al. Randomized trial of studer pouch versus T-pouch orthotopic ileal neobladder in patients with bladder cancer. J Urol 2015;194(2):433–9.

13. Furrer MA, Roth B, Kiss B, et al. Patients with an orthotopic low pressure bladder substitute enjoy long-term good function. J Urol 2016;196(4):1172–80.

14. Hautmann RE, de Petriconi RC, Volkmer BG. 25 years of experience with 1,000 neobladders: long-term complications. J Urol 2011;185(6):2207–12.

15. Hautmann RE, de Petriconi R, Gottfried HW, et al. The ileal neobladder: complications and functional results in 363 patients after 11 years of followup. J Urol 1999;161(2):422–7 [discussion: 7–8].

16. Henningsohn L, Steven K, Kallestrup EB, et al. Distressful symptoms and well-being after radical cystectomy and orthotopic bladder substitution compared with a matched control population. J Urol 2002;168(1):168–74 [discussion: 74–5].

17. Hart S, Skinner EC, Meyerowitz BE, et al. Quality of life after radical cystectomy for bladder cancer in patients with an ileal conduit, cutaneous or urethral kock pouch. J Urol 1999;162(1):77–81.

18. Mansson A, Caruso A, Capovilla E, et al. Quality of life after radical cystectomy and orthotopic bladder substitution: a comparison between Italian and Swedish men. BJU Int 2000;85(1):26–31.

19. Bihrle R. The Indiana pouch continent urinary reservoir. Urol Clin North Am 1997;24(4):773–9.

20. Chan Y, Fisher P, Tilki D, et al. Urethral recurrence after cystectomy: current preventative measures, diagnosis and management. BJU Int 2016;117(4): 563–9.

21. Studer UE, Burkhard FC, Schumacher M, et al. Twenty years experience with an ileal orthotopic low pressure bladder substitute–lessons to be learned. J Urol 2006;176(1):161–6.

22. Hardeman SW, Soloway MS. Urethral recurrence following radical cystectomy. J Urol 1990;144(3): 666–9.

23. Stein JP, Clark P, Miranda G, et al. Urethral tumor recurrence following cystectomy and urinary diversion: clinical and pathological characteristics in 768 male patients. J Urol 2005;173(4):1163–8.

24. Soukup V, Babjuk M, Bellmunt J, et al. Follow-up after surgical treatment of bladder cancer: a critical analysis of the literature. Eur Urol 2012;62(2): 290–302.

25. Hautmann RE, Simon J. Ileal neobladder and local recurrence of bladder cancer: patterns of failure and impact on function in men. J Urol 1999;162(6): 1963–6.

26. Bowyer GW, Davies TW. Methotrexate toxicity associated with an ileal conduit. Br J Urol 1987; 60(6):592.

27. Fossa SD, Heilo A, Bormer O. Unexpectedly high serum methotrexate levels in cystectomized bladder cancer patients with an ileal conduit treated with intermediate doses of the drug. J Urol 1990;143(3): 498–501.

28. Davidsson T, Akerlund S, White T, et al. Mucosal permeability of ileal and colonic reservoirs for urine. Br J Urol 1996;78(1):64–8.

29. Ekman I, Mansson W, Nyberg L. Absorption of drugs from continent caecal reservoir for urine. Br J Urol 1989;64(4):412–6.

30. Alhasso A, Bryden AA, Neilson D. Lithium toxicity after urinary diversion with ileal conduit. BMJ 2000; 320(7241):1037.

31. Basic DT, Hadzi-Djokic J, Ignjatovic I. The history of urinary diversion. Acta Chir Iugosl 2007;54(4):9–17.

32. Barre PH, Herve JM, Botto H, et al. Update on the Camey II procedure. World J Urol 1996;14(1):27–8.

33. Studer UE, Danuser H, Merz VW, et al. Experience in 100 patients with an ileal low pressure bladder substitute combined with an afferent tubular isoperistaltic segment. J Urol 1995;154(1):49–56.

34. Rowland RG, Mitchell ME, Bihrle R, et al. Indiana continent urinary reservoir. J Urol 1987;137(6):1136–9.

35. Lampel A, Fisch M, Stein R, et al. Continent diversion with the Mainz pouch. World J Urol 1996;14(2):85–91.

36. Ghoneim MA, Shaaban AA, Mahran MR, et al. Further experience with the urethral Kock pouch. J Urol 1992;147(2):361–5.

37. D'Elia G, Pahernik S, Fisch M, et al. Mainz Pouch II technique: 10 years' experience. BJU Int 2004;93(7):1037–42.

38. Weijerman PC, Schurmans JR, Hop WC, et al. Morbidity and quality of life in patients with orthotopic and heterotopic continent urinary diversion. Urology 1998;51(1):51–6.

39. Goodwin WE, Winter CC, Barker WF. Cup-patch technique of ileocystoplasty for bladder enlargement or partial substitution. Surg Gynecol Obstet 1959;108(2):240–4.

40. Studer UE, Turner WH. The ileal orthotopic bladder. Urology 1995;45(2):185–9.

41. Flohr P, Hefty R, Paiss T, et al. The ileal neobladder–updated experience with 306 patients. World J Urol 1996;14(1):22–6.

42. Studer UE, Danuser H, Hochreiter W, et al. Summary of 10 years' experience with an ileal low-pressure bladder substitute combined with an afferent tubular isoperistaltic segment. World J Urol 1996;14(1):29–39.

43. LEADBETTER WF. Surgical treatment of bladder cancer. Proc Natl Cancer Conf 1960;4:477–82.

44. Mills RD, Studer UE. Female orthotopic bladder substitution: a good operation in the right circumstances. J Urol 2000;163(5):1501–4.

45. Ali-el-Dein B, el-Sobky E, Hohenfellner M, et al. Orthotopic bladder substitution in women: functional evaluation. J Urol 1999;161(6):1875–80.

46. Smith E, Yoon J, Theodorescu D. Evaluation of urinary continence and voiding function: early results in men with neo-urethral modification of the Hautmann orthotopic neobladder. J Urol 2001;166(4):1346–9.

47. Mikuma N, Hirose T, Yokoo A, et al. Voiding dysfunction in ileal neobladder. J Urol 1997;158(4):1365–8.

48. Aboseif SR, Borirakchanyavat S, Lue TF, et al. Continence mechanism of the ileal neobladder in women: a urodynamics study. World J Urol 1998;16(6):400–4.

49. Arai Y, Okubo K, Konami T, et al. Voiding function of orthotopic ileal neobladder in women. Urology 1999;54(1):44–9.

50. Ankem MK, Han KR, Hartanto V, et al. Routine pouchograms are not necessary after continent urinary diversion. Urology 2004;63(3):435–7.

51. Hautmann RE. Urinary diversion: ileal conduit to neobladder. J Urol 2003;169(3):834–42.

52. Varol C, Studer UE. Managing patients after an ileal orthotopic bladder substitution. BJU Int 2004;93(3):266–70.

53. Steven K, Poulsen AL. The orthotopic Kock ileal neobladder: functional results, urodynamic features, complications and survival in 166 men. J Urol 2000;164(2):288–95.

54. Alcini E, D'Addessi A, Racioppi M, et al. Results of 4 years of experience with bladder replacement using an ileocecal segment with multiple transverse teniamyotomies. J Urol 1993;149(4):735–8.

55. Lee KS, Montie JE, Dunn RL, et al. Hautmann and Studer orthotopic neobladders: a contemporary experience. J Urol 2003;169(6):2188–91.

56. Stein JP, Lieskovsky G, Ginsberg DA, et al. The T pouch: an orthotopic ileal neobladder incorporating a serosal lined ileal antireflux technique. J Urol 1998;159(6):1836–42.

57. Stein JP, Grossfeld GD, Freeman JA, et al. Orthotopic lower urinary tract reconstruction in women using the Kock ileal neobladder: updated experience in 34 patients. J Urol 1997;158(2):400–5.

58. Beduk Y, Turkolmez K, Baltaci S, et al. Comparison of clinical and urodynamic outcome in orthotopic ileocaecal and ileal neobladder. Eur Urol 2003;43(3):258–62.

59. Stein JP, Dunn MD, Quek ML, et al. The orthotopic T pouch ileal neobladder: experience with 209 patients. J Urol 2004;172(2):584–7.

60. Steers WD. Voiding dysfunction in the orthotopic neobladder. World J Urol 2000;18(5):330–7.

61. Simon J, Bartsch G Jr, Kufer R, et al. Neobladder emptying failure in males: incidence, etiology and therapeutic options. J Urol 2006;176(4 Pt 1):1468–72 [discussion: 72].

62. Thurairaja R, Studer UE. How to avoid clean intermittent catheterization in men with ileal bladder substitution. J Urol 2008;180(6):2504–9.

63. Clifford TG, Shah SH, Bazargani ST, et al. Prospective evaluation of continence following radical cystectomy and orthotopic urinary diversion using a validated questionnaire. J Urol 2016;196(6):1685–91.

64. Pantuck AJ, Han KR, Perrotti M, et al. Ureteroenteric anastomosis in continent urinary diversion: long-term results and complications of direct versus nonrefluxing techniques. J Urol 2000;163(2):450–5.

65. Schwaibold H, Friedrich MG, Fernandez S, et al. Improvement of ureteroileal anastomosis in continent urinary diversion with modified Le Duc procedure. J Urol 1998;160(3 Pt 1):718–20.

66. Roth S, van Ahlen H, Semjonow A, et al. Does the success of ureterointestinal implantation in orthotopic bladder substitution depend more on surgeon level of experience or choice of technique? J Urol 1997;157(1):56–60.

67. Wood DP Jr, Bianco FJ Jr, Pontes JE, et al. Incidence and significance of positive urine cultures in patients with an orthotopic neobladder. J Urol 2003;169(6):2196–9.

68. Keegan SJ, Graham C, Neal DE, et al. Characterization of Escherichia coli strains causing urinary tract infections in patients with transposed intestinal segments. J Urol 2003;169(6):2382–7.

69. Van der Aa F, Joniau S, Van Den Branden M, et al. Metabolic changes after urinary diversion. Adv Urol 2011;2011:764325.

70. McDougal WS. Metabolic complications of urinary intestinal diversion. J Urol 1992;147(5):1199–208.

71. Sagalowsky AI, Frenkel EP. Cobalamin profiles in patients after urinary diversion. J Urol 2002;167(4):1696–700.

72. Yakout H, Bissada NK. Intermediate effects of the ileocaecal urinary reservoir (Charleston pouch 1) on serum vitamin B12 concentrations: can vitamin B12 deficiency be prevented? BJU Int 2003;91(7):653–5 [discussion: 5–6].

73. Pfitzenmaier J, Lotz J, Faldum A, et al. Metabolic evaluation of 94 patients 5 to 16 years after ileocecal pouch (Mainz pouch 1) continent urinary diversion. J Urol 2003;170(5):1884–7.

74. Bettice JA, Gamble JL Jr. Skeletal buffering of acute metabolic acidosis. Am J Physiol 1975;229(6):1618–24.

75. McDougal WS, Koch MO, Shands C 3rd, et al. Bony demineralization following urinary intestinal diversion. J Urol 1988;140(4):853–5.

76. Lee SW, Russell J, Avioli LV. 25-hydroxycholecalciferol to 1,25-dihydroxycholecalciferol: conversion impaired by systemic metabolic acidosis. Science 1977;195(4282):994–6.

77. Arnett TR, Dempster DW. Effect of pH on bone resorption by rat osteoclasts in vitro. Endocrinology 1986;119(1):119–24.

78. Gupta A, Atoria CL, Ehdaie B, et al. Risk of fracture after radical cystectomy and urinary diversion for bladder cancer. J Clin Oncol 2014;32(29):3291–8.

79. Hossain M. The osteomalacia syndrome after colocystoplasty; a cure with sodium bicarbonate alone. Br J Urol 1970;42(2):243–5.

80. Siklos P, Davie M, Jung RT, et al. Osteomalacia in ureterosigmoidostomy: healing by correction of the acidosis. Br J Urol 1980;52(1):61–2.

81. Perry W, Allen LN, Stamp TC, et al. Vitamin D resistance in osteomalacia after ureterosigmoidostomy. N Engl J Med 1977;297(20):1110–2.

Orthotopic Urinary Diversion for Women

Dimitar V. Zlatev, MD, Eila C. Skinner, MD*

KEYWORDS

- Neoblader • Orthotopic urinary diversion • Urinary bladder • Urinary incontinence
- Urinary obstruction • Vesicovaginal fistula

KEY POINTS

- Female patients with an intact functioning urethra are potential candidates for orthotopic diversion because the urethra is rarely involved with cancer in women with bladder cancer.
- The primary risk factors for urethral tumor involvement at cystectomy are tumor at the bladder neck and invasion into the cervix or vagina.
- The orthotopic neoblader relies on the rhabdosphincter for continence; in women, this structure is primarily around the portion of the urethra that is below the endopelvic fascia.
- The benefits of uterine preservation include decreased risk of vaginal fistula formation, improved sexual function, and possible decreased risk of late urinary retention.
- A vesicovaginal fistula is a unique complication for women that may be difficult to diagnose and treat. An omental flap between the vagina and neoblader can decrease the risk.

INTRODUCTION

After nearly 30 years of widespread experience with orthotopic urinary diversion for patients with bladder cancer, this form of diversion can no longer be considered experimental. Nonetheless, the adoption of orthotopic neoblader diversion for women has lagged behind that for men, in part because the urethra was routinely removed in women as part of the cystectomy, because it was commonly believed that the bladder neck itself was required for continence in women. Neobladers were occasionally performed for women with nonurothelial malignancies with promising results. Then in 1995, Stein and colleagues and Stenzl and associations each published pathologic studies suggesting the urethra was involved with cancer in only a relatively small percentage of women with urothelial bladder cancer, and thus could safely be retained in the majority.[1,2] These findings were subsequently confirmed in

prospective series of women undergoing orthotopic diversion,[3,4] which led to additional centers starting to offer neoblader reconstruction to women. Today, in many institutions this option is discussed with every patient who is a potential candidate. Patient selection, technical factors that impact functional outcomes, and reported results after orthotopic urinary diversion for women are discussed in this article.

PATIENT SELECTION

There are patient-specific and cancer-specific factors that must be considered in deciding who might be a candidate for an orthotopic diversion. Many of these factors are the same in men and women. The only absolute contraindications to orthotopic diversion are poor renal function (an estimated glomerular filtration rate of <40 mL/min), lack of available bowel, or poorly functioning urethral sphincter. Other patient

Disclosure Statement: D.V. Zlatev and E.C. Skinner have nothing they wish to disclose.
Department of Urology, Stanford University School of Medicine, Stanford University Hospital and Clinics, 300 Pasteur Drive, Room S287, Stanford, CA 94304, USA
* Corresponding author.
E-mail address: skinnere@stanford.edu

urologic.theclinics.com

factors include age, general health and fitness, and significant comorbidities such as poor cardiac or pulmonary function that may require an expeditious surgery. Additionally, patient motivation and social support are important considerations. Female cystectomy patients tend to be older and are more likely to live alone than males, which may impact these decisions. In addition, women are more likely than men to have preexisting pelvic floor relaxation that causes stress incontinence. Women also have experience wearing pads; thus, leakage is less a theoretic concern than it is for men facing a cystectomy. Therefore, women may elect to not risk incontinence. Finally, prior high-dose pelvic radiation for gynecologic or pelvic malignancy may cause severe scarring around the vagina and urethra that likely would make a neobladder impossible. These considerations can easily be assessed on careful history assessment and physical examination.

Self-catheterization may be required in 50% or more of women undergoing neobladder reconstruction; therefore, patients must be willing and able to potentially do this before surgery.[3,5] In questionable cases, it is prudent to teach the patient self-catheterization before they make a decision on the type of diversion.

Many oncologic factors are also similar between men and women. Tumor bulk, presence of lymph node metastases, and the presence of carcinoma in situ within the bladder have all been shown not to be critical contraindications to orthotopic diversion.[6] Local pelvic recurrence is a rare after a properly performed cystectomy, and even when it occurs it does not generally affect neobladder function.[6] Conversely, a patient with disease invading the sidewall, palpable extension into the vaginal wall, or with extensive lymphadenopathy is a poor candidate for neobladder construction and may be best managed with a cutaneous diversion.

Risk of Urethral Recurrence in Women

The primary oncologic factor that is unique to the female patients is the risk of subsequent recurrence in the urethral stump when the urethra is preserved. The initial studies by Stein, Stenzl, and others in the 1990s showed that the primary risk factors for urethral tumor involvement at the time of cystectomy were tumor at the bladder neck and invasion into the cervix or vagina.[1,2,7–9] Fortunately, these neoplasms are straightforward to diagnose through cystoscopy and a careful pelvic examination, and using these criteria approximately 70% of women with muscle-invasive bladder cancer are potential candidates for orthotopic diversion. When these criteria are used for patient selection, along with a frozen section of the urethral margin at the time of cystectomy, urethral recurrence has been extremely rare. Ali-el-Dien[10] reported on 180 women with a 57-month median follow-up and found only 2 urethral recurrences. Stein and colleagues[3] found only 1 urethral recurrence in 120 women who underwent radical cystectomy and orthotopic neobladder with a 103-month median follow-up.

Preoperative Evaluation

A careful pelvic examination is critical in planning cystectomy in women. The urethra and bladder neck are easily palpable and can be evaluated for palpable tumor, presence of vaginal atrophy or prolapse, and pelvic floor muscle strength. This is also an opportunity to teach the patient how to do proper Kegel exercises and self-catheterization.

Gross and colleagues[11] have suggested that preoperative urodynamics with measurement of the urethral pressure profile, functional urethral length, and maximum urethral pressure could predict women who may have worse continence or higher risk of urinary retention with neobladder construction. These measures of urethral function correlated with age and whether patients had a prior or concomitant hysterectomy. However, there was considerable overlap in the groups and this finding has not been confirmed in another prospective series; thus, it is unclear if urodynamics have a definite role in choosing the type of urinary diversion. If a patient does have stress incontinence, she should expect that it will likely get worse after cystectomy. A concomitant Burch procedure at the time of cystectomy can decrease the risk of incontinence, but with a trade-off of increasing the risk of urinary retention.

SURGICAL TECHNIQUE
Anatomy of the Urethra

Although it was long believed that the bladder neck was required for continence in females, it now seems that the rhabdosphincter in the midurethra is adequate for continence after a cystectomy. Very elegant neuroanatomic studies of the urethra in female cadavers established that the rhabdosphincter exists as an omega-shaped structure around the urethra, most robust anteriorly and thinned out posteriorly.[12] This structure is primarily around the portion of the urethra that is below the endopelvic fascia, whereas the more proximal urethra and bladder neck are above that fascia. There is a smooth muscle component innervated by branches of the autonomic plexus that run longitudinally along the lateral posterior vagina and rectum. These nerves seem to provide important innervation of the bladder neck and most proximal urethra, which are removed with the cystectomy. The importance of preserving this plexus in women undergoing neobladder reconstruction is somewhat controversial.[11,13] However, the rhabdosphincter, which is innervated by branches of the pudendal nerve, seems to be more critical for continence. These nerve branches run under the endopelvic fascia from the pudendal nerve and enter the caudal portion of the urethra laterally.[12,14] It is, therefore, of paramount importance for continence function to avoid dissection around the urethra below the endopelvic fascia that could damage these nerves and weaken the sphincter.

Technique of Cystectomy in the Female Undergoing Neobladder Reconstruction

In women undergoing cystectomy with planned orthotopic diversion, the posterior pedicles and apical dissection must be adapted to preserve the urethra and as much of the vaginal wall as possible. The lymph node dissection and more proximal dissection do not need to be altered. The tissue posterior and lateral along the vagina should be avoided when feasible from an oncologic perspective to preserve the autonomic plexus running there. Most critically, the dissection around the urethra is kept above the endopelvic fascia to avoid injury to the rhabdosphincter (**Fig. 1**).

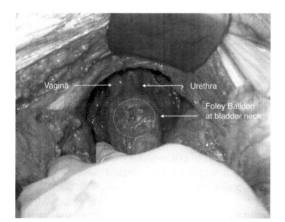

Fig. 1. Dissection around the female urethra in preparation for an orthotopic neobladder. The fatty tissue overlying the anterior urethra is swept off the endopelvic fascia. The vesicourethral junction is identified by positioning the inflated balloon of the urethral catheter at the bladder neck. The endopelvic fascia below the dissection is not disturbed to avoid injury to the rhabdosphincter. (*From* Skinner EC, Daneshmand S. Orthotopic Urinary Diversion. In: Wein AJ, Kavoussi LR, Partin AW, et al. eds. Campbell-Walsh Urology. 11th ed. Philadelphia, PA: Elsevier; 2016. p. 2344–68; with permission.)

Management of the Uterus

There are some observations suggesting that preservation of the uterus in women who have not undergone prior hysterectomy may have advantages in functional outcomes after neobladder construction. A number of studies have shown that direct involvement of the uterus or cervix with malignancy is quite unusual in women who underwent standard anterior exenteration for bladder cancer.[15,16] The benefits of uterine preservation include decreased risk of vaginal fistula formation, improved sexual function, and a possible decreased risk of urinary retention.[17,18] In the authors' experience, it is unclear if uterine-sparing cystectomy really impacts the potential need for self-catheterization. However, because the other benefits have been shown more definitively, we offer the option of uterine-sparing orthotopic diversion routinely to younger women without bulky posterior tumors.

If uterine-sparing is planned, the infundibulopelvic and round ligaments are preserved to provide support to the uterus and preserve the ovaries. The uterine artery bilaterally is preserved, taking the branches of the internal iliac artery coursing to the bladder distal to the uterine branch. The ureteral stump must be passed under the uterine artery to keep it attached to the bladder. The peritoneum is incised just anterior to the cervix and the white plane along the anterior vaginal wall is carefully and sharply developed using superior traction to avoid inadvertent entry into the bladder. Dissection lateral to the cervix should be avoided, because that maneuver will result in considerable bleeding. The vascular tissue coming around the vagina coursing toward the bladder is taken down, staying as far anterior as possible to preserve the autonomic nerves. This dissection is continued down to just distal to the bladder neck, which can be identified by tugging and palpation of the urethral catheter balloon (see **Fig. 1**). The fat is then removed around the proximal urethra, staying above the endopelvic fascia. If there is a well-developed dorsal venous complex, it can be ligated above the endopelvic fascia with a vessel-sealing device. Once the bladder is attached only by the urethra, the planned incision in the urethra just outside the bladder neck is identified and marked with a suture or light cautery. The catheter is then removed, a clamp placed across the bladder neck to avoid spillage, and the urethra is divided with a knife. The urethral sutures can be placed later, because they are straightforward in the female patient. An absorbable suture placed at 5 o'clock and 7 o'clock lateral to the urethral stump is helpful for hemostasis and can be kept to use later to tack an omental flap behind the urethral anastomosis.

If the patient has had a prior hysterectomy, the vaginal apex may be identified with a sponge stick in the vagina and the same plane developed along the anterior vaginal wall. If the patient has a large tumor on the posterior bladder wall, it may be necessary to excise a portion of the anterior vaginal wall with the tumor. In that case, we try to preserve the more distal anterior vagina to avoid having the vaginal closure in close proximity behind the urethral anastomosis. A careful, water-tight closure of the vagina is critical and the omental flap particularly helpful in this scenario. We often also do a sacrocolpopexy with mesh to provide additional support to the vagina when the uterus is absent or is removed.

The specific type of neobladder constructed and the perioperative management are not unique to the female patient and are not discussed in detail here.

RESULTS AND MANAGEMENT OF COMPLICATIONS

Most early and late complications are similar in men and women and are managed in a similar manner. Vesicovaginal fistula is a unique complication for women that may be difficult to diagnose and treat. Women who require a concomitant hysterectomy or partial vaginectomy are at increased risk for this complication. We routinely place a flap of omentum between the repaired vagina and the neobladder as a preventive maneuver.

Any woman who has persistent total incontinence 2 to 3 months after a cystectomy neobladder should have an evaluation to rule out a fistula, because this complication will not resolve spontaneously. The easiest way to diagnose this entity is to place saline with a few drops of methylene blue through a catheter into the bladder and then use a speculum to evaluate the vaginal apex to look for the blue dye. It can also be diagnosed on delayed views of a computed tomography urogram or computed tomography cystogram with full lateral views.

If a fistula is diagnosed, generally catheter drainage is not effective. Most authors have described a transvaginal approach to repair, which may require a Martius flap or other advanced techniques. We often call on our female pelvic medicine colleagues to assist with these challenging cases. Transvaginal success rates are variable, and if attempted repair fails consideration is made for transabdominal exploration and conversion to a cutaneous form of urinary diversion.[19–22]

Urinary Retention

Urinary retention (so-called hypercontinence) is significantly more common in women than in men, with a reported rate of 20% to 60% in women and only 4% to 10% in men.[23–25] The reasons for this discrepancy remain somewhat obscure. Monitoring of postvoid residual with ultrasound imaging is reasonable as a part of routine follow-up, with encouragement to start intermittent catheterization for large residual volumes or symptoms. Patients often complain of recurrent symptomatic urinary infections or worsening incontinence, especially at night. Occasionally, patients go into complete retention, but this scenario is relatively rare. Often, retention develops a year or more after surgery.

Cystoscopy with a careful pelvic examination and urinary cytology should be performed to rule out urethral cancer recurrence. Pharmacologic intervention does not seem to be effective for urinary retention in this setting.[25] In the authors' opinion, there is not much of a role for attempted surgical treatment of this problem. We generally will encourage the patient to accept intermittent catheterization and avoid spending a lot of time straining to empty.

Incontinence

Continence results in female patients with orthotopic urinary diversion are summarized in **Table 1**. The wide range of outcomes is partly due to how the data were collected. Few studies have used the gold standard patient-completed outcomes using a standardized questionnaire.[3,5,23,26] Generally, however, daytime continence has been reported in the 80% to 90% range and nighttime continence around 70%. Approximately 60% of women in the 2 largest series using a patient questionnaire reported needing to perform self-catheterization at least occasionally.[3,26]

Evaluation of persistent incontinence that is not due to a vaginal fistula should be delayed 6 to 12 months after surgery to ensure adequate time for the neobladder to expand.[27] The best treatment for incontinence is prevention of the complication by careful patient selection and surgical technique. Pelvic floor physical therapy is recommended and can help some patients to attain continence.[28] Bulking agents may be successful.[29,30] A midurethral sling may be performed, but extreme care must be taken if passing blind needles through the pelvis because the neobladder and loops of small and large bowel may be adherent to the pelvic sidewall. Bone anchor systems might be safer in this setting.[31] A patient undergoing a sling procedure should expect to

Table 1
Continence results of orthotopic diversion in series limited to female patients

Author	No. of Patients	Mean Follow-up (mo)	Mean Age (y)	Continence Day (%)	Night (%)	IC (%)
Stenzl et al,[35] 2001	102	26	59	82	72	12
Granberg et al,[36] 2008	59	29	62	90	57	35
Ali-el-Dein et al,[20] 2008	192	51	54	92	72	16
Stein et al,[3] 2009	56	103	66	77[a]	66[a]	61[a] (39% dependent on IC to void)
Jentzmik et al,[26] 2012	131	56	61	82.4[a]	75.9[a]	58[a]
Anderson et al,[37] 2012	49	37	60	57	45	31
Bartsch et al,[5] 2014	56	63	64	30[a]	35[a]	62[a] (45% dependent on IC to void)

Abbreviation: IC, intermittent catheterization to empty neobladder.
[a] Continence results from validated patient-completed questionnaires.

require intermittent catheterization to empty. No large series of these interventions have been reported.

QUALITY OF LIFE

Quality-of-life studies of patients after orthotopic urinary diversion have been limited by methodologic problems and study design. One recent study reported better quality of life after an orthotopic neobladder, but only as long as continence was preserved.[32] There are no data to suggest a clear difference in quality of life for women undergoing neobladder construction compared with other methods of urinary diversion. It seems that the majority of patients report good overall quality of life and little emotional distress after urinary diversion.[33,34]

SUMMARY

Orthotopic neobladder is a viable option for women undergoing cystectomy for bladder cancer, with excellent oncologic outcomes and low incidence of urethral recurrence. Careful patient selection is important, as is developing a clear understanding by the patient and her family in what to expect with an orthotopic diversion. Surgical technique is important in optimizing functional outcomes such as continence, sexual function, and a decreased rate of vaginal fistula formation and urinary retention.

REFERENCES

1. Stein JP, Cote RJ, Freeman JA, et al. Indications for lower urinary tract reconstruction in women after cystectomy for bladder cancer: a pathological review of female cystectomy specimens. J Urol 1995;154(4):1329–33.
2. Stenzl A, Draxl H, Posch B, et al. The risk of urethral tumors in female bladder cancer: can the urethra be used for orthotopic reconstruction of the lower urinary tract? J Urol 1995;153(3 Pt 2):950–5.
3. Stein JP, Penson DF, Lee C, et al. Long-term oncological outcomes in women undergoing radical cystectomy and orthotopic diversion for bladder cancer. J Urol 2009;181(5):2052–8 [discussion: 2058–9].
4. Stenzl A, Colleselli K, Poisel S, et al. Anterior exenteration with subsequent ureteroileal urethrostomy in females. Anatomy, risk of urethral recurrence, surgical technique, and results. Eur Urol 1998;33(Suppl 4):18–20.
5. Bartsch G, Daneshmand S, Skinner EC, et al. Urinary functional outcomes in female neobladder patients. World J Urol 2014;32(1):221–8.
6. Hautmann RE, Abol-Enein H, Davidsson T, et al. ICUD-EAU International consultation on bladder cancer 2012: urinary diversion. Eur Urol 2013;63(1):67–80.
7. Chen ME, Pisters LL, Malpica A, et al. Risk of urethral, vaginal and cervical involvement in patients undergoing radical cystectomy for bladder cancer: results of a contemporary cystectomy series from M. D. Anderson Cancer Center. J Urol 1997;157(6):2120–3.
8. Coloby PJ, Kakizoe T, Tobisu K, et al. Urethral involvement in female bladder cancer patients: mapping of 47 consecutive cysto-urethrectomy specimens. J Urol 1994;152(5 Pt 1):1438–42.
9. De Paepe ME, Andre R, Mahadevia P. Urethral involvement in female patients with bladder cancer. A study of 22 cystectomy specimens. Cancer 1990;65(5):1237–41.

10. Ali-El-Dein B. Oncological outcome after radical cystectomy and orthotopic bladder substitution in women. Eur J Surg Oncol 2009;35(3):320–5.

11. Gross T, Meierhans Ruf SD, Meissner C, et al. Orthotopic ileal bladder substitution in women: factors influencing urinary incontinence and hypercontinence. Eur Urol 2015;68(4):664–71.

12. Colleselli K, Stenzl A, Eder R, et al. The female urethral sphincter: a morphological and topographical study. J Urol 1998;160(1):49–54.

13. Skinner EC, Comiter CV. Can we improve the functional outcomes of orthotopic diversion in women? Eur Urol 2015;68(4):672–3.

14. Hinata N, Murakami G, Abe S, et al. Detailed histological investigation of the female urethra: application to radical cystectomy. J Urol 2012;187(2):451–6.

15. Chang SS, Cole E, Smith JA Jr, et al. Pathological findings of gynecologic organs obtained at female radical cystectomy. J Urol 2002;168(1):147–9.

16. Djaladat H, Bruins HM, Miranda G, et al. Reproductive organ involvement in female patients undergoing radical cystectomy for urothelial bladder cancer. J Urol 2012;188(6):2134–8.

17. Ali-El-Dein B, Mosbah A, Osman Y, et al. Preservation of the internal genital organs during radical cystectomy in selected women with bladder cancer: a report on 15 cases with long term follow-up. Eur J Surg Oncol 2013;39(4):358–64.

18. Zippe CD, Nandipati KC, Agarwal A, et al. Female sexual dysfunction after pelvic surgery: the impact of surgical modifications. BJU Int 2005;96(7):959–63.

19. Ali-El-Dein B, Ashamallah A. Vaginal repair of pouch-vaginal fistula after orthotopic bladder substitution in women. Urology 2013;81(1):198–202.

20. Ali-el-Dein B, Shaaban AA, Abu-Eideh RH, et al. Surgical complications following radical cystectomy and orthotopic neobladders in women. J Urol 2008;180(1):206–10 [discussion: 210].

21. Rapp DE, O'Connor RC, Katz EE, et al. Neobladder-vaginal fistula after cystectomy and orthotopic neobladder construction. BJU Int 2004;94(7):1092–5 [discussion: 1095].

22. Smith JA Jr. Neobladder-vaginal fistula after cystectomy and orthotopic neobladder construction. J Urol 2005;174(3):970–1.

23. Ahmadi H, Skinner EC, Simma-Chiang V, et al. Urinary functional outcome following radical cystoprostatectomy and ileal neobladder reconstruction in male patients. J Urol 2013;189(5):1782–8.

24. Nagele U, Kuczyk M, Anastasiadis AG, et al. Radical cystectomy and orthotopic bladder replacement in females. Eur Urol 2006;50(2):249–57.

25. Steers WD. Voiding dysfunction in the orthotopic neobladder. World J Urol 2000;18(5):330–7.

26. Jentzmik F, Schrader AJ, de Petriconi R, et al. The ileal neobladder in female patients with bladder cancer: long-term clinical, functional, and oncological outcome. World J Urol 2012;30(6):733–9.

27. Studer UE, Burkhard FC, Schumacher M, et al. Twenty years experience with an ileal orthotopic low pressure bladder substitute–lessons to be learned. J Urol 2006;176(1):161–6.

28. Parekh AR, Feng MI, Kirages D, et al. The role of pelvic floor exercises on post-prostatectomy incontinence. J Urol 2003;170(1):130–3.

29. Tchetgen MB, Sanda MG, Montie JE, et al. Collagen injection for the treatment of incontinence after cystectomy and orthotopic neobladder reconstruction in women. J Urol 2000;163(1):212–4.

30. Wilson S, Quek ML, Ginsberg DA. Transurethral injection of bulking agents for stress urinary incontinence following orthotopic neobladder reconstruction in women. J Urol 2004;172(1):244–6.

31. Quek ML, Stein JP, Daneshmand S, et al. A critical analysis of perioperative mortality from radical cystectomy. J Urol 2006;175(3 Pt 1):886–9 [discussion: 889–90].

32. Zahran MH, Taha DE, Harraz AM, et al. Health related quality of life after radical cystectomy in women: orthotopic neobladder versus ileal loop conduit and impact of incontinence. Minerva Urol Nefrol 2017;69(3):262–70.

33. Hart S, Skinner EC, Meyerowitz BE, et al. Quality of life after radical cystectomy for bladder cancer in patients with an ileal conduit, cutaneous or urethral Kock pouch. J Urol 1999;162(1):77–81.

34. Rouanne M, Legrand G, Neuzillet Y, et al. Long-term women-reported quality of life after radical cystectomy and orthotopic ileal neobladder reconstruction. Ann Surg Oncol 2014;21(4):1398–404.

35. Stenzl A, Jarolim L, Coloby P, et al. Urethra-sparing cystectomy and orthotopic urinary diversion in women with malignant pelvic tumors. Cancer 2001;92(7):1864–71.

36. Granberg CF, Boorjian SA, Crispen PL, et al. Functional and oncological outcomes after orthotopic neobladder reconstruction in women. BJU Int 2008;102(11):1551–5.

37. Anderson CB, Cookson MS, Chang SS, et al. Voiding function in women with orthotopic neobladder urinary diversion. J Urol 2012;188(1):200–4.

Continent Cutaneous Diversion

Shane M. Pearce, MD, Siamak Daneshmand, MD*

KEYWORDS

- Urinary diversion • Continent cutaneous • Bladder cancer • Indiana pouch • Right colon pouch

KEY POINTS

- Appropriate selection of patients for continent cutaneous diversion is a key factor to successful outcomes. Indications and contraindications are discussed in the context of extirpative surgery for bladder cancer.
- The 2 most common forms of urinary diversion, the Indiana Pouch and the right colon pouch with appendicoumbilicostomy, are illustrated in detail.
- Components of enhanced recovery after surgery are described, including the incidence of early and late complications and tips on how to minimize them.
- Continence rates and health-related quality of life from various series are summarized.

INTRODUCTION

Continent cutaneous urinary diversion (CCUD) was introduced in the United States after Kock's report of clinical results with an ileal reservoir in a 12 patient series.[1] Rowland's description of a right colon reservoir with a reinforced ileocecal valve for continence (Indiana pouch) in 1987 further aided acceptance of CCUD as a reasonable option for urinary diversion.[2] The University of Southern California reported excellent outcomes using the Kock reservoir for urinary diversion in the first large American series of 531 patients from 1982 to 1988.[3] CCUD provides an excellent option for patients who are not candidates for orthotopic neobladder (ONB), yet desire continence and are capable of intermittent catheterization. However, with the widespread adoption of orthotopic diversion in the 1990s (1% before 1990 and 16% between 200 and 2008), there was a significant decline in the percent of patients undergoing CCUD.[4] Among experienced surgeons who routinely offer CCUD to appropriately selected patients, the percent of patients choosing CCUD is as high as 20% to 30% compared with just 9% in population-based data.[5]

The principal advantages of CCUD over orthotopic diversion are excellent early daytime and nighttime continence. Some surgeons prefer CCUD over ONB in women because of the 20% to 30% risk of hypercontinence associated with ONB[6]; additionally, CCUD is well suited for patients with a diseased urethra from either benign damage or malignancy. CCUD are constructed with adherence to basic principles of continent urinary diversion, including the use of detubularized bowel in a spherical conformation for pouch creation with either ileum or the right colon. Construction of a robust and stable continent catheterizable channel remains the most critical aspect of the operation with a variety of methods and approaches largely based on individual surgeon experience and preference. Additional considerations include the use of a refluxing versus anti-refluxing techniques for the afferent limb or ureteroenteric anastomoses. Although there is no

Disclosure Statement: The authors have nothing they wish to disclose.
Department of Urology, USC/Norris Comprehensive Cancer Center, Institute of Urology, 1441 Eastlake Avenue, Suite 7416, Los Angeles, CA 90089, USA
* Corresponding author.
E-mail address: daneshma@med.usc.edu

Urol Clin N Am 45 (2018) 55–65
https://doi.org/10.1016/j.ucl.2017.09.004

evidence for impact on renal function,[7] the risk of reflux is balanced against a potentially higher risk of ureteral obstruction with anti-reflexing techniques.[8,9] This article reviews the history, patient selection, preoperative evaluation, surgical technique, and outcomes of CCUD.

HISTORICAL BACKGROUND

The first description of a catheterizable reservoir for urinary diversion was by Verhoogen in 1908,[10] who reported early results after creation of a cecal reservoir. Initial attempts permitted catheterization but did not provide continence. The first series describing a continent channel was from Gilchrist and Merricks[11] at Presbyterian Hospital in Chicago beginning in 1949.[11] In the 1980s, further refinements of continent diversion by Kock, Skinner, Rowland, and others led to improved functional outcomes and reduced complications through the use of detubularized bowel for the pouch and description of numerous plication and intussusception strategies for creation of a flap valve between the pouch and catheterizable channel to provide adequate continence. These techniques form the armamentarium of urologists performing urinary diversion in the current era.[1–3]

PATIENT SELECTION AND PREOPERATIVE EVALUATION

Before counseling a patient about options for continent diversion, it is important to consider the contraindications. Absolute contraindications include significant renal insufficiency (glomerular filtration rate <50 mL/min), pelvic extension of disease, gastrointestinal disorders affecting the segment intended for urinary diversion, hepatic dysfunction, or neuromuscular disorders that could impede one's ability to self-catheterize. Most eligible patients will likely elect for continent diversion with appropriate counseling.[12] Most patients who are candidates for continent diversion tend to prefer ONB; however, there are patients who prefer CCUD. There are also many situations wherein CCUD may be encouraged as a favorable alternative to ONB, such as in patients with preexisting incontinence or malignancy at the bladder neck, prostate, or urethral margin.[13] Women considering ONB must be counseled regarding the known risk of urinary retention and need to perform clean intermittent catheterization after orthotopic diversion.[14–16]

Assessment of past medical and surgical history must include particular attention to preexisting neurologic disease, renal dysfunction, liver disease, and prior abdominal surgery. Laboratory evaluation is performed with a focus on renal function, electrolytes, and nutritional parameters. Colonoscopy may be considered to rule out bowel disease in clinically appropriate scenarios and computerized tomography to assess anatomy. Patients should see an ostomy nurse for selection of an optimal stoma site, typically the lower abdomen or umbilicus, and many stoma nurses will also mark the patient for an ileal conduit as a backup. The site should be in a location that is easy to conceal, locate, and manage. At the authors' institution, they use the umbilicus as the site for the vast majority of stomas given its consistency and for the aforementioned criteria.

Although enhanced recovery after surgery (ERAS) protocols for radical cystectomy and urinary diversion have improved return of bowel function and length of stay, most current data focus on patients undergoing ileal conduit or ONB.[17,18] Elimination of a mechanical bowel preparation (MBP) is advocated by most ERAS pathways as part of a multifaceted strategy to speed return of bowel function. Most recent evidence suggests that MBP may have negative consequences on bowel motility through electrolyte and fluid imbalances, and there are no data to suggest it reduces the rate of wound infection, anastomotic leak, reoperation, or mortality.[19,20] However, because of the frank stool load and high bacterial count in the colon, most urologists continue to use an MBP when planning a urinary diversion with colon, which is the current practice at the authors' institution. They do not recommend routine oral antibiotic bowel preparation because of the risk for selection of resistant, pathogenic bacterial strains.[21]

TECHNIQUE

This section outlines the basic aspects of CCUD creation. There are a variety of approaches to CCUD. Many technical modifications have focused on creation of continence mechanisms and anti-reflux strategies such as tunneled ureteral anastomoses, the ileocecal valve, the Kock nipple valve, or an extraserosal tunnel. These techniques are not discussed here in detail, and there is some evidence that anti-reflexing ureteroenteric anastomosis techniques may have a higher risk of late upper tract obstruction and stenosis compared with direct reflexing techniques, leading to favor for the latter currently among most urologists.[8,9] The Indiana pouch is probably the most common approach to CCUD, which involves a right colon pouch with the tapered terminal ileum functioning as the catheterizable channel and a reinforced ileocecal valve providing continence (**Fig. 1**). Following completion of a side-to-side ileocolic bowel anastomosis, the ileal segment is tapered

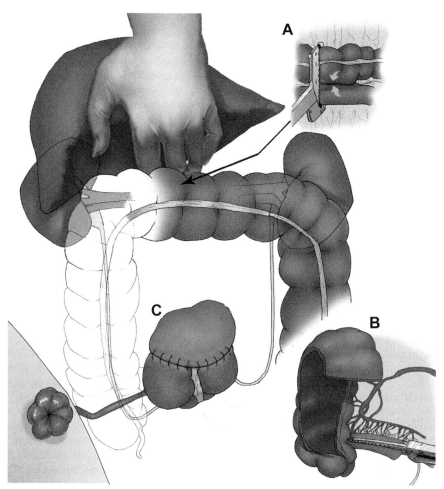

Fig. 1. Indiana pouch: a right colon pouch with the tapered terminal ileum functioning as the catheterizable channel, and a reinforced ileocecal valve providing continence. (A) A side-to-side ileocolic bowel anastomosis completed after the right colon segment has been isolated. (B) The isolated right colon segment is incised along the taeniae coli and then folded into a U-configuration; the back wall of the pouch is closed with a running, absorbable suture. The colon pouch is then closed to create a spherical reservoir. (C) The efferent catheterizable ileal segment is tapered over a 16-French red rubber catheter using a GIA stapler. Imbricating sutures are placed at the ileocecal valve, and the efferent limb is matured to the skin. (*From* Pearce SM, Cohn JA, Steinberg Z, et al. Patient selection, operative technique, and contemporary outcomes of continent catheterizable diversion: the Indiana pouch. Curr Bladder Dysfunct Rep 2014;9(4):294; with permission.)

over a 16-French red rubber catheter using a GIA stapler. Imbricating sutures are placed at the ileo-cecal valve, and it is critical to ensure the catheterization of the channel remains smooth and easy following this step. The isolated right colon segment is incised along the taeniae coli and then folded into a U-configuration, and the back wall of the pouch is closed with a running, absorbable suture. Bilateral ureteroenteric anastomoses are then completed in a direct, end-to-side, freely refluxing manner. The anastomoses are stented with a 7-French single J urinary diversion stent. Following completion of the ureteroenteric anastomoses, the suprapubic tube site is selected, and a large Malecot catheter is brought from outside in through the abdominal wall and into the pouch and secured with a purse-string suture. The stents are tied to the suprapubic tube to facilitate removal in the future. The remainder of the colon pouch is now closed to create a spherical reservoir. A surgical drain is placed near the reservoir. Finally, the stoma site is selected and a V-flap skin incision is made. After incision of the fascia, the tapered ileum is passed through the abdominal wall. Any redundant ileum is resected, and spatulation is performed if needed. Ease of catheterization is confirmed, and the cutaneous stoma is matured. A 14-French Foley catheter is placed in the efferent limb and capped. A variety of combined laparoscopic and open techniques have been applied to Indiana pouch creation, including a recently published initial experience of 10 patients undergoing robotic completely intracorporeal Indiana pouch diversion.[22]

The remainder of this section focuses on the right colon pouch with a tunneled appendicoumbilicostomy, which is the authors' preferred method of CCUD. Advantages to this technique are multiple and include the use of the terminal ileum as an afferent limb permitting uretero-ileal as opposed to uretero-colic anastomoses facilitating ease of ureteroenteric anastomosis with a theoretic decreased risk of stricture. The ileocecal valve provides a natural anti-reflux mechanism. The appendix is embedded in the submucosa of the colon to achieve continence using the Mitrofanoff principle (**Figs. 2** and **3**). Continence rates using this technique are excellent, reported as high as 100% with 33 months mean follow-up.[23] In addition, the appendix does not tend to elongate over time compared with ileal channels and avoids potential difficulty catheterizing due to kinks and tortuosity. Although the appendix is not always suitable for use as the efferent limb when its length (at least 5–6 cm) or caliber (at least 12 French) is inadequate, a 2- to 3-cm segment of ileum can be retubularized using the Yang-Monti principle and fashioned as a neo-appendicoumbilicostomy with acceptable outcomes.[24] Higher rates of stomal stenosis have been reported with the use of appendiceal stoma representing an important disadvantage of this approach; however, most of these patients can be managed with minor procedures in clinic or as outpatient surgery.[23,25]

When any type of right colon reservoir is planned, the right colon must be mobilized completely along the line of Toldt distal to the hepatic flexure. The terminal ileum is divided 5 to 10 cm proximal to the ileocecal valve, and the right colon is typically divided just proximal to the middle colic artery. Approximately 30 cm of right colon is required to create a reservoir of adequate capacity. If the appendix is deemed suitable for use, the appendix and its mesentery are carefully mobilized, and the appendix is incised to allow cannulation with at least a 12-French catheter. Several windows are created in the appendiceal mesentery (see **Fig. 2**), followed by a 4- to 5-cm incision through the anterior tenia of the colon down to the level of the mucosa (see **Fig. 3**). The appendix is then flipped into the submucosal tunnel, and the incised tenia is reapproximated to fashion a seromuscular tunnel. The colon is detubularized with an incision along its antimesenteric border with deviation away from the appendix near the cecum (**Fig. 4**). The colon is then folded to create and inverted "U", and the posterior wall is

closed with an absorbable suture (**Fig. 5**). Following closure of the remainder of the pouch, bilateral end-to-side ureteroileal anastomosis is performed over a double J stent, which is tied to the pouchostomy tube to facilitate later removal (**Fig. 6**). Finally, the stoma site is selected, and absorbable sutures are used to secure the cecum to the posterior rectus fascia on either side of the stoma. The appendix is passed through the anterior abdominal wall and matured. When the appendix is surgically absent or not usable for an efferent limb, a Yang-Monti channel can be created as described previously (**Figs. 7** and **8**).[24]

POSTOPERATIVE CARE AND FOLLOW-UP

Postoperative care provided follows the authors' previously published ERAS pathway, which has been shown to reduce length of hospital stay and rates of gastrointestinal complications.[18,26] The authors start all patients on a peripherally acting μ-opioid antagonist, alvimopan, 1 hour preoperatively and continue it postoperatively until occurrence of the first bowel movement because this has been shown to reduce the time to bowel recovery after abdominal surgery in 5 well-designed, randomized controlled trials.[27] Intraoperative fluids are minimized; narcotics are avoided if possible, and a nasogastric tube is used intraoperatively and removed at the end of the procedure. Early ambulation is encouraged, and patients are started on a liquid diet on the evening of the procedure followed by solids on postoperative day (POD) 1. Extended thromboembolic prophylaxis with low-molecular-weight heparin is continued until POD 28 because of the reduced risk of venous thromboembolic events associated with extended prophylaxis.[28] Patients with a serum bicarbonate less than 22 mmol/L are started on an alkalinizing agent. Surgical drains are typically removed on the day of discharge. Prophylactic oral antibiotics are administered until the indwelling tubes are removed. Irrigation of the pouch every 6 hours with normal saline is initiated on POD 1. The patients and/or caregivers are instructed on how to perform irrigations after discharge. General postoperative follow-up includes a clinic visit 1 week after discharge. The authors begin teaching patients to perform clean intermittent catheterization 3 weeks postoperatively. The suprapubic tube and attached stents are removed once the patient has demonstrated the ability to adequately catheterize.

COMPLICATIONS

Most studies examining complication rates after urinary diversion focus on patients undergoing

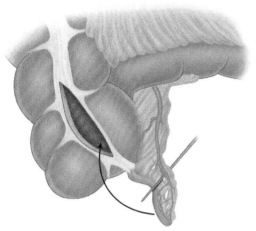

Fig. 2. A channel in the tenia of the cecum is created that will hold the proximal appendix. (*From* Warner JN, Chan KG. Continent cutaneous urinary diversion. In: Daneshmand S, editor. Urinary diversion. Cham (Switzerland): Springer; 2017. p. 46; with permission.)

radical cystectomy for bladder cancer. More than 75% of complications following cystectomy are related to the urinary diversion, and the types of complications are specific to the type of diversion.[29,30] The perioperative morbidity of radical cystectomy and urinary diversion is consistently reported in the range of 40% to 80%, which is particularly important considering the typically elderly and frail patient population at greatest risk for bladder cancer.[31,32] The complication rate following CCUD has been reported as high as 89% to 94% and may actually be higher compared

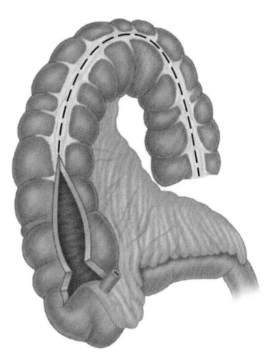

Fig. 4. The colonic segment is detubularized along its antimesenteric border. (*From* Warner JN, Chan KG. Continent cutaneous urinary diversion. In: Daneshmand S, editor. Urinary diversion. Cham (Switzerland): Springer; 2017. p. 47; with permission.)

with complication rates after ileal conduit or ONB.[33,34] Complications following urinary diversion must be categorized as either early (typically within 90 days of surgery) or late, which can occur years or decades after surgery. In addition, utilization of the modified Clavien system allows for discussion of complications using a standardized and validated grading system, which has aided objective outcomes assessment.[35,36] Broadly speaking, Clavien grade 1 and 2 are considered minor complications that can be treated with bedside procedures or medications, such as opening a superficial wound infection or giving a blood transfusion. Clavien grade 3 to 5 are considered major complications and include interventions under local anesthesia or sedation (grade 3a), interventions under general anesthesia (grade 3b), life-threatening postoperative events such as intensive care unit admission (grade 4), and death (grade 5).

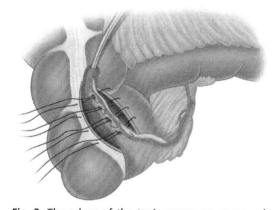

Fig. 3. The edges of the tenia serosa are reapproximated through the appendiceal mesenteric windows using 3-0 silk sutures. (*From* Warner JN, Chan KG. Continent cutaneous urinary diversion. In: Daneshmand S, editor. Urinary diversion. Cham (Switzerland): Springer; 2017. p. 46; with permission.)

EARLY COMPLICATIONS

Types of early postoperative complications are similar with all types of urinary diversion and principally include catheter problems, infections, urine leak, gastrointestinal problems, and death. For the

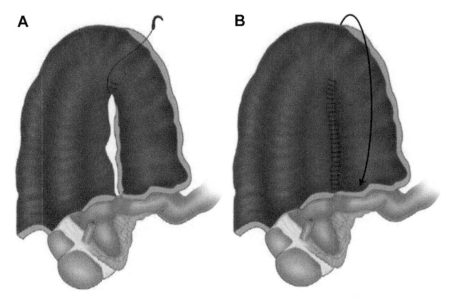

Fig. 5. The back wall of the colonic pouch reapproximated with a running 3-0 polyglactin suture. The pouch is then closed in a Heineke-Mikulicz fashion with a running 3-0 polyglactin suture. (*A*) The back wall of the colonic pouch reapproximated with a running 3-0 polyglactin suture. (*B*) The pouch is then closed in a Heineke-Mikulicz fashion with a running 3-0 polyglactin suture. (*From* Warner JN, Chan KG. Continent cutaneous urinary diversion. In: Daneshmand S, editor. Urinary diversion. Cham (Switzerland): Springer; 2017. p. 48; with permission.)

purposes of discussion, early complications are considered as those occurring within 90 days of surgery because this definition is thought to capture a more complete picture of perioperative morbidity following cystectomy and urinary diversion.[37] It is important to recognize that patients with a history of pelvic radiation experience higher

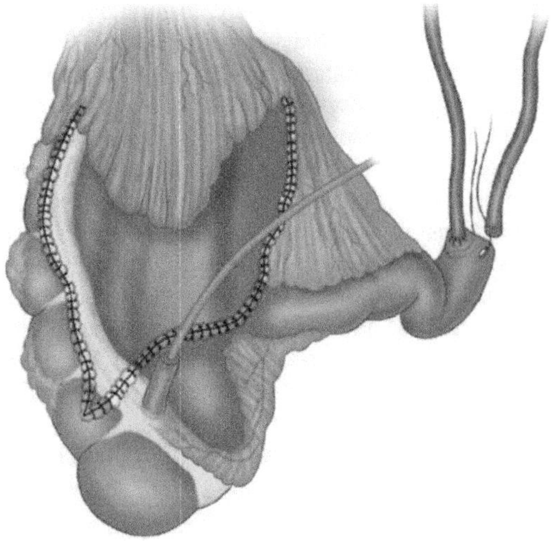

Fig. 6. Ureteroileal anastomoses are completed, and the appendix is matured to the umbilicus. (*From* Warner JN, Chan KG. Continent cutaneous urinary diversion. In: Daneshmand S, editor. Urinary diversion. Cham (Switzerland): Springer; 2017. p. 48; with permission.)

complication rates after ileal conduit and Indiana pouch (IP) diversion.[38–40] This association is critical because pelvic radiation is a common indication for CCUD, due to concerns about placing an ONB in an irradiated field or in women who have suffered complications of pelvic radiotherapy for gynecologic malignancy. Reports of complications following CCUD need to be interpreted in this context. In addition, rates of complication may be higher with CCUD compared with ONB and ileal conduit,[31] and there are several complications unique to CCUD, including efferent limb necrosis and pouch rupture that must be discussed specifically.

Shabsigh and colleagues[41] detailed the 90-day perioperative morbidity following radical cystectomy and urinary diversion (any type) in a cohort of 1142 patients. They report a 64% overall complication rate, most commonly gastrointestinal or infectious-type complications, with Clavien grade 3 to 5 complications accounting for 21% of all complications. The 30- and 90-day mortalities in this cohort were 1.5% and 2.7%, respectively. It is worth noting that most deaths occurred after hospital discharge secondary to cardiopulmonary events. Multivariable analysis in this cohort identified continent diversion (ONB or IP) as a predictor of grade 1 to 2 but not grade 3 to 5 complications.

Indiana University examined their own institution's complication rates following various forms of urinary diversion using National Surgical Quality Improvement Project data.[42] Their final sample

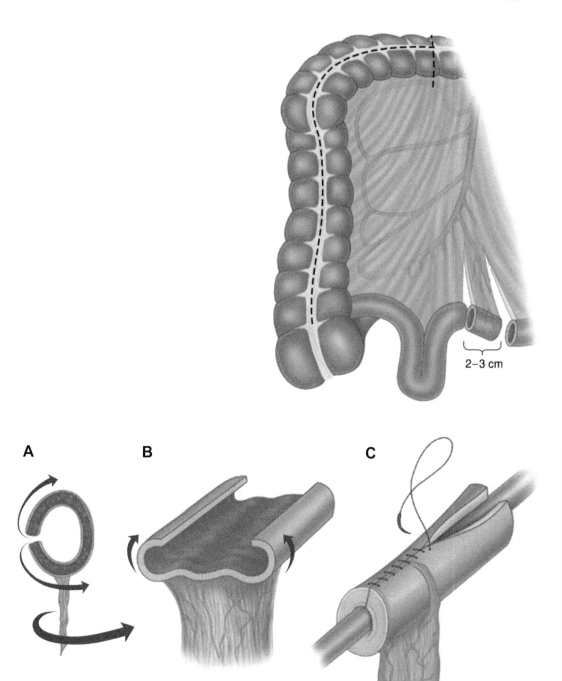

A   B   C

Fig. 7. For the Yang-Monti channel, a 2- to 3-cm segment small bowel, proximal to the initial ileal division, is utilized. (*A*) The 2- to 3-cm ileal segment is detubularized halfway to its antimesenteric border to allow more tubular distance on one side of the mesentery. (*B*) The detubularized segment is now ready to be rolled on its perpendicular axis. (*C*) The reoriented ileal segment is retubularized with 3-0 absorbable suture. (*From* Warner JN, Chan KG. Continent cutaneous urinary diversion. In: Daneshmand S, editor. Urinary diversion. Cham (Switzerland): Springer; 2017. p. 49; with permission.)

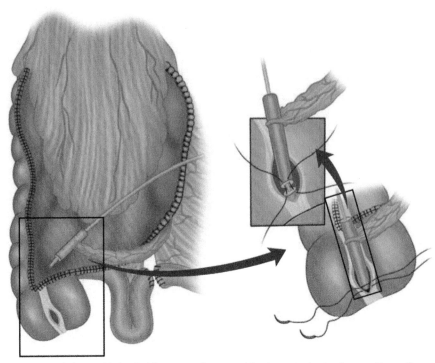

Fig. 8. The Yang-Monti channel is buried in a trough created in the anterior tenia, creating a flap-valve mechanism. (*From* Warner JN, Chan KG. Continent cutaneous urinary diversion. In: Daneshmand S, editor. Urinary diversion. Cham (Switzerland): Springer; 2017. p. 50; with permission.)

included 39 patients who underwent Indiana pouch diversion and demonstrated a 13% rate of Clavien 3 or higher complications. This rate was similar to the rate of major complications after ileal conduit and ONB; however, Indiana pouch was associated with a higher rate of infectious complications. Patients undergoing Indiana pouch were also at higher risk for fascial dehiscence, which could be related to the increased incidence of infections. Higher infection rates may be due to bacterial contamination related to the colon being open in the wound during pouch construction. Longer operative times associated with CCUD construction compared with ileal conduit or ONB may also predispose patients to surgical site infections. Another cohort study included 48 patients undergoing robotic cystectomy followed by extracorporeal IP urinary diversion. They report an 88% 90-day complication rate with a 29% risk of grade 3 to 5 complications. Indiana pouch was an independent risk factor for infectious complications, most commonly urinary tract infection.[31] These results are consistent with other single institutional CCUD series, including the largest series of 125 patients.[33,34,43]

Early stoma-related complications are important to consider. Efferent limb necrosis is a feared complication that is caused by ischemia of the catheterizable channel. Careful surgical technique and preservation of the mesenteric blood supply

should prevent this. Should there be clinical suspicion, flexible cystoscopy can help delineate if the channel appears abnormal just at the skin level or more proximally. Ischemia at or below the level of the fascia would warrant either immediate or delayed exploration with construction of a new catheterizable channel. A series of patients who underwent CCUD with an appendiceal efferent limb experienced a 17% and 21% rate of stomal complications within 90 days in nonirradiated and irradiated groups, respectively.[44] Operative stoma revision was required in 17% of the irradiated patients versus 9% of the nonirradiated patients. Spontaneous perforation of a CCUD is a rare complication that requires prompt diagnosis and management. A multinational survey of performing surgeons in Scandinavia estimated a 1.5% incidence of perforation.[45] Readmission rate following CCUD has been reported at 39%, and the rate of reoperation in currently available literature ranges from 1% to 32%.[34,46]

LATE COMPLICATIONS

Late complications can be classified as general if related to the use of a bowel segment for diversion or specific if the complication relates to the continent catheterizable reservoir. Examples of general complications include decline in renal function, metabolic abnormalities, kidney stones, ureteral stricture, or bowel obstruction. Specific complications can be pouch- or efferent limb-related, including stones in the reservoir, fistula, incontinence, difficulty catheterizing, stomal stenosis, and parastomal hernia. The overall rate of late complications and reoperation has been reported at 23% to 90% and 8% to 69%, respectively.[8,25,33,47]

Holmes and colleagues[33] study is a single surgeon series of 125 modified Indiana pouches completed over a 14-year period with a mean follow-up of 41 months and excellent characterization of late postoperative complications. Notable findings include a 15% rate of stomal stenosis, the vast majority of which required operative revision. Published rates of stomal stenosis range from 4% to 36%.[48] Formation of pouch stones incidence in the literature ranges from 5% to 42%.[48] Treatment approach to pouch stones is dependent on the number and size of the stones, with most stones managed endoscopically, and large or numerous stones requiring open removal. Frequent catheterization and avoidance of metal staples may reduce the risk of stone formation. Very few studies report late complications after CCUD; additionally, reporting is highly variable. When counseling patients regarding CCUD, it is important to note that there is a significant rate of additional procedures and surgical intervention following CCUD, including revision procedure for ureteral stenosis, stomal stenosis, fistula repair, deep revision of the catheterizable channel, treatment of stones, and hernia repair.

Rate and type of general complications following CCUD are similar to ONB. There is no evidence for a difference in renal function decline comparing conduit diversion to CCUD, and other studies have demonstrated that patients with CCUD experience a decline in renal function similar to age-matched controls.[7,49] Rates of ureteroenteric strictures following CCUD are comparable to rates observed in other types of diversion. Patients who have undergone a right colon pouch creation may be more susceptible to hyperchloremic metabolic acidosis because of exaggerated chloride absorption and bicarbonate excretion observed in the colon compared with ileum. Chronic acidosis can predispose patients to bone demineralization and associated sequelae.[50] It is also important to monitor for vitamin B12 deficiency and its associated neurologic and hematologic consequences if the ileocecal segment is used for diversion.[51]

FUNCTIONAL OUTCOMES

Incontinence rates after CCUD are generally low at an average of 15% and compare favorably to orthotopic diversion.[52] Reporting of continence and urinary function is hampered by a lack of standardized questionnaire for assessment of function outcomes after CCUD. Persistent leakage from a CCUD is likely due to failure of the continence mechanism; however, for colon pouches, urodynamics should be considered because reservoirs from colon can generate high-pressure waves. Endoscopic bulking agents have been used with some success in this population; however, many patients ultimately require an open surgical repair of the efferent limb.[53]

Health-related quality of life (HRQOL) may be impacted by a patient's choice of urinary diversion; however, the published literature is conflicting. A recent study with a mean follow-up of 11 years reported that urinary function, but not bother, was significantly better for ileal conduit and Indiana pouch compared with ONB.[54] This study has the longest follow-up in the HRQOL literature to the authors' knowledge. These findings conflict with results reported by Large and colleagues[55] that found no difference in any HRQOL domains comparing a cohort of ONB in 47 women and Indiana pouch in 45; however, this study was hampered by a small sample size and limited follow-up. A recent review article compared HRQOL after ONB and ileal conduit. Most of the included studies found no difference between the 2 types of diversion in terms of HRQOL.[56] Additional well-designed prospective trials are needed to assess differences in HRQOL with long-term follow-up so that patients may be counseled effectively regarding the pros and cons of various options for urinary diversion.

SUMMARY

Techniques in CCUD have evolved significantly over the last 30 years resulting in several well-established techniques. Urinary diversion is consistently associated with significant morbidity and a high complication rate. CCUD is associated with some specific complications related to the catheterizable channel and stoma that lead to a significant risk for surgical revision. However, CCUD can offer patients good urinary function and excellent continence with HRQOL measures that compare favorably with other types of urinary diversion.

REFERENCES

1. Kock NG, Nilson AE, Nilsson LO, et al. Urinary diversion via a continent ileal reservoir: clinical results in 12 patients. J Urol 1982;128(3):469–75.
2. Rowland RG, Mitchell ME, Bihrle R, et al. Indiana continent urinary reservoir. J Urol 1987;137(6): 1136–9.

3. Skinner DG, Lieskovsky G, Boyd SD. Continent urinary diversion. A 5 1/2 year experience. Ann Surg 1988;208(3):337–44.

4. Van Hemelrijck M, Thorstenson A, Smith P, et al. Risk of in-hospital complications after radical cystectomy for urinary bladder carcinoma: population-based follow-up study of 7608 patients. BJU Int 2013; 112(8):1113–20.

5. Skinner EC. Continent cutaneous diversion. Curr Opin Urol 2015;25(6):555–61.

6. Smith AB, Crowell K, Woods ME, et al. Functional outcomes following radical cystectomy in women with bladder cancer: a systematic review. Eur Urol Focus 2017;3(1):136–43.

7. Kristjánsson A, Wallin L, Månsson W. Renal function up to 16 years after conduit (refluxing or anti-reflux anastomosis) or continent urinary diversion. 1. Glomerular filtration rate and patency of uretero-intestinal anastomosis. Br J Urol 1995;76(5):539–45.

8. Wilson TG, Moreno JG, Weinberg A, et al. Late complications of the modified Indiana pouch. J Urol 1994;151(2):331–4.

9. Webster C, Bukkapatnam R, Seigne JD, et al. Continent colonic urinary reservoir (Florida pouch): long-term surgical complications (greater than 11 years). J Urol 2003;169(1):174–6.

10. Verhoogen J. Neostomie uretero-cecale. Formation d'une poche vesicale et d'un noveau uretre. Assoc Franc d'Urol 1908;12:352–65.

11. Gilchrist RK, Merricks JW. Construction of a substitute bladder and urethra. Surg Clin North Am 1956;36(4):1131–43.

12. Ashley MS, Daneshmand S. Factors influencing the choice of urinary diversion in patients undergoing radical cystectomy. BJU Int 2010;106(5):654–7.

13. Hautmann RE. Urinary diversion: ileal conduit to neobladder. J Urol 2003;169(3):834–42.

14. Granberg CF, Boorjian SA, Crispen PL, et al. Functional and oncological outcomes after orthotopic neobladder reconstruction in women. BJU Int 2008;102(11):1551–5.

15. Jentzmik F, Schrader AJ, de Petriconi R, et al. The ileal neobladder in female patients with bladder cancer: long-term clinical, functional, and oncological outcome. World J Urol 2012;30(6):733–9.

16. Stein JP, Penson DF, Lee C, et al. Long-term oncological outcomes in women undergoing radical cystectomy and orthotopic diversion for bladder cancer. J Urol 2009;181(5):2052–8 [discussion: 2058–9].

17. Azhar RA, Bochner B, Catto J, et al. Enhanced recovery after urological surgery: a contemporary systematic review of outcomes, key elements, and research needs. Eur Urol 2016;70(1):176–87.

18. Daneshmand S, Ahmadi H, Schuckman AK, et al. Enhanced recovery protocol after radical cystectomy for bladder cancer. J Urol 2014;192(1):50–6.

19. Large MC, Kiriluk KJ, DeCastro GJ, et al. The impact of mechanical bowel preparation on postoperative complications for patients undergoing cystectomy and urinary diversion. J Urol 2012;188(5):1801–5.

20. Güenaga KF, Matos D, Wille-Jørgensen P. Mechanical bowel preparation for elective colorectal surgery. Cochrane Database Syst Rev 2011;(9): CD001544.

21. Maffezzini M, Campodonico F, Canepa G, et al. Current perioperative management of radical cystectomy with intestinal urinary reconstruction for muscle-invasive bladder cancer and reduction of the incidence of postoperative ileus. Surg Oncol 2008;17(1):41–8.

22. Desai MM, Simone G, de Castro Abreu AL, et al. Robotic intracorporeal continent cutaneous diversion. J Urol 2017. https://doi.org/10.1016/j.juro.2017.01.091.

23. Stein JP, Daneshmand S, Dunn M, et al. Continent right colon reservoir using a cutaneous appendicostomy. Urology 2004;63(3):577–80 [discussion: 580–1].

24. Wagner M, Bayne A, Daneshmand S. Application of the Yang-Monti channel in adult continent cutaneous urinary diversion. Urology 2008;72(4):828–31.

25. Wiesner C, Bonfig R, Stein R, et al. Continent cutaneous urinary diversion: long-term follow-up of more than 800 patients with ileocecal reservoirs. World J Urol 2006;24(3):315–8.

26. Bazargani ST, Djaladat H, Ahmadi H, et al. Gastrointestinal complications following radical cystectomy using enhanced recovery protocol. Eur Urol Focus 2017. https://doi.org/10.1016/j.euf.2017.04.003.

27. Vaughan-Shaw PG, Fecher IC, Harris S, et al. A meta-analysis of the effectiveness of the opioid receptor antagonist alvimopan in reducing hospital length of stay and time to GI recovery in patients enrolled in a standardized accelerated recovery program after abdominal surgery. Dis Colon Rectum 2012;55(5):611–20.

28. Pariser JJ, Pearce SM, Anderson BB, et al. Extended duration enoxaparin decreases the rate of venous thromboembolic events after radical cystectomy compared to inpatient only subcutaneous heparin. J Urol 2017;197(2):302–7.

29. Hautmann RE, de Petriconi RC, Volkmer BG. Lessons learned from 1,000 neobladders: the 90-day complication rate. J Urol 2010;184(3):990–4 [quiz: 1235].

30. Shimko MS, Tollefson MK, Umbreit EC, et al. Long-term complications of conduit urinary diversion. J Urol 2011;185(2):562–7.

31. Nazmy M, Yuh B, Kawachi M, et al. Early and late complications of robot-assisted radical cystectomy: a standardized analysis by urinary diversion type. J Urol 2014;191(3):681–7.

32. Nieuwenhuijzen JA, de Vries RR, Bex A, et al. Urinary diversions after cystectomy: the association of

clinical factors, complications and functional results of four different diversions. Eur Urol 2008;53(4):834–42 [discussion: 842–4].

33. Holmes DG, Thrasher JB, Park GY, et al. Long-term complications related to the modified Indiana pouch. Urology 2002;60(4):603–6.

34. Torrey RR, Chan KG, Yip W, et al. Functional outcomes and complications in patients with bladder cancer undergoing robotic-assisted radical cystectomy with extracorporeal Indiana pouch continent cutaneous urinary diversion. Urology 2012;79(5):1073–8.

35. Dindo D, Demartines N, Clavien P-A. Classification of surgical complications: a new proposal with evaluation in a cohort of 6336 patients and results of a survey. Ann Surg 2004;240(2):205–13.

36. Morgan M, Smith N, Thomas K, et al. Is Clavien the new standard for reporting urological complications? BJU Int 2009;104(4):434–6.

37. Hollenbeck BK, Miller DC, Taub D, et al. Identifying risk factors for potentially avoidable complications following radical cystectomy. J Urol 2005;174(4 Pt 1):1231–7 [discussion: 1237].

38. Eisenberg MS, Dorin RP, Bartsch G, et al. Early complications of cystectomy after high dose pelvic radiation. J Urol 2010;184(6):2264–9.

39. Kim HL, Steinberg GD. Complications of cystectomy in patients with a history of pelvic radiation. Urology 2001;58(4):557–60.

40. Wilkin M, Horwitz G, Seetharam A, et al. Long-term complications associated with the Indiana pouch urinary diversion in patients with recurrent gynecologic cancers after high-dose radiation. Urol Oncol 2005;23(1):12–5.

41. Shabsigh A, Korets R, Vora KC, et al. Defining early morbidity of radical cystectomy for patients with bladder cancer using a standardized reporting methodology. Eur Urol 2009;55(1):164–74.

42. Monn MF, Kaimakliotis HZ, Cary KC, et al. Short-term morbidity and mortality of Indiana pouch, ileal conduit, and neobladder urinary diversion following radical cystectomy. Urol Oncol 2014;32(8):1151–7.

43. Maffezzini M, Campodonico F, Capponi G, et al. Fast-track surgery and technical nuances to reduce complications after radical cystectomy and intestinal urinary diversion with the modified Indiana pouch. Surg Oncol 2012;21(3):191–5.

44. Bochner BH, Karanikolas N, Barakat RR, et al. Ureteroileocecal appendicostomy based urinary reservoir in irradiated and nonirradiated patients. J Urol 2009;182(5):2376–80.

45. Månsson W, Bakke A, Bergman B, et al. Perforation of continent urinary reservoirs. Scandinavian experience. Scand J Urol Nephrol 1997;31(6):529–32.

46. Myers JB, Lenherr SM. Perioperative and long-term surgical complications for the Indiana pouch and similar continent catheterizable urinary diversions. Curr Opin Urol 2016;26(4):376–82.

47. Ahlering TE, Weinberg AC, Razor B. A comparative study of the ileal conduit, Kock pouch and modified Indiana pouch. J Urol 1989;142(5):1193–6.

48. Rink M, Kluth L, Eichelberg E, et al. Continent catheterizable pouches for urinary diversion. Eur Urol Suppl 2010;9(10):754–62.

49. Abol-Enein H, Salem M, Mesbah A, et al. Continent cutaneous ileal pouch using the serous lined extramural valves. The Mansoura experience in more than 100 patients. J Urol 2004;172(2):588–91.

50. Koch MO, McDougal WS. Bone demineralization following ureterosigmoid anastomosis: an experimental study in rats. J Urol 1988;140(4):856–9.

51. Yakout H, Bissada NK. Intermediate effects of the ileocaecal urinary reservoir (Charleston pouch 1) on serum vitamin B12 concentrations: can vitamin B12 deficiency be prevented? BJU Int 2003;91(7):653–5 [discussion: 655–6].

52. Ardelt PU, Woodhouse CRJ, Riedmiller H, et al. The efferent segment in continent cutaneous urinary diversion: a comprehensive review of the literature. BJU Int 2012;109(2):288–97.

53. Kass-iliyya A, Rashid TG, Citron I, et al. Long-term efficacy of polydimethylsiloxane (Macroplastique) injection for Mitrofanoff leakage after continent urinary diversion surgery. BJU Int 2015;115(3):461–5.

54. Gellhaus PT, Cary C, Kaimakliotis HZ, et al. Long-term health-related quality of life outcomes following radical cystectomy. Urology 2017;106:82–6.

55. Large MC, Katz MH, Shikanov S, et al. Orthotopic neobladder versus Indiana pouch in women: a comparison of health related quality of life outcomes. J Urol 2010;183(1):201–6.

56. Ali AS, Hayes MC, Birch B, et al. Health related quality of life (HRQoL) after cystectomy: comparison between orthotopic neobladder and ileal conduit diversion. Eur J Surg Oncol 2015;41(3):295–9.

Robotic Cystectomy with Intracorporeal Urinary Diversion

Review of Current Techniques and Outcomes

Tyler M. Thress, MD[a], Michael S. Cookson, MD, MMHC[b],*,
Sanjay Patel, MD[c]

KEYWORDS

- Bladder cancer • Cystectomy • Robotic • Intracorporeal • Diversion • Neobladder

KEY POINTS

- Robotic cystectomy is increasing in use nationwide.
- Surgeons are looking toward totally intracorporeal urinary diversion to maximize the minimally invasive benefit of robot-assisted radical cystectomy (RARC).
- There are multiple different methods of performing RARC with intracorporeal urinary diversion.

INTRODUCTION

Radical cystectomy is well accepted as the gold standard for muscle invasive bladder cancer. Incorporation of robotic technology has been shown to offer equivalent oncologic and technical outcomes.[1,2] It seemed that the crux of the operation remained the urinary diversion, with many physicians electing to perform the cystectomy robotically and then opening for a traditional extracorporeal diversion. This approach came under some criticism, which suggested that conversion to extracorporeal diversion did away with any benefit of the robotic approach.[3]

As the use of robotic-assisted radical cystectomy (RARC) increased, surgeons began moving toward totally intracorporeal urinary diversions in an attempt to maximize the benefits of this minimally invasive approach, though the widespread use of this technique has been slow due to the technical complexity of these cases and the increased operative time required. The first RARC with totally intracorporeal urinary diversion was described in 2003.[4] Almost a decade later, a multiinstitutional review revealed that only 3% of robotic cystectomies were being performed with completely intracorporeal diversion.

This article describes the available operative approaches to RARC with intracorporeal diversion techniques and provides analysis of postoperative outcomes.

GENERAL TECHNICAL CONSIDERATIONS
Port Placement

There is a general consensus on port placement for robotic cystectomy with intracorporeal diversion, though small variations exist. Goh and colleagues[5]

Disclosure: The authors have nothing they wish to disclose.
[a] PGY-4, Department of Urology, University of Oklahoma Health Sciences Center, Oklahoma City, OK, USA;
[b] Department of Urology, University of Oklahoma Health Sciences Center, Oklahoma City, OK, USA;
[c] Department of Urology, University of Oklahoma Health Sciences Center, 920 Stanton L Young Boulevard, Suite 3150, Oklahoma City, OK 73104, USA
* Corresponding author.
E-mail address: michael.cookson@mac.com

Urol Clin N Am 45 (2018) 67–77
https://doi.org/10.1016/j.ucl.2017.09.009
0094-0143/18/© 2017 Elsevier Inc. All rights reserved.

describe what is perhaps the most common port placement template. The camera is placed approximately 2 finger breadths above the umbilicus with the 3 robotic trocars lateral to and at the level of the umbilicus spaced approximately 8 cm apart from each other. A 15-mm assistant port, used to pass the bowel stapler, is on the lateral abdominal wall opposite the third robotic arm. A 12-mm assistant port is superior to and halfway between the camera port and the first robotic trocar (**Fig. 1**).

The City of Hope group describes a template that places trocars from the pubic bone as a common reference point. The camera and trocars are all placed within 20 to 25 cm from the pubic bone (**Fig. 2**).[6] The Karolinska group, Stockholm, Sweden places the camera 5 cm above the umbilicus with the assistant and robotic trocars at the level of the umbilicus (**Fig. 3**).[7] Pruthi and colleagues[8] place their camera port in a similar fashion, though they place a 12-mm assistant port below the level of the umbilicus in line with the camera port, the robotic trocar, and the anterior superior iliac spine (ASIS) (**Fig. 4**).

Tan and colleagues[9] place their camera port 5 cm above the umbilicus, with the robotic trocars at the level of the umbilicus on each side. Two assistant ports are placed 5 cm above and 5 cm lateral to each ASIS, with a 5-mm assistant port between the camera port and the right robotic trocar (**Fig. 5**).

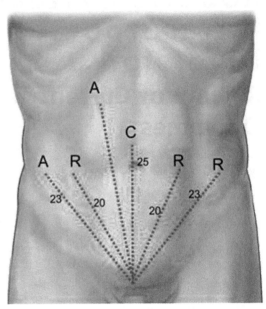

Fig. 2. City of Hope port placement (*A*)assistant trocar, (*R*) = robotic trocar, (*C*)camera trocar. (*From* Chan KG, Guru K, Wiklund P, et al. Robot-assisted radical cystectomy and urinary diversion: technical recommendations from the Pasadena Consensus Panel. Eur Urol 2015;67:425; with permission.)

Bowel Measurement

A premeasured Penrose drain, suture, or umbilical tape can be used to measure the bowel segment that will form the urinary diversion. It is the practice at the authors' institution to measure the bowel using a 20-cm length of umbilical tape marked at 5 cm intervals. When moistened, the tape gently adheres to the bowel and prevents sliding during measuring.

Bowel Manipulation

As is the case in open surgery, careful handling of the bowel is paramount. It is therefore important to use robotic instruments with low grip strength to avoid injury to the bowel during manipulation.

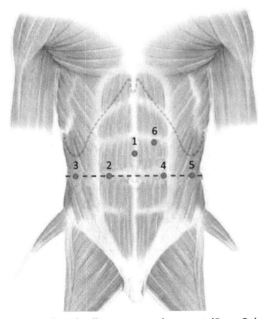

Fig. 1. Goh and colleagues port placement. (*From* Goh AC, Gill IS, Lee DJ, et al. Robotic intracorporeal orthotopic ileal neobladder: replicating open surgical principles. Eur Urol 2012;62:893; with permission.)

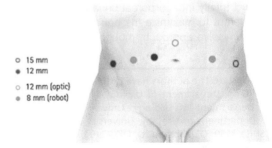

○ 15 mm
● 12 mm
○ 12 mm (optic)
● 8 mm (robot)

Fig. 3. Karolinska group port placement. (*From* Wiklund NP, Poulakis V. Robotic neobladder. BJU Int 2011;107:1516; with permission.)

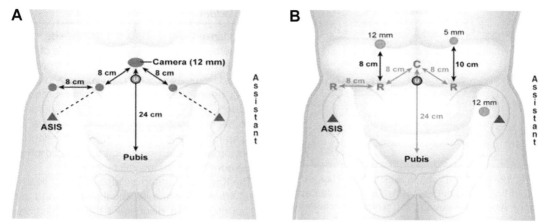

Fig. 4. Pruthi and colleagues port placement. (*From* Pruthi RS, Nix J, McRackan D, et al. Robotic-assisted laparoscopic intracorporeal urinary diversion. Eur Urol 2010;57:1015; with permission.)

Cadiére forceps and double fenestrated robotic graspers have the lowest grip strength among the robotic instruments. Two techniques for manipulation of the bowel for urinary diversion have been described. The first technique involves passage of vessel loop strings at the border of the mesentery and the intestine that are then manipulated with the robotic instruments.[10] The second technique, perhaps more common, is the marionette technique. This technique involves measuring and dividing the desired segment of bowel for the ileal conduit in the standard fashion. After the desired conduit is divided from the small bowel a 60-in silk suture is passed through the abdominal wall on a Keith needle and passed through the distal end of the conduit. The silk suture is then passed through the assistant port and is used to manipulate the bowel (like a marionette puppet) to assist in further dissection.[11] Colorized sutures have been used to preserve the orientation of the remaining bowel to easily and efficiently restore continuity.

Division of the Mesentery

After selection of the desired bowel segment, incision of the mesentery is needed to provide sufficient length and mobility for conduit or neobladder creation. Use of robotic or assistant-controlled bowel staplers to incise both the bowel and its associated mesentery is common. Bipolar electrocautery, hook electrocautery, or the LigaSure device can be used to divide the small bowel mesentery with careful attention paid to maintain hemostasis. A technique to transilluminate the mesentery and identify vessels has been described through use of a lighted cystoscope from the urethral stump.[12] Though it has been criticized for being costly, use indocyanine green fluorescence imagery to identify mesenteric vasculature has been described.[13]

An efficient means of bowel detubularization for continent urinary diversions involves use of a lubricated catheter or chest tube, which is placed in the lumen of the bowel. The antimesenteric side can then be easily and quickly incised while the tube protects the mesenteric bowel wall (**Fig. 6**).[14]

Irrigation of Conduit

Irrigation of the bowel segment can be performed to prevent gross spillage of bowel contents. A small opening in the distal end of the conduit or neobladder is made and a 22-French (F) 3-way catheter is placed via the assistant port into the lumen of the bowel. The bowel segment is then irrigated until clear and the catheter is removed.[11] It should be noted that the Roswell Park Cancer

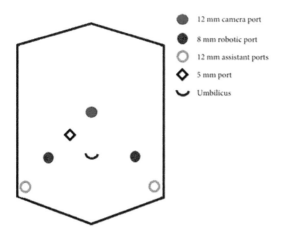

Fig. 5. Tan and colleagues port placement. (*From* Tan WS, Sridhar A, Goldstraw M, et al. Robot-assisted intracorporeal pyramid neobladder. BJU Int 2015;116:772; with permission.)

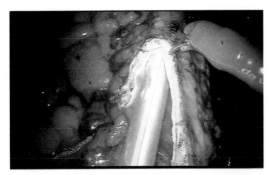

Fig. 6. Use of a chest tube to assist with detubulariza-tion of bowel. (*From* Desai MM, Simone G, de Castro Abreu AL, et al. Robotic intracorporeal continent cutaneous diversion. J Urol 2017; with permission.)

Group that first described this technique has since abandoned its use with no significant change in infectious complications.[15]

Ureteral Anastomosis

The left ureter is passed under the sigmoid mesentery and anterior to the aortic bifurcation.[16] Both Wallace-type and Bricker-type ureterointestinal anastomoses have been described. Prior studies comparing the techniques have revealed no appreciable difference in stricture rate.[17] Analysis of robotic cystectomies with intracorporeal versus extracorporeal diversion did not analyze for postoperative ureteral stricture rate.[18]

DIVERSION-SPECIFIC TECHNICAL CONSIDERATIONS
Ileal Conduit

The ileal conduit is the quickest and simplest means of performing an intracorporeal urinary diversion. At the authors' institution, after completion of the cystectomy, a 20-cm length of ileum is selected no closer than 15 cm from the ileocecal junction. Staplers are passed via the assistant ports to divide the conduit and stay sutures are placed to preserve the orientation of the remaining bowel to easily restore continuity. The previously described marionette technique is used to manipulate the conduit. The left ureter is tunneled under the sigmoid mesentery as first described by Dr Canda and colleagues.[16] Bricker ureterointestinal anastomoses are performed and single-J stents are placed over wires that are passed via the assistant port. A stapler is used to return the bowel to continuity via side-to-side stapled anastomosis.[15] The robot is undocked and the specimen bag is removed by widening the camera port until the bag can pass from the abdomen. The conduit is matured to the skin at the stomal site and a drain is left in 1 of the robotic trocar sites.

Neobladder

Detubularized ileal reservoirs have been described in numerous variations. The most notable of which include the Karolinska-modified Studer neobladder, the University of Southern California–modified Studer neobladder, the pyramid pouch, and the Y-pouch. Other techniques and configurations have been described but not in large series. The descriptions presented here may not reflect the exact order of each operation but should offer a good concept of the overall technique.

The Karolinska group isolates 40 cm of ileum at least 40 cm from the ileocecal junction and uses bowel staplers to disconnect the segment from continuity. All but the proximal 10 cm of ileum are detubularized. The remaining proximal 10 cm is preserved for a Wallace ureterointestinal anastomosis. Two stents are passed through 2 separate abdominal incisions in the Seldinger fashion. A 20-F ureterointestinal anastomosis is performed in the van Velthoven fashion with 2-0 barbed, self-retaining sutures. The posterior and anterior portions of the neobladder are closed with running 3-0 V-lock sutures. A catheter remains in the neobladder for 21 days postoperatively (**Fig. 7**).[19]

The University of Southern California group isolates a total of 60 cm of ileum for their version of the Studer neobladder. A total of 44 cm of the loop is detubularized using a chest tube as previously described; 16 cm remains as an afferent limb. The posterior plate is sewn together and the pouch is subsequently rotated 90° before sewing the anterior suture line vertically to create a spherical configuration of pouch. A Bricker-type ureterointestinal anastomosis is performed over a 7-F double-J ureteral stent (**Fig. 8**).[20]

The pyramid neobladder is constructed from 50 cm of ileum, the most dependent portion of which is secured to the urethral stump over a 16-F catheter. The bowel is detubularized using robotic scissors leaving 2-cm tubular segments on each end. The posterior plate is closed using 3-0 barbed, self-retaining sutures. A Bricker ureterointestinal anastomosis is performed over 8-F feeding tubes, which are externalized from the neobladder. The remaining anterior portion of the neobladder is folded from lateral to medial in a coronal plane. An 18-F suprapubic tube is placed in the suture line (**Fig. 9**).[9]

The Y-pouch is similar in initial construction to the pyramid pouch. It differs in that both the anterior and posterior portion of the reservoir are closed in a vertical running fashion. This technique has been criticized due to its similarity the U-pouch, which has been long abandoned due to its increased intraluminal filling pressures and risk of upper tract deterioration[21] (**Fig. 10**).

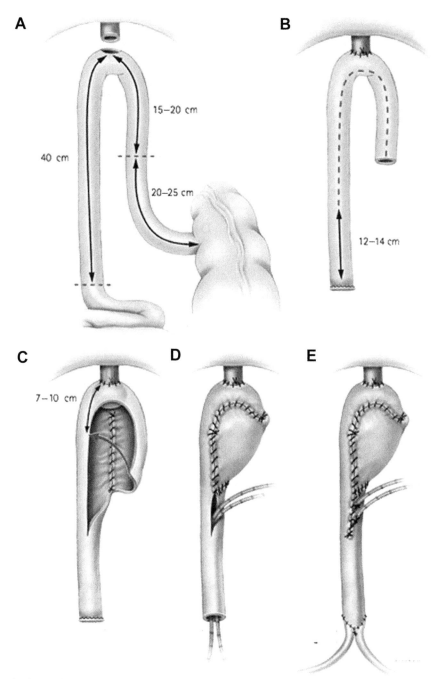

A

15–20 cm

40 cm

20–25 cm

B

12–14 cm

C

7–10 cm

D

E

Fig. 7. Karolinska-modified Studer neobladder. (*From* Collins JW, Hosseini A, Sooriakumaran P, et al. Tips and tricks for intracorporeal robot-assisted urinary diversion. Current Urology Reports 2014;15:17; with permission.)

Indiana Pouch

One continent cutaneous diversion has been described in the literature. Dr Goh and colleagues[22] have described a robotic creation of an Indiana pouch. Port placement is modified from the traditional radical cystectomy layout. Three additional port sites are changed from the traditional robotic cystectomy template. This layout allows improved access to the right abdomen for large bowel mobilization and pouch creation. The pouch itself consists of the cecum and 30 cm of detubularized distal colon. The efferent catheterizable channel is formed from 10 cm of distal ileum. A Bricker-type ureterointestinal anastomosis is created. Development

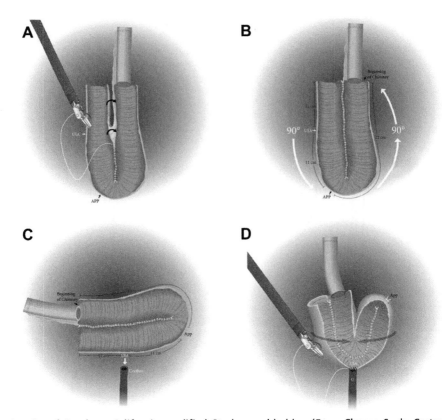

Fig. 8. University of Southern California–modified Studer neobladder. (*From* Chopra S, de Castro Abreu AL, Berger AK, et al. Evolution of robot-assisted orthotopic ileal neobladder formation: a step-by-step update to the University of Southern California (USC) technique. BJU Int 2017;119:189; with permission.)

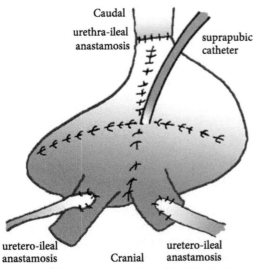

Fig. 9. Pyramid neobladder. (*From* Tan WS, Sridhar A, Goldstraw M, et al. Robot-assisted intracorporeal pyramid neobladder. BJU Int 2015;116:774; with permission.)

of the continence mechanism was performed via the specimen extraction site, and the stoma was matured via a port site. One year follow-up finds their patient catheterizing without issue.

LEARNING CURVE

As with any laparoscopic procedure, an improvement in operative parameters with increasing repetition can be expected. This is especially true when dealing with such technically challenging surgeries as intracorporeal urinary diversion. Several investigators have established correlations between number of cases performed and surgical outcomes.

In what is currently thought to be the largest study based on cohort volume, Hayn and colleagues[23] describe a multiinstitution, multisurgeon review of 496 patients undergoing RARC. Surgeons were grouped into 3 divisions based on RARC volume: those with fewer than 30 cases, those with between 30 and 50 cases, and those with more than 50 cases. Retrospective review found a significant decrease in operative time and an increase in total lymph node yield with

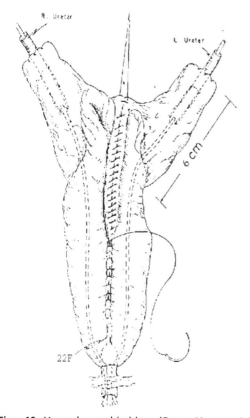

Fig. 10. Y-pouch neobladder. (*From* Hassan AA, Elgamal SA, Sabaa MA, et al. Evaluation of direct versus non-refluxing technique and functional results in orthotopic Y-ileal neobladder after 12 years of follow up. Int J Urol 2007;14:301; with permission.)

increasing experience. The group with fewer than 30 cases had a mean operative time of 454 minutes and gathered an average of 13 lymph nodes. The group with between 30 and 50 cases had a mean operative time of 392 minutes and averaged 18 lymph nodes. Finally, the group with more than 50 cases had a mean operative time of 339 minutes and harvested an average of 20 lymph nodes. Estimated blood loss (EBL) was paradoxically lowest in the 30 to 50 case group. No significant difference in length of stay (LOS), transfusion rate, positive margins, or pathologic stage was identified. Although the type of urinary diversion and whether it was performed intracorporeally or extracorporeally could not be determined in the design of this study, the investigators go on to suggest that surgeons achieve "an acceptable level of proficiency by the 30th case" when dealing with RARC.

Similarly, the Karolinska group describes a cohort of 45 patients split into groups of 15 each.[24] These sections represent an early, middle, and late phase of the learning curve at their institution. They found a statistically significant decrease in operative time, as well as a significant increase in positive node yield with increasing case numbers. An increased number of cases was not associated with a significant change in EBL or total lymph node yield.[24]

Two years later, the same institution released a study comparing the learning curve of 2 different surgeons. Both surgeons performed RARC with totally intracorporeal neobladders. Surgeon A performed a total of 47 of these procedures, whereas Surgeon B performed a total of 20. The cases were divided into 10-patient sections to better define the learning curve. As with the earlier study, increasing case volume was associated with a decrease in total operative time. For surgeon A, the average case time was approximately 600 minutes among his first 10 cases, whereas his final group of cases averaged around 350 minutes. Surgeon B, who performed fewer overall cases, saw his average decrease from 420 minutes to 395 minutes. The investigators report that increased experience results not only in improved surgeon performance but in improved performance of the entire operative team. There were no significant changes in EBL, LOS, or total lymph node yield.[25]

Desai and colleagues[14] describe a 37-patient cohort consisting of 19 intracorporeal ileal conduits and 18 intracorporeal neobladders. They compared operative data between their first 9 and last 10 patients in both the ileal conduit and neobladder group. They found that ureterointestinal anastomosis in their ileal conduit group was significantly shortened between their first and last groups of patients. Time for the anastomosis was 95 minutes in the first 9 patients, compared with only 50 minutes in their last 10 patients.

Azzouni and colleagues[15] reported a 100-patient, single-surgeon, all intracorporeal ileal conduit study. Patients were divided into groups of 25 each. Interestingly, total operative time and EBL were not found to have changed significantly throughout the learning curve. However, time to create the diversion did significantly decrease with increasing surgeon experience.

OUTCOMES

Studies limited specifically to intracorporeal diversion are limited to single-institution series with limited sample sizes. As such, it remains challenging to draw broad, detailed conclusions about operative outcomes. Small series exist to provide a glimpse of early operative data in this still-developing field. The authors identified and included 16 studies that specified use of cystectomy with a totally intracorporeal urinary diversion. A varying amount of information was included among these studies related to various operative and postoperative outcomes.

For the purposes of this article, outcomes were subdivided into operative and postoperative outcomes. Operative outcomes included EBL, operative time, and LOS, whereas postoperative data included major and minor Clavien complications in both early (<30 postoperative days) and late (31–90 postoperative days) groups, as well as continence rate of neobladders when disclosed. These groups were stratified into ileal conduit and neobladder series, when appropriate (**Table 1**). Due to the paucity of data available on intracorporeal continent catheterizable channels, this diversion is not included in this review.

Operative Outcomes

Operative times

Operative times for creation of neobladders range from 330 minutes to 720 minutes (see **Table 1**). This is compared with an expectedly shorter ileal conduit range of 292 minutes to 691 minutes. This difference is expected given the extensive bowel manipulation and suturing required for neobladder creation and fixation to the native urethra. When comparing operative times for intracorporeal diversion versus extracorporeal diversion, Ahmed and colleagues[18] found no significant difference in operative time between the 2 groups. They quoted an average operative time of

414 minutes for both intracorporeal and extracorporeal approaches.

Estimated blood loss

EBL ranged from 100 to 500 mL for neobladders. The ileal conduit series ranged from 200 to 430 mL. A large difference in EBL between the 2 diversion types is not to be expected, given that the type of diversion should not alter blood loss from the prior dissection. However, one could assume that the longer overall operative time could lead to a slightly larger blood loss. Randomized controlled trials comparing open cystectomy to robotic cystectomy reveal a significantly lower blood loss when compared with standard open cystectomy.[2,26] This lower blood loss is likely due to the benefits of magnified surgical view, instruments with cautery features, and the hemostatic benefits of pneumoperitoneum. Ahmed and colleagues[18] found no significant difference in EBL between extracorporeal diversion and intracorporeal diversion.

Transfusion

Where reported, transfusion rates ranged from 10% to 71% with ileal conduits. This is compared with 17% to 56% transfusion rate with neobladders. Hayn and colleagues[23] reviewed a total of 496 RARCs at 14 separate institutions and reported an overall transfusion rate of 17%. Meta-analysis shows transfusion following RARC is associated with a 1.86 odds ratio of any

Table 1
Operative outcomes with intracorporeal neobladders and intracorporeal ileal conduits

	Author, Year	Patients	Operating Time (min)	EBL (mL)	Transfusion Rate (%)	Conversion Rate (%)
Neobladders	Schwentner et al, 2015	62	477	385	NR	0
	Atmaca et al, 2015	32	586	412.5	56	NR
	Collins et al,[19] 2014	80	420	475	NR	5.7
	Desai et al,[14] 2014	18	387	200	17	0
	Goh et al,[5] 2012	8	450	225	38	0
	Kang et al, 2012	1	585	500	NR	0
	Canda et al,[16] 2012	25	594	429.5	NR	4
	Pruthi et al,[8] 2010	3	330	221	NR	NR
	Sala et al, 2006	1	720	100	NR	NR
	Beechen et al, 2003	1	510	200	NR	NR
Ileal Conduits	Desai et al,[14] 2014	19	386	250	32	0
	Collins et al,[19] 2013	43	292	200	NR	2.3
	Azzouni et al,[15] 2013	100	352	300	10	0
	Goh et al,[5] 2012	7	450	225	71	0
	Kang et al, 2012	3	510	400	NR	0
	Canda et al,[16] 2011	2	594	429.5	NR	0
	Pruthi et al,[8] 2010	9	318	221	NR	NR
	Balaji et al, 2004	3	691	250	NR	NR

Abbreviations: EBL, estimated blood loss; NR, not reported.

complication (Clavien 1–5), and a 3.86 odds ratio of 90-day mortality.[18]

Open conversion

Open conversion ranges from 0% to 5.7% with neobladders and 0% to 2.3% with ileal conduits.

Postoperative Outcomes

Length of stay

LOS ranged from an average of 5 days to 17.4 days in the neobladder cohort (**Table 2**). This is compared with a range of 4.5 to 10.5 days in the ileal conduit group. The overall longer LOS in the neobladder cohort is certainly due to the increased complexity and longer bowel segments harvested and manipulated.

Complications

All of the neobladder papers in this series, with the exception of 1, included data on early (<30 postoperative days) and late (31–90 postoperative days) complications. These complications were further subdivided into minor (Clavien I–II) and major (Clavien III–V). In the neobladder studies included, the early, minor complication rate ranged from 0 to 100%. A focus on the studies

with larger cohorts shows that those with more than 30 patients have a range of early, minor complications from 17% to 62.5%. These same 3 larger series quote a range of early, major complications from 19% to 27%.

Late minor and major complication rates were reported by only 2 studies with cohorts larger than 30 patients. They reported late minor complications at a range of 11% to 15.6%. Late major complications rates ranged from 6.3% to 19%.

The ileal conduit series report an early low-grade complication rate ranging from 0% to 71%. Early high-grade complications ranged from 0% to 39%. Late low-grade complications ranged from 0% to 66%, with late high-grade complications ranging from 0% to 32%.

A metaanalysis reveals no statistically significant difference in 30-day and 90-day complication rates between intracorporeal urinary diversion and extracorporeal urinary diversion. The early complication rate for both groups combined was 41%, whereas the late complication rate for both groups combined was 47%. The extracorporeal group had a 43% early complication rate and a 49% late complication rate. The

Table 2
Postoperative outcomes with intracorporeal neobladders and intracorporeal ileal conduits

	Author, Year	Patients	LOS (days)	Early (<30 d) Clavien I–II (%)	Early (<30 d) Clavien III–V (%)	Late (31–90 d) Clavien I–II (%)	Late (31–90 d) Clavien III–V (%)	Continence
Neobladders	Schwentner et al, 2015	62	16.7	24.2	25.8	NR	NR	88% overall
	Atmaca et al, 2015	32	17.4	62.5	19	15.6	6.3	84.6% day, 46.1% night
	Collins et al,[19] 2014	80	9	17	27	11	19	87% day, 80% night
	Goh et al,[5] 2012	8	8	63	25	0	13	75% day
	Kang et al, 2012	1	14	100	0	0	0	NR
	Canda et al, 2012	25	10.5	33	15	15	11	65% day, 17% night
	Pruthi et al,[8] 2010	3	5	NR	NR	NR	NR	NR
	Sala et al, 2006	1	5	0	0	0	0	NR
	Beechen et al, 2003	1	10	0	0	0	0	NR
Ileal Conduits	Collins et al,[19] 2013	43	9	24	39	0	20	—
	Azzouni et al,[15] 2013	100	9	50	13	66	15	—
	Goh et al,[5] 2012	7	8	71	0	14	0	—
	Kang et al, 2012	3	NR	0	0	0	0	—
	Canda et al, 2011	2	10.5	33	15	15	11	—
	Pruthi et al,[8] 2010	9	4.5	NR	NR	NR	NR	—
	Balaji et al, 2004	3	7.3	33	0	NR	NR	—

intracorporeal diversion group had a 35% early complication rate and a 41% late complication rate.[18] The most common type of complication was gastrointestinal followed by infectious. These represented 20% and 17% of the combined intracorporeal and extracorporeal groups, respectively. In a statistically significant finding, the extracorporeal diversion group reported a 23% gastrointestinal complication rate compared with only 10% gastrointestinal complications with the intracorporeal group. In another statistically significant finding, the rates of infectious complications were 18% in the extracorporeal group and 12% in the intracorporeal group.[18]

Continence

Five of the neobladder studies in this review included information on continence following neobladder creation. Three of those studies further divided continence to specify daytime and nighttime continence rates. Daytime continence ranged from 65% to 87%, whereas nighttime continence ranged from 17% to 80%.

Readmission

Ahmed and colleagues[18] revealed that 13% of all robotic cystectomies were readmitted within 30 days, with 18% being readmitted within 90 days. When stratified between groups, the comparisons between the intracorporeal and extracorporeal groups were statistically significant in both the 30-day and 90-day readmission rates. The 30-day readmission rates were 15% in the extracorporeal group and just 5% in the intracorporeal group. The 90-day readmission rate was 19% in the extracorporeal group and 12% in the intracorporeal group.

Current Clinical Trial

At the time of this publication, there is an ongoing clinical trial with the goal of providing further information about the potential benefits of radical cystectomy with totally intracorporeal urinary diversion. NCT02252393 intends to randomize cystectomy patients between intracorporeal and extracorporeal diversion arms. The primary endpoint is the 90-day complication rate. Secondary endpoints are many and include operative time, EBL, LOS, readmission, ureteral stricture rate, stomal stenosis, disease recurrence, and many other metrics (available at https://clinicaltrials.gov/ct2/show/NCT02252393).

Further studies such as this will be needed to determine the optimal manner of urinary diversion for these complex patients.

SUMMARY

With increased surgeon familiarity with robotic surgery in urology, several techniques have been developed to perform intracorporeal continent and incontinent urinary diversion after RARC while replicating open techniques. As with any new surgical technique, there is a learning curve that can be overcome with diligence to refinement of surgical technique and increased surgical volumes. Review of existing literature suggests comparable and, in some cases, improved operative, postoperative, and functional outcomes. Until randomized clinical trials comparing intracorporeal and extracorporeal diversion are performed, larger series with longer follow-up will be needed to define the advantages and disadvantages of intracorporeal urinary diversions.

REFERENCES

1. Hellenthal NJ, Hussain A, Andrews PE, et al. Surgical margin status after robot assisted radical cystectomy: results from the International Robotic Cystectomy Consortium. J Urol 2010;184:87–91.
2. Bochner BH, Dalbagni G, Sjoberg DD, et al. Comparing open radical cystectomy and robot-assisted laparoscopic radical cystectomy: a randomized clinical trial. Eur Urol 2015;67:1042–50.
3. Hautmann RE, Herr HW, Pruthi RS, et al. Robotic radical cystectomy—is the diversion the Achilles' heel? J Urol 2014;192:1601–3.
4. Beecken WD, Wolfram M, Engl T, et al. Robotic-assisted laparoscopic radical cystectomy and intra-abdominal formation of an orthotopic ileal neobladder. Eur Urol 2003;44:337–9.
5. Goh AC, Gill IS, Lee DJ, et al. Robotic intracorporeal orthotopic ileal neobladder: replicating open surgical principles. Eur Urol 2012;62:891–901.
6. Chan KG, Guru K, Wiklund P, et al. Robot-assisted radical cystectomy and urinary diversion: technical recommendations from the Pasadena Consensus Panel. Eur Urol 2015;67:423–31.
7. Wiklund NP, Poulakis V. Robotic neobladder. BJU Int 2011;107:1514–37.
8. Pruthi RS, Nix J, McRackan D, et al. Robotic-assisted laparoscopic intracorporeal urinary diversion. Eur Urol 2010;57:1013–21.
9. Tan WS, Sridhar A, Goldstraw M, et al. Robot-assisted intracorporeal pyramid neobladder. BJU Int 2015;116:771–9.
10. Jonsson MN, Adding LC, Hosseini A, et al. Robot-assisted radical cystectomy with intracorporeal urinary diversion in patients with transitional cell carcinoma of the bladder. Eur Urol 2011;60:1066–73.
11. Guru K, Seixas-Mikelus SA, Hussain A, et al. Robot-assisted intracorporeal ileal conduit: marionette

technique and initial experience at Roswell Park Cancer Institute. Urology 2010;76:866–71.

12. Dal Moro F, Zattoni F. Lighting from the urethral cystoscope side: A novel technique to safely manage bowel division during intracorporeal robotic urinary diversion. Int J Urol 2016;23:344–5.

13. Manny TB, Hemal AK. Fluorescence-enhanced robotic radical cystectomy using unconjugated indocyanine green for pelvic lymphangiography, tumor marking, and mesenteric angiography: the initial clinical experience. Urology 2014;83:824–9.

14. Desai MM, de Abreu AL, Goh AC, et al. Robotic intracorporeal urinary diversion: technical details to improve time efficiency. J Endourol 2014;28:1320–7.

15. Azzouni FS, Din R, Rehman S, et al. The first 100 consecutive, robot-assisted, intracorporeal ileal conduits: evolution of technique and 90-day outcomes. Eur Urol 2013;63:637–43.

16. Canda AE, Atmaca AF, Altinova S, et al. Robot-assisted nerve-sparing radical cystectomy with bilateral extended pelvic lymph node dissection (PLND) and intracorporeal urinary diversion for bladder cancer: initial experience in 27 cases. BJU Int 2012;110:434–44.

17. Evangelidis A, Lee EK, Karellas ME, et al. Evaluation of ureterointestinal anastomosis: Wallace vs Bricker. J Urol 2006;175:1755–8 [discussion: 1758].

18. Ahmed K, Khan SA, Hayn MH, et al. Analysis of intracorporeal compared with extracorporeal urinary diversion after robot-assisted radical cystectomy: results from the International Robotic Cystectomy Consortium. Eur Urol 2014;65:340–7.

19. Collins JW, Sooriakumaran P, Sanchez-Salas R, et al. Robot-assisted radical cystectomy with intracorporeal neobladder diversion: the Karolinska experience. Indian J Urol 2014;30:307.

20. Abreu AL, Chopra S, Azhar RA, et al. Robotic radical cystectomy and intracorporeal urinary diversion: the USC technique. Indian J Urol 2014;30:300–6.

21. Dal Moro F, Haber GP, Wiklund P, et al. Robotic intracorporeal urinary diversion: practical review of current surgical techniques. Minerva Urol Nefrol 2017;69(1):14–25.

22. Goh AC, Aghazadeh MA, Krasnow RE, et al. Robotic intracorporeal continent cutaneous urinary diversion: primary description. J Endourol 2015;29:1217–20.

23. Hayn MH, Hussain A, Mansour AM, et al. The learning curve of robot-assisted radical cystectomy: results from the International Robotic Cystectomy Consortium. Eur Urol 2010;58:197–202.

24. Schumacher MC, Jonsson MN, Hosseini A, et al. Surgery-related complications of robot-assisted radical cystectomy with intracorporeal urinary diversion. Urology 2011;77:871–6.

25. Collins JW, Tyritzis S, Nyberg T, et al. Robot-assisted radical cystectomy (RARC) with intracorporeal neobladder - what is the effect of the learning curve on outcomes? BJU Int 2013;113:100–7.

26. Nix J, Smith A, Kurpad R, et al. Prospective randomized controlled trial of robotic versus open radical cystectomy for bladder cancer: perioperative and pathologic results. Eur Urol 2010;57:196–201.

Surgical Complications of Urinary Diversion

Christopher B. Anderson, MD, MPH*, James M. McKiernan, MD

KEYWORDS

- Urinary diversion • Ileal conduit • Orthotopic neobladder • Continent catheterizable pouch
- Complication

KEY POINTS

- Complications are common after urinary diversion.
- Patients are at risk for early and late complications after urinary diversion, and the risk increases over time.
- Patients with urinary diversions require long-term surveillance for anatomic, infectious, and metabolic complications.

INTRODUCTION

Urinary diversion (UD) is most commonly performed after radical cystectomy (RC), but can also be used in patients with nonmalignant conditions.[1–3] Most diversions are performed using ileum, although ileocecal and colonic segments are also used in some patients. Regardless of the surgical indication, bowel segment used, or type of diversion constructed, UDs are associated with significant risks of short- and long-term complications. Because most studies using contemporary reporting criteria of complications in patients with UD are in the setting of RC, these are the primary sources for this review. Still, RC and UD for noncancerous indications likely have a similar morbidity profile.[3,4]

RC with UD is generally performed on elderly patients with extensive comorbidities, requires operating times of 4 to 7 hours, and a hospital stay of 4 to 17 days.[5–15] Given the length and complexity of the procedure and the overall health and age of the patient, most patients experience early postoperative complications and up to 10% suffer mortality within 90 days of surgery.[5–8,10–26]

It is estimated that at least 60% of complications after RC occur as a result of the UD and, importantly, the risk of UD-related complications increases over time.[27,28]

The fidelity of reporting postoperative complications in recent years has improved. There are now several criteria to assess the quality of reporting for surgical complications, such as whether the report captured outpatient information, described the mortality and morbidity rates, and defined and graded all complications.[29,30] Using contemporary reporting methodology and stratification of complications by organ system, one is better able to standardize and compare postoperative complication rates across institutions.[31] Institutional series that use modern reporting methods are able to describe postoperative complications more accurately than less granular population-level studies, and this increases the number of complications described.[7,11,20,21]

Postoperative complications after UD are classified as early (less than 90 days) or late, and the types and frequencies of complications that occur during time periods differ. Any physician that performs UD or follows these patients postoperatively must understand the prevalence, presentation,

Disclosure Statement: The authors have nothing they wish to disclose.
Department of Urology, Columbia University Medical Center, 161 Fort Washington Avenue, 11th Floor, New York, NY 10032, USA
* Corresponding author.
E-mail address: cba2125@cumc.columbia.edu

Urol Clin N Am 45 (2018) 79–90
https://doi.org/10.1016/j.ucl.2017.09.008
0094-0143/18/Published by Elsevier Inc

and timing of complications after UD. This article reviews the complications partially or completely attributable to UD that are either associated with surgical technique or require surgical intervention to treat.

EARLY COMPLICATIONS
Prevalence and Risk Factors

Up to two-thirds of patients experience at least one complication within the first 90 days after surgery (**Table 1**).[5,7,10,14,15] Approximately half of these complications occur within the first few weeks after initial hospital discharge, but nearly 20% occur after 30 days.[7,32] Most postoperative complications are minor (Clavien grade I-II); however, up to 20% of patients experience a major complication (Clavien grade III-V) (see **Table 1**). Complications can lead to additional interventions, a longer hospital length of stay (LOS), added morbidity, and higher costs.[6,7,10,14]

There are several risk factors for postoperative complications, including patient comorbidity, age, frailty, longer operating room time, female gender, higher tumor stage, worse mental health, more intraoperative blood loss, and a higher body mass index (BMI).[5,7,14,15,20–22,33,34] It is reasonable to suspect that patients with a continent diversion have more postoperative complications because of the longer segment of bowel and higher complexity procedure, although data on this are mixed.[7,10,11,14,35] Higher surgeon and hospital volume are protective against postoperative morbidity and mortality.[6,20,36,37] There is no evidence that neoadjuvant chemotherapy in properly selected patients impacts risk of perioperative complications.[38,39]

Early Complications by Organ System

Recent high-quality institutional series that use modern reporting criteria group early postoperative complications into 1 of 11 organ-systems (see **Table 1**): gastrointestinal, infectious, wound, genitourinary, cardiac, pulmonary, bleeding, thromboembolic, neurologic, miscellaneous, and surgical. Although this discussion does not comprehensively cover all possible postoperative complications, we highlight select organ systems whose complications may be more attributable to UD rather than RC.

Gastrointestinal

Because of the use of bowel for UDs, gastrointestinal complications are common after RC and UD, seen in up to 30% of patients (see **Table 1**). The most common gastrointestinal complication is paralytic ileus, although patients are at risk for a

Table 1 Early complication rates after radical cystectomy and urinary diversion based on several large contemporary institutional cohorts	
Complication	**Percent**
Overall	49–64
Minor[a]	34–51
Major[a]	13–22
By organ system	
Gastrointestinal	15–29
Infectious	7–30
Wound	5–21
Genitourinary	7–17
Cardiac	<1–11
Pulmonary	1–9
Bleeding	<1–16
Thromboembolic	<1–8
Neurologic	2–5
Miscellaneous	1–9
Surgical	0–1
Secondary procedure	7–14
Mortality	2–5

[a] Minor complications are Clavien grades I-II. Major complications are Clavien grades III-V.
Data from Refs.[5,7,10,14,15]

variety of other complications, such as bowel obstruction, anastomotic leak, gastrointestinal bleeding, and *Clostridium difficile* colitis (CDC).

Ileus is caused by the temporary of impairment of small bowel peristalsis causing a functional bowel obstruction. Although somewhat variable, the definition of an ileus is the absence of bowel function by postoperative day 5; need for nasogastric tube; or conversion to NPO status because of nausea, vomiting, or abdominal distention.[5,7] Depending on the definition used, nearly one-quarter of patients with RC experience postoperative ileus and it is the most common cause of prolonged LOS following RC.[5,7,14,15,40] Paralytic ileus is likely caused by an insult to small bowel innervation secondary to irritation, inflammation, or medication effects. There are several proposed inciting factors including intraoperative bowel manipulation; medications, such as opioids and anticholinergics; and metabolic abnormalities including hypokalemia, hypocalcemia, hypomagnesemia, and hyponatremia.[41]

Patients who develop an ileus are best treated supportively with hydration, nasogastric tubes, treatment of electrolyte imbalances, and cessation of offending medications. Prokinetics, such as metoclopramide and erythromycin, have been studied to prevent ileus, although there are limited data to support their use for this indication.[42–45] Alvimopan is a peripheral opioid μ-receptor antagonist that blocks the effect of opioids on the gastrointestinal tract and has been approved by the US Food and Drug Administration to accelerate gastrointestinal recovery following a bowel resection and primary anastomosis. A recent randomized trial demonstrated that use of perioperative alvimopan during RC and UD is associated with faster return of bowel function, shorter hospital stay, and less ileus-related morbidity with a favorable safety profile and lower hospitals costs.[46,47] Because ileus may occur from an imbalance of parasympathetic innervation to the small bowel, some centers have used neostigmine, although this medication has not been studied in patients with UD.[42,48]

Avoidance of bowel edema from fluid overload may also enhance the recovery of bowel function.[49] A recent randomized trial of standard versus restricted intraoperative hydration demonstrated that restricted hydration was associated with a significantly lower risk of postoperative gastrointestinal complications.[50] Additional interventions, such as gum chewing, coffee drinking, early enteral feeding, and peritoneal readaptation over the pelvic sidewalls, may lessen gastrointestinal morbidity after RC.[51–55] There is no evidence that routine use of mechanical bowel preparations decreases postoperative gastrointestinal complications.[56,57]

Perioperative enhanced recovery protocols have become widely popularized to decrease complications after RC and UD. One of the main goals of such protocols is to reduce gastrointestinal morbidity by using several evidence-based interventions known to impact bowel recovery.[58] Enhanced recovery protocols are associated with decreased LOS and faster return of bowel function, but may not decrease overall complication rates.[9,43,59,60] In fact, recent data suggest shortening hospital stay may actually increase postoperative complication rates, necessitating closer outpatient surveillance.[61] Further study is needed to understand the trade-offs of shifting postoperative care out of the inpatient setting at an earlier time.

Other less common gastrointestinal complications include small bowel obstruction, CDC, and anastomotic bowel leak. Small bowel obstruction is seen in approximately 7% of patients with RC and usually occurs secondary to internal adhesions or bowel edema.[7] Initial treatment is similar to that of an ileus, although it is critical to monitor for signs of ischemia or perforation. If the obstruction does not resolve with supportive care, abdominal exploration may be required. CDC is caused by the gram-positive spore-forming bacterium *C difficile* and has historically been seen in fewer than 3% of patients after RC and UD, although rates seem to be on the rise and were nearly 9% in a recent series.[7,15,62–64] The diagnosis of CDC is made in the presence of diarrhea, abdominal pain, and leukocytosis, and a positive fecal *C difficile* toxin. The primary risk factor for CDC is exposure to antibiotics, which can disrupt normal bowel flora, but additional risks include older patient age, immunosuppression, chronic antacid therapy, and longer LOS.[62,64–66] Prevention of disease transmission is critical, namely through use of antibiotic stewardship and hand hygiene. Depending on disease severity, CDC is usually treated with up to 2 weeks of oral metronidazole or vancomycin.[66] Patients who develop toxic megacolon may require a colectomy. An anastomotic bowel leak is rare, but can be lethal.[5,7,10,11,15,67] Risk factors include active smoking, obesity, and immunosuppression and creation of a tension-free and well-vascularized anastomosis is necessary to avoid leaks.[68] Some patients are managed with conservative measures; however, many require exploration.

Infectious

Infections can also be seen in up to 30% of patients after RC and UD, most commonly in the urinary tract (see **Table 1**). Because of the exposure to enteric contents, patients can also develop intra-abdominal and wound infections. Patients must be carefully monitored for postoperative infection and signs or symptoms of infection should prompt a full infectious work-up, including blood and urine cultures; chest imaging; and, when indicated, abdominal imaging. Treatment includes the early initiation of intravenous fluids, broad-spectrum antibiotics and source control. Professional guidelines recommend administration of prophylactic antibiotics within 1 hour of incision and not continued for longer than 24 hours postoperatively in the absence of a known infection.[69,70] First-line antimicrobial prophylaxis includes either a second- or third-generation cephalosporin, or aztreonam plus metronidazole or clindamycin.[69] Antibiotic choices can also be informed by prior culture data and the local antibiogram.

Genitourinary

Genitourinary complications are nearly always related to the UD, with ureteral obstruction and urinary leak being the most common ones in the early postoperative period.[7,14,15] A urine leak occurs in less than 5% of patients after RC and UD and can originate from any suture or staple line including the ureterointestinal anastomosis, the butt end of an ileal conduit, the wall of a continent diversion, or the urethroneovesical anastomosis of a neo-bladder.[7,15] Early leaks can present with high intra-peritoneal drain output with elevated fluid creatinine; elevated serum creatinine caused by urine reabsorption; or even chemical peritonitis, ileus, and abdominal distention. Maximal urinary tract drainage, using percutaneous drains, neph-rostomy tubes, or Foley catheters, effectively treats most leaks. Ureteral stents placed at the time of surgery may help avoid urine leaks, but do not necessarily reduce early ureteral obstruc-tion.[71,72] Early ureteral obstruction can occur in up to 10% of patients.[7,15] Importantly, although some patients may present with flank pain, obstruction can also present with pyelonephritis or worsening renal function in the absence of pain. Early ureteral obstruction most commonly occurs because of edema or scarring at the ureter-ointestinal anastomosis, and can generally be pre-vented by meticulous surgical technique with avoidance of tissue ischemia. Treatment requires relief of the obstruction, usually with a percuta-neous nephrostomy tube. After patients are fully recovered from surgery, the ureterointestinal anastomosis should be investigated for a possible stricture.

Patients with an ileal conduit can have early sto-mal complications, including hyperemia, retrac-tion, and necrosis. Stomal retraction is problematic if it leads to subcutaneous or subfas-cial urinary extravasation. Stomal necrosis most commonly involves the stoma alone, but rarely the entire conduit can necrose. Looposcopy is required to differentiate the two, and an ischemic conduit often requires urgent surgical revision. If treatment is required for stomal retraction or ne-crosis, it usually entails conduit drainage with a catheter, or diversion with nephrostomy tubes for particularly severe cases, with a delayed repair af-ter several months.

Wound

Around one in five patients experience a postoper-ative wound complication after RC and UD, most commonly a wound infection.[7,15] The estimated risk for a wound infection after a clean-contaminated procedure is 4% to 10%, but this in-creases to 10% to 15% with spillage of gastroin-testinal contents.[70] Wound infections can present with incisional pain, redness, purulent drainage, fevers, and leukocytosis. Several patient- and procedure-related factors increase the risk of a postoperative wound infection, such as patient

comorbidity, obesity, malignancy, malnutrition, diabetes, and smoking, as well as longer proced-ure duration, open surgery, wound classification, and need for a blood transfusion.[73-77]

Many techniques have been shown to reduce the risk of a wound infection, including use of anti-biotic prophylaxis, skin sterilization with chlorhexi-dine, avoidance of hyperglycemia and hypothermia, and abdominal closure techniques including wound irrigation and elimination of dead space.[74,78-80] Perioperative care bundles to reduce wound infections have been pioneered in colo-rectal surgery that include many of the previously mentioned techniques, in addition to other wound closure techniques, such as the changing of gown and gloves and use of a clean set of instru-ments.[81] Treatment of wound infections includes opening and packing of the wound and initiation of antibiotics. Noninfectious wound complications include superficial skin separation and subcutane-ous seromas, which are usually treated with local wound care and healing by secondary intention.

Fascial dehiscence can occur in up to 3% of pa-tients after RC and UD.[7,10,15,82] A recent study re-ported that early dehiscence occurred at a median of 11 days after surgery and was universally accompanied by a concomitant wound infec-tion.[82] Other risk factors for dehiscence included obesity and chronic obstructive pulmonary dis-ease. Although there are patient risk factors for dehiscence, it is strongly related to technical fac-tors during fascial closure. Dehiscence is often a surgical emergency that requires reoperation given the risk of evisceration. However, if the skin is closed, the patient is stable, and there is no exposed bowel or bowel obstruction, patients may be managed conservatively with a hernia repair at a later date.

Thromboembolic

Between 1% and 8% patients experience a venous thromboembolism (VTE) within 90 days of surgery, most of which are deep venous throm-bosis.[7,10,14,15] There are several well-known pa-tient risk factors for VTE include older age, increased comorbidity, higher BMI, personal or family history of VTE, malignancy, smoking, and immobility.[83-85] Long procedures and open ap-proaches also increase the risk of VTE. A recent study using a large, population-based dataset observed a 6% risk of VTE within 30 days of RC, approximately 50% of which occurred after hospi-tal discharge.[86] A similarly high rate of postdi-scharge VTE was reported using large institutional cohorts.[87,88]

Patients with RC are at high-risk for VTE and benefit from chemoprophylaxis and/or mechanical prophylaxis during their hospital stay.[84] Chemo-prophylaxis with subcutaneous low-dose unfrac-tionated heparin or low-molecular-weight heparin is associated with a decreased risk of VTE, including fatal pulmonary embolism and death, whereas mechanical prophylaxis with sequential compression devices or compression stockings reduces deep venous thrombosis but not fatal pul-monary embolism or death.[84] Chemoprophylaxis is more effective at reducing VTE than mechanical prophylaxis, but does increase the risk of nonfatal bleeding.[84] Patients at particularly high risk of VTE, such as those having RC and UD, likely benefit from the combination of chemoprophylaxis and mechanical prophylaxis.

Given the increased risk of outpatient VTE for high-risk patients, there is growing use of extended courses of chemoprophylaxis after hos-pital discharge.[84] Continuing low-molecular-weight heparin for up to a month after RC and UD has demonstrated effectiveness at reducing VTEs after hospital discharge and is recommen-ded by the American College of Chest Physicians.[84,88,89]

Surgical

Intraoperative complications are rare in the hands of experienced surgeons, but can include acci-dental injury to surrounding viscera, vasculature, or nerves. Many such complications occur during the course of RC and pelvic lymphadenectomy rather than during UD. Rectal injuries are uncom-mon during RC, but may occur more frequently in the postradiation setting.[90] Small rectal injuries with minimal fecal contamination can often be pri-marily closed in several layers. If a rectal injury oc-curs during an orthotopic neobladder (ONB), vascularized interposition flaps are required to avoid a rectal-neobladder fistula. If a rectal injury is large, associated with significant fecal contami-nation, or in a radiated patient, fecal diversion may be required.

Other Early Complications

Up to 14% of patients require a secondary pro-cedure within 90 days of RC either with a return trip to the operating room or by the interventional radiologists.[7,15] Common reasons for reoperation are wound dehiscence, bowel obstruction, wound infection, and ileus, whereas most indications for an interventional radiology procedure are drainage of an abscess or lymphocele, and placement of a percutaneous nephrostomy tube.[7,10,11,91]

Up to one-third of patients return for emergency evaluation within 90 days of RC, and nearly as many require readmission, usually within the first several weeks following surgery.[7,10,18,25,92]

Common causes of readmission include ileus, urinary tract infection, urinary obstruction, and fail-ure to thrive.[18,25,92] Patients who have more comorbidities, experience postoperative compli-cations, and are discharged to a nursing facility are more likely to get readmitted.[18,25,92]

Finally, 3% to 9% of patients experience a mor-tality within 90 days of surgery, and most deaths occur after initial hospital discharge.[7,20,23,24,93] The most common causes of death are cardiovas-cular complications and sepsis with multiorgan system failure.[5,10,14,15,67] Risk factors for postop-erative mortality include advanced tumor stage, nutritional deficiency, multiple comorbidities, and older age.[23,26,94] There is a protective effect on mortality with higher hospital volume.[36] Patients with multiple risk factors may have a 90-day mor-tality risk of 25%, and prediction tools can help quantify this risk during preoperative counseling.[24,26]

Robotic Radical Cystectomy

Robotic-assisted RC was popularized as a means of decreasing the morbidity of RC and UD, and several randomized studies have examined early postoperative complications compared with open RC.[95–99] In short, most randomized trials agree that robotic-assisted RC is associated with less blood loss and may be associated with faster return of bowel function, but it is unclear if the ro-botic approach is associated with fewer early complications overall. Some institutional reports suggest improved outcomes with robotic-assisted RC, but these reports are subject to se-lection bias.[95,100] Further research is needed to determine whether the growing experience with intracorporeal UD will further impact the risk profile of surgery.

LATE COMPLICATIONS

The presence of bowel in continuity with the urinary tract can predispose patients to several types of surgical complications that occur after 90 days. Most patients with a UD experience a complication over time, some of which occur many years after surgery (**Fig. 1**).[27,28]

Ureterointestinal Anastomotic Stricture

Strictures at the ureteroenteric anastomosis are a troublesome problem after UD. Although reports of prevalence vary, stricture rates of around 10% have been reported by several high-volume cen-ters with experienced surgeons.[28,101–103] Stric-tures are more common on the left side and usually occur within the first year after

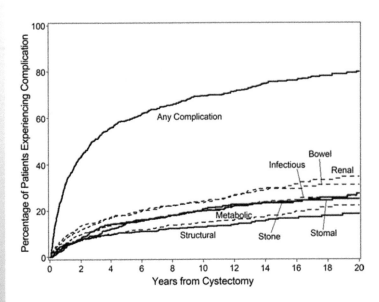

Fig. 1. Risk of complications over time for patients with ileal conduit urinary diversion. (*From* Shimko MS, Tollefson MK, Umbreit EC, et al. Long-term complications of conduit urinary diversion. J Urol 2011;185(2):562–7; with permission.)

surgery.[28,101,103] Presentation can include flank pain, infection, and worsening renal function, but some may be asymptomatic. Asymptomatic strictures can demonstrate hydronephrosis on imaging and the presence and location of obstruction is confirmed with a retrograde contrast study (loopogram, pouchogram, cystogram) or nuclear renogram with furosemide (Lasix). Initial management includes placement of a percutaneous nephrostomy tube or antegrade nephroureteral stent. Endoscopic techniques to incise or dilate strictures are effective in some patients, although open reconstruction is usually required for durable repair.[104,105] Strictures can often be prevented by meticulous surgical technique, including the creation of a tension-free, well-vascularized, freely refluxing ureteroenteric anastomosis. An interrupted suture technique and avoidance of postoperative urine leak seems to be protective against strictures.[103,106] Whereas it is our practice to perform a high ureteral transection so as to avoid distal ureteral ischemia, it is unclear if excision of a longer distal ureteral segment reduces stricture rates.[103]

Parastomal Hernia

Although patients with ileal conduits are at risk for several problems with their stomas, including stenosis, difficulty pouching, skin irritation, and leakage, parastomal hernia (PH) is common and particularly problematic. Among large cohorts of patients with ileal conduits, the prevalence of PH reaches up to 50% within 2 years of surgery with the median time to occurrence of 1 year.[107,108] Although many PHs are asymptomatic and

detected on imaging, approximately 28% to 40% of hernias are clinically evident and some were associated with symptoms, such as bulge, discomfort, bowel symptoms, and pouching difficulties.[107,108] Risk factors for PH include female gender, increasing BMI, and lower preoperative albumin.[107] Patients can often be conservatively managed with hernia belts in consultation with an ostomy nurse, although between 9% and 30% are ultimately referred for surgical repair. There are ongoing studies to investigate the use of prophylactic mesh at the time of ileal conduit to prevent hernias in high-risk patients, a technique that has shown to be beneficial in the colorectal literature.[109]

Incisional Hernia

Incisional hernias occur in up to 20% of patients after RC and UD with a median time to presentation of approximately 1 year.[108] Most patients present with a symptomatic bulge in their incision. One series found that patients with longer (supraumbilical) incisions, older patients, higher BMI, male gender, and an orthotopic UD all increased the risk of an incisional hernia.[108] Still, similar to fascial dehiscence, technical factors may also influence incisional hernia risk. A tension-free fascial closure with approximation of healthy tissue is required to minimize hernia risk. In addition, the choice of suture and suture technique (running vs interrupted) are also important. Fascial closure with a continuous absorbable suture is associated with lower hernia rates compared with several interrupted absorbable sutures.[110] Obtaining smaller fascial bites (5 mm every 5 mm) is associated with a lower hernia risk at 1 year compared with larger fascial bites (1 cm every 1 cm).[111]

Orthotopic Neobladder Bladder Neck Obstruction

Urinary retention after ONB occurs in 10% to 30% of patients. This is a functional problem, because of overdistention of the pouch, or from obstruction or kinking at the bladder neck.[112,113] It is possible that preservation or restoration of pelvic support can avoid kinking and posterior displacement of the neobladder, particularly in females.[114] Bladder neck stenosis occurs in fewer than 2% of patients, but is likely related to technical factors.[102] Creation of a tension-free, well-vascularized urethroneovesical anastomosis is critical to avoid stenosis. Patients with anastomotic stenosis can often be treated endoscopically.[112]

Continent Catheterizable Pouch Efferent Limb Complications

Most patients with continent catheterizable pouches (CCP) have efferent limbs constructed of either appendix or tubularized ileum, and up to half of patients with CCPs have efferent limb complications over time.[115] The main surgical complications of the efferent limb are incontinence and stenosis. Although use of appendix has a lower incontinence rate than ileum, it has a higher risk of stenosis.[116–118] Up to 30% of patients with a CCP can develop stenosis, which can sometimes be managed with dilation but many require surgical revision.[116,117] Incontinence is seen in approximately 15% to 30% of patients and may be caused by shorter functional length of the efferent segment, an incompetent valve mechanism, or a poorly compliant reservoir.[115,116,119] Urodynamics may help differentiate the cause of incontinence, and treatment ranges from injecting bulking agents into the efferent limb to surgical revision of the efferent limb or augmentation of the pouch.

Urolithiasis

Patients with UDs have multiple risk factors for upper- and lower-tract urolithiasis, such as metabolic changes, chronic infections, urinary stasis, and presence of foreign bodies, including mucous and exposed staple lines.[120,121] Lower urinary tract stones can present with infections, pain, hematuria, obstruction, or difficulty emptying CCP, and they have a high risk of recurrence.[120]

Patients with continent diversions have a higher risk of lower-tract stones, likely caused by more urinary stasis and metabolic changes from a greater surface of exposed bowel in the urinary tract.[122] Among 1057 patients with an ileal conduit followed for a median 6.3 years, 13.4% developed upper tract stones and 4.5% developed conduit stones.[28] Conduit stones were diagnosed 2 to 3 years postoperatively, and about half of the patients with conduit stones also had upper tract stones. Patients with continent CCPs have a 5% to 10% risk of stones, although this is much higher in stapled pouches.[115,118] Similarly, the risk of stone formation in stapled ONBs is considerably higher than hand-sewn ones.[102,123,124] Importantly, the risk of stones in continent pouches increases over time.[123]

Methods to prevent recurrent stones in patients with continent diversions include improved pouch drainage; correction of metabolic abnormalities, such as dehydration, acidosis, hypocitraturia, and hyperoxaluria; and regular pouch irrigations.[125] Most stones are managed endoscopically, although some require open removal.[121] Patients with UDs are also at risk for upper tract stones because of similar risk factors, the management of which usually requires percutaneous nephrolithotomy or extracorporeal shock wave lithotripsy.

RARE COMPLICATIONS

Certain rare complications of UD require urgent treatment or surgical repair. Rupture of continent pouches can occur in around 2% of patients and may present with acute abdominal pain, distention, and decreased urine output.[102,126] This is caused by abdominal trauma or failure to empty, particularly in patients with compromised sensation. If a pouch rupture is suspected, contrasted imaging studies should be obtained to confirm the diagnosis. Patients with small leaks may be treated conservatively with catheter drainage, but large pouch injuries usually require surgical repair. Fistulas to bowel, skin, or vagina can occur, particularly with CCPs and ONBs. Fistula between the diversion and bowel can manifest with frequent urinary infections, fecaluria, and pneumaturia. Conservative management with urinary drainage and bowel rest with parenteral nutrition may effectively treat smaller enteral fistula, but surgical repair may be required. Approximately 5% to 11% of women with ONBs can develop fistulae to the vagina and present with worsening or severe incontinence.[114] An ONB-vaginal fistula can occur if the anterior vaginal wall is damaged during surgery and is overlapped with an ONB suture line. Reconstruction with interposition flaps is effective, but incontinence can persist.[127] Patients with ileal conduits can rarely develop conduit strictures and stomal stenosis, which sometimes requires surgical revision.[28]

SUMMARY

UD has a significant risk of complications. The frequency and type of complication is associated with time from surgery. The most common early surgical complications are ileus and infection, whereas late complications include strictures, hernias, and urolithiasis. Long-term surveillance after UD is required to identify and treat patients with complications in a timely fashion.

REFERENCES

1. Bassett MR, Santiago-Lastra Y, Stoffel JT, et al. Urinary diversion for severe urinary adverse events of prostate radiation: results from a multi-institutional study. J Urol 2017;197(3 Pt 1):744–50.
2. Norus T, Fode M, Nordling J. Ileal conduit without cystectomy may be an appropriate option in the treatment of intractable bladder pain syndrome/interstitial cystitis. Scand J Urol 2014;48(2):210–5.
3. Brown ET, Osborn D, Mock S, et al. Temporal trends in conduit urinary diversion with concomitant cystectomy for benign indications: a population-based analysis. Urology 2016;98:70–4.
4. Deboudt C, Perrouin-Verbe MA, Le Normand L, et al. Comparison of the morbidity and mortality of cystectomy and ileal conduit urinary diversion for neurogenic lower urinary tract dysfunction according to the approach: laparotomy, laparoscopy or robotic. Int J Urol 2016;23(10):848–53.
5. Hautmann RE, de Petriconi RC, Volkmer BG. Lessons learned from 1,000 neobladders: the 90-day complication rate. J Urol 2010;184(3):990–4 [quiz: 1235].
6. Leow JJ, Reese S, Trinh QD, et al. Impact of surgeon volume on the morbidity and costs of radical cystectomy in the USA: a contemporary population-based analysis. BJU Int 2015;115(5): 713–21.
7. Shabsigh A, Korets R, Vora KC, et al. Defining early morbidity of radical cystectomy for patients with bladder cancer using a standardized reporting methodology. Eur Urol 2009;55(1):164–74.
8. Novotny V, Hakenberg OW, Wiessner D, et al. Perioperative complications of radical cystectomy in a contemporary series. Eur Urol 2007;51(2):397–401 [discussion: 401–2].
9. Daneshmand S, Ahmadi H, Schuckman AK, et al. Enhanced recovery protocol after radical cystectomy for bladder cancer. J Urol 2014;192(1):50–5.
10. Novara G, De Marco V, Aragona M, et al. Complications and mortality after radical cystectomy for bladder transitional cell cancer. J Urol 2009; 182(3):914–21.
11. Jerlstrom T, Gardmark T, Carringer M, et al. Urinary bladder cancer treated with radical cystectomy: perioperative parameters and early complications prospectively registered in a national population-based database. Scand J Urol 2014;48(4):334–40.
12. Lowrance WT, Rumohr JA, Chang SS, et al. Contemporary open radical cystectomy: analysis of perioperative outcomes. J Urol 2008;179(4): 1313–8 [discussion: 1318].
13. Prasad SM, Ferreria M, Berry AM, et al. Surgical Apgar outcome score: perioperative risk assessment for radical cystectomy. J Urol 2009;181(3): 1046–52 [discussion: 1052–3].
14. Schiavina R, Borghesi M, Guidi M, et al. Perioperative complications and mortality after radical cystectomy when using a standardized reporting methodology. Clin Genitourin Cancer 2013;11(2):189–97.
15. Takada N, Abe T, Shinohara N, et al. Peri-operative morbidity and mortality related to radical cystectomy: a multi-institutional retrospective study in Japan. BJU Int 2012;110(11 Pt B):E756–64.
16. Fairey AS, Jacobsen NE, Chetner MP, et al. Associations between comorbidity, and overall survival and bladder cancer specific survival after radical cystectomy: results from the Alberta Urology Institute Radical Cystectomy database. J Urol 2009; 182(1):85–92 [discussion: 93].
17. Trinh VQ, Trinh QD, Tian Z, et al. In-hospital mortality and failure-to-rescue rates after radical cystectomy. BJU Int 2013;112(2):E20–7.
18. Hu M, Jacobs BL, Montgomery JS, et al. Sharpening the focus on causes and timing of readmission after radical cystectomy for bladder cancer. Cancer 2014;120(9):1409–16.
19. Lee KL, Freiha F, Presti JC Jr, et al. Gender differences in radical cystectomy: complications and blood loss. Urology 2004;63(6):1095–9.
20. Kim SP, Boorjian SA, Shah ND, et al. Contemporary trends of in-hospital complications and mortality for radical cystectomy. BJU Int 2012;110(8):1163–8.
21. Lavallee LT, Schramm D, Witiuk K, et al. Peri-operative morbidity associated with radical cystectomy in a multicenter database of community and academic hospitals. PLoS One 2014;9(10):e111281.
22. Svatek RS, Fisher MB, Matin SF, et al. Risk factor analysis in a contemporary cystectomy cohort using standardized reporting methodology and adverse event criteria. J Urol 2010;183(3):929–34.
23. Isbarn H, Jeldres C, Zini L, et al. A population based assessment of perioperative mortality after cystectomy for bladder cancer. J Urol 2009;182(1):70–7.
24. Aziz A, May M, Burger M, et al. Prediction of 90-day mortality after radical cystectomy for bladder cancer in a prospective European multicenter cohort. Eur Urol 2014;66(1):156–63.
25. Porter MP, Gore JL, Wright JL. Hospital volume and 90-day mortality risk after radical cystectomy: a population-based cohort study. World J Urol 2011;29(1):73–7.

26. Schiffmann J, Gandaglia G, Larcher A, et al. Contemporary 90-day mortality rates after radical cystectomy in the elderly. Eur J Surg Oncol 2014; 40(12):1738–45.

27. Madersbacher S, Schmidt J, Eberle JM, et al. Long-term outcome of ileal conduit diversion. J Urol 2003;169(3):985–90.

28. Shimko MS, Tollefson MK, Umbreit EC, et al. Long-term complications of conduit urinary diversion. J Urol 2011;185(2):562–7.

29. Martin RC 2nd, Brennan MF, Jaques DP. Quality of complication reporting in the surgical literature. Ann Surg 2002;235(6):803–13.

30. Dindo D, Demartines N, Clavien PA. Classification of surgical complications: a new proposal with evaluation in a cohort of 6336 patients and results of a survey. Ann Surg 2004;240(2):205–13.

31. Donat SM. Standards for surgical complication reporting in urologic oncology: time for a change. Urology 2007;69(2):221–5.

32. Sood A, Kachroo N, Abdollah F, et al. An evaluation of the timing of surgical complications following radical cystectomy: data from the American College of Surgeons National Surgical Quality Improvement Program. Urology 2017; 103:91–8.

33. Chappidi MR, Kates M, Patel HD, et al. Frailty as a marker of adverse outcomes in patients with bladder cancer undergoing radical cystectomy. Urol Oncol 2016;34(6):256.e1-6.

34. Sharma P, Henriksen CH, Zargar-Shoshtari K, et al. Preoperative patient reported mental health is associated with high grade complications after radical cystectomy. J Urol 2016;195(1):47–52.

35. Antonelli A, Belotti S, Cristinelli L, et al. Comparison of perioperative morbidity of radical cystectomy with neobladder versus ileal conduit: a matched pair analysis of 170 patients. Clin Genitourin Cancer 2016;14(3):244–8.

36. Birkmeyer JD, Siewers AE, Finlayson EV, et al. Hospital volume and surgical mortality in the United States. N Engl J Med 2002;346(15):1128–37.

37. Birkmeyer JD, Stukel TA, Siewers AE, et al. Surgeon volume and operative mortality in the United States. N Engl J Med 2003;349(22):2117–27.

38. Johnson DC, Nielsen ME, Matthews J, et al. Neoadjuvant chemotherapy for bladder cancer does not increase risk of perioperative morbidity. BJU Int 2014;114(2):221–8.

39. Tyson MD 2nd, Bryce AH, Ho TH, et al. Perioperative complications after neoadjuvant chemotherapy and radical cystectomy for bladder cancer. Can J Urol 2014;21(3):7259–65.

40. Chang SS, Cookson MS, Baumgartner RG, et al. Analysis of early complications after radical cystectomy: results of a collaborative care pathway. J Urol 2002;167(5):2012–6.

41. Batke M, Cappell MS. Adynamic ileus and acute colonic pseudo-obstruction. Med Clin North Am 2008;92(3):649–70, ix.

42. Traut U, Brugger L, Kunz R, et al. Systemic prokinetic pharmacologic treatment for postoperative adynamic ileus following abdominal surgery in adults. Cochrane Database Syst Rev 2008;(1): CD004930.

43. Pruthi RS, Nielsen M, Smith A, et al. Fast track program in patients undergoing radical cystectomy: results in 362 consecutive patients. J Am Coll Surg 2010;210(1):93–9.

44. Donat SM, Slaton JW, Pisters LL, et al. Early nasogastric tube removal combined with metoclopramide after radical cystectomy and urinary diversion. J Urol 1999;162(5):1599–602.

45. Lightfoot AJ, Eno M, Kreder KJ, et al. Treatment of postoperative ileus after bowel surgery with low-dose intravenous erythromycin. Urology 2007; 69(4):611–5.

46. Lee CT, Chang SS, Kamat AM, et al. Alvimopan accelerates gastrointestinal recovery after radical cystectomy: a multicenter randomized placebo-controlled trial. Eur Urol 2014;66(2):265–72.

47. Kauf TL, Svatek RS, Amiel G, et al. Alvimopan, a peripherally acting mu-opioid receptor antagonist, is associated with reduced costs after radical cystectomy: economic analysis of a phase 4 randomized, controlled trial. J Urol 2014;191(6):1721–7.

48. Hautmann RE. Surgery illustrated: surgical atlas ileal neobladder. BJU Int 2010;105(7):1024–35.

49. Lobo DN, Bostock KA, Neal KR, et al. Effect of salt and water balance on recovery of gastrointestinal function after elective colonic resection: a randomised controlled trial. Lancet 2002;359(9320): 1812–8.

50. Wuethrich PY, Burkhard FC, Thalmann GN, et al. Restrictive deferred hydration combined with preemptive norepinephrine infusion during radical cystectomy reduces postoperative complications and hospitalization time: a randomized clinical trial. Anesthesiology 2014;120(2):365–77.

51. de Vries RR, Kauer P, van Tinteren H, et al. Short-term outcome after cystectomy: comparison of two different perioperative protocols. Urol Int 2012;88(4):383–9.

52. Kouba EJ, Wallen EM, Pruthi RS. Gum chewing stimulates bowel motility in patients undergoing radical cystectomy with urinary diversion. Urology 2007;70(6):1053–6.

53. Muller SA, Rahbari NN, Schneider F, et al. Randomized clinical trial on the effect of coffee on postoperative ileus following elective colectomy. Br J Surg 2012;99(11):1530–8.

54. Roth B, Birkhauser FD, Zehnder P, et al. Readaptation of the peritoneum following extended pelvic lymphadenectomy and cystectomy has a

significant beneficial impact on early postoperative recovery and complications: results of a prospective randomized trial. Eur Urol 2011;59(2):204–10.

55. Deibert CM, Silva MV, RoyChoudhury A, et al. A prospective randomized trial of the effects of early enteral feeding after radical cystectomy. Urology 2016;96:69–73.

56. Large MC, Kiriluk KJ, DeCastro GJ, et al. The impact of mechanical bowel preparation on postoperative complications for patients undergoing cystectomy and urinary diversion. J Urol 2012; 188(5):1801–5.

57. Raynor MC, Lavien G, Nielsen M, et al. Elimination of preoperative mechanical bowel preparation in patients undergoing cystectomy and urinary diversion. Urol Oncol 2013;31(1):32–5.

58. Cerantola Y, Valerio M, Persson B, et al. Guidelines for perioperative care after radical cystectomy for bladder cancer: enhanced recovery after surgery (ERAS((R))) society recommendations. Clin Nutr 2013;32(6):879–87.

59. Karl A, Buchner A, Becker A, et al. A new concept for early recovery after surgery for patients undergoing radical cystectomy for bladder cancer: results of a prospective randomized study. J Urol 2014;191(2):335–40.

60. Djaladat H, Katebian B, Bazargani ST, et al. 90-Day complication rate in patients undergoing radical cystectomy with enhanced recovery protocol: a prospective cohort study. World J Urol 2017; 35(6):907–11.

61. Osawa T, Ambani SN, Olugbade K Jr, et al. Potential Implications of shortening length of stay following radical cystectomy in a Pre-ERAS population. Urology 2017;102:92–9.

62. Calvert JK, Holt SK, Mossanen M, et al. Use and outcomes of extended antibiotic prophylaxis in urological cancer surgery. J Urol 2014;192(2):425–9.

63. Kim SP, Shah ND, Karnes RJ, et al. The implications of hospital acquired adverse events on mortality, length of stay and costs for patients undergoing radical cystectomy for bladder cancer. J Urol 2012;187(6):2011–7.

64. Liu NW, Shatagopam K, Monn MF, et al. Risk for *Clostridium difficile* infection after radical cystectomy for bladder cancer: analysis of a contemporary series. Urol Oncol 2015;33(12):503.e17-22.

65. Brown KA, Khanafer N, Daneman N, et al. Meta-analysis of antibiotics and the risk of community-associated *Clostridium difficile* infection. Antimicrob Agents Chemother 2013;57(5):2326–32.

66. Cohen SH, Gerding DN, Johnson S, et al. Clinical practice guidelines for *Clostridium difficile* infection in adults: 2010 update by the Society for Healthcare Epidemiology of America (SHEA) and the Infectious Diseases Society of America (IDSA). Infect Control Hosp Epidemiol 2010;31(5):431–55.

67. Quek ML, Stein JP, Daneshmand S, et al. A critical analysis of perioperative mortality from radical cystectomy. J Urol 2006;175(3 Pt 1):886–9 [discussion: 889–90].

68. McDermott FD, Heeney A, Kelly ME, et al. Systematic review of preoperative, intraoperative and postoperative risk factors for colorectal anastomotic leaks. Br J Surg 2015;102(5):462–79.

69. The American Urological Association: Best practice policy statement on urologic surgery antimicrobial prophylaxis. Available at: https://www.auanet.org/common/pdf/education/clinical-guidance/Antimicrobial-Prophylaxis.pdf. Accessed December 14, 2015.

70. European Association of Urology: Guidelines on urological infections. Available at: http://uroweb.org/wp-content/uploads/17_Urological-infections_LR-II.pdf. Accessed December 14, 2015.

71. Mattei A, Birkhaeuser FD, Baermann C, et al. To stent or not to stent perioperatively the ureteroileal anastomosis of ileal orthotopic bladder substitutes and ileal conduits? Results of a prospective randomized trial. J Urol 2008;179(2):582–6.

72. Mullins JK, Guzzo TJ, Ball MW, et al. Ureteral stents placed at the time of urinary diversion decreases postoperative morbidity. Urol Int 2012;88(1):66–70.

73. Grabe M, Botto H, Cek M, et al. Preoperative assessment of the patient and risk factors for infectious complications and tentative classification of surgical field contamination of urological procedures. World J Urol 2012;30(1):39–50.

74. Darouiche RO, Wall MJ Jr, Itani KM, et al. Chlorhexidine-alcohol versus povidone-iodine for surgical-site antisepsis. N Engl J Med 2010;362(1):18–26.

75. Sorensen LT, Karlsmark T, Gottrup F. Abstinence from smoking reduces incisional wound infection: a randomized controlled trial. Ann Surg 2003; 238(1):1–5.

76. Tang R, Chen HH, Wang YL, et al. Risk factors for surgical site infection after elective resection of the colon and rectum: a single-center prospective study of 2,809 consecutive patients. Ann Surg 2001;234(2):181–9.

77. Liu JJ, Mullane P, Kates M, et al. Infectious complications in transfused patients after radical cystectomy. Can J Urol 2016;23(4):8342–7.

78. Hirose Y, Naiki T, Ando R, et al. Novel closing method using subcutaneous continuous drain for preventing surgical site infections in radical cystectomy. ISRN Urol 2014;2014:897451.

79. Mohan S, Kaoutzanis C, Welch KB, et al. Postoperative hyperglycemia and adverse outcomes in patients undergoing colorectal surgery: results from the Michigan surgical quality collaborative database. Int J Colorectal Dis 2015;30(11):1515–23.

80. Forbes SS, Eskicioglu C, Nathens AB, et al. Evidence-based guidelines for prevention of

perioperative hypothermia. J Am Coll Surg 2009; 209(4):492–503.e1.

81. Tanner J, Padley W, Assadian O, et al. Do surgical care bundles reduce the risk of surgical site infections in patients undergoing colorectal surgery? A systematic review and cohort meta-analysis of 8,515 patients. Surgery 2015;158(1):66–77.

82. Meyer CP, Rios Diaz AJ, Dalela D, et al. Wound dehiscence in a sample of 1 776 cystectomies: identification of predictors and implications for outcomes. BJU Int 2015;117(6B):E95–101.

83. Pannucci CJ, Laird S, Dimick JB, et al. A validated risk model to predict 90-day VTE events in postsurgical patients. Chest 2014;145(3):567–73.

84. Gould MK, Garcia DA, Wren SM, et al. Prevention of VTE in nonorthopedic surgical patients: antithrombotic therapy and prevention of thrombosis, 9th ed: American College of Chest Physicians Evidence-Based Clinical Practice Guidelines. Chest 2012;141(2 Suppl):e227S–277S.

85. Prevention of Deep vein Thrombosis in Patients Undergoing Urologic Surgery: American Urological Association Best Practice Statement. Available at: https://www.auanet.org/common/pdf/education/clinical-guidance/Deep-Vein-Thrombosis.pdf.

86. VanDlac AA, Cowan NG, Chen Y, et al. Timing, incidence and risk factors for venous thromboembolism in patients undergoing radical cystectomy for malignancy: a case for extended duration pharmacological prophylaxis. J Urol 2014;191(4):943–7.

87. Sun AJ, Djaladat H, Schuckman A, et al. Venous thromboembolism following radical cystectomy: significant predictors, comparison of different anticoagulants and timing of events. J Urol 2015; 193(2):565–9.

88. Pariser JJ, Pearce SM, Anderson BB, et al. Extended duration enoxaparin decreases the rate of venous thromboembolic events after radical cystectomy compared to inpatient only subcutaneous heparin. J Urol 2017;197(2):302–7.

89. Bergqvist D, Agnelli G, Cohen AT, et al. Duration of prophylaxis against venous thromboembolism with enoxaparin after surgery for cancer. N Engl J Med 2002;346(13):975–80.

90. Kozminski M, Konnak JW, Grossman HB. Management of rectal injuries during radical cystectomy. J Urol 1989;142(5):1204–5.

91. Varkarakis IM, Chrisofos M, Antoniou N, et al. Evaluation of findings during re-exploration for obstructive ileus after radical cystectomy and ileal-loop urinary diversion: insight into potential technical improvements. BJU Int 2007;99(4):893–7.

92. Stimson CJ, Chang SS, Barocas DA, et al. Early and late perioperative outcomes following radical cystectomy: 90-day readmissions, morbidity and mortality in a contemporary series. J Urol 2010; 184(4):1296–300.

93. Taylor JM, Feifer A, Savage CJ, et al. Evaluating the utility of a preoperative nomogram for predicting 90-day mortality following radical cystectomy for bladder cancer. BJU Int 2012;109(6):855–9.

94. Gregg JR, Cookson MS, Phillips S, et al. Effect of preoperative nutritional deficiency on mortality after radical cystectomy for bladder cancer. J Urol 2011; 185(1):90–6.

95. Novara G, Catto JW, Wilson T, et al. Systematic review and cumulative analysis of perioperative outcomes and complications after robot-assisted radical cystectomy. Eur Urol 2015;67(3):376–401.

96. Bochner BH, Dalbagni G, Sjoberg DD, et al. Comparing open radical cystectomy and robot-assisted laparoscopic radical cystectomy: a randomized clinical trial. Eur Urol 2015;67(6):1042–50.

97. Khan MS, Gan C, Ahmed K, et al. A single-centre early phase randomised controlled three-arm trial of open, robotic, and laparoscopic radical cystectomy (CORAL). Eur Urol 2016;69(4):613–21.

98. Nix J, Smith A, Kurpad R, et al. Prospective randomized controlled trial of robotic versus open radical cystectomy for bladder cancer: perioperative and pathologic results. Eur Urol 2010;57(2): 196–201.

99. Parekh DJ, Messer J, Fitzgerald J, et al. Perioperative outcomes and oncologic efficacy from a pilot prospective randomized clinical trial of open versus robotic assisted radical cystectomy. J Urol 2013;189(2):474–9.

100. Ng CK, Kauffman EC, Lee MM, et al. A comparison of postoperative complications in open versus robotic cystectomy. Eur Urol 2010;57(2):274–81.

101. Anderson CB, Morgan TM, Kappa S, et al. Ureteroenteric anastomotic strictures after radical cystectomy-does operative approach matter? J Urol 2013;189(2):541–7.

102. Hautmann RE, de Petriconi RC, Volkmer BG. 25 years of experience with 1,000 neobladders: long-term complications. J Urol 2011;185(6): 2207–12.

103. Richards KA, Cohn JA, Large MC, et al. The effect of length of ureteral resection on benign ureterointestinal stricture rate in ileal conduit or ileal neobladder urinary diversion following radical cystectomy. Urol Oncol 2015;33(2):65.e1-8.

104. Laven BA, O'Connor RC, Gerber GS, et al. Long-term results of endoureterotomy and open surgical revision for the management of ureteroenteric strictures after urinary diversion. J Urol 2003; 170(4 Pt 1):1226–30.

105. Wolf JS Jr, Elashry OM, Clayman RV. Long-term results of endoureterotomy for benign ureteral and ureteroenteric strictures. J Urol 1997;158(3 Pt 1): 759–64.

106. Large MC, Cohn JA, Kiriluk KJ, et al. The impact of running versus interrupted anastomosis on

ureterointestinal stricture rate after radical cystectomy. J Urol 2013;190(3):923–7.

107. Donahue TF, Bochner BH, Sfakianos JP, et al. Risk factors for the development of parastomal hernia after radical cystectomy. J Urol 2014;191(6): 1708–13.

108. Movassaghi K, Shah SH, Cai J, et al. Incisional and parastomal hernia following radical cystectomy and urinary diversion: the University of Southern California experience. J Urol 2016;196(3):777–81.

109. Donahue TF, Cha EK, Bochner BH. Rationale and early experience with prophylactic placement of mesh to prevent parastomal hernia formation after ileal conduit urinary diversion and cystectomy for bladder cancer. Curr Urol Rep 2016;17(2):9.

110. Diener MK, Voss S, Jensen K, et al. Elective midline laparotomy closure: the INLINE systematic review and meta-analysis. Ann Surg 2010;251(5):843–56.

111. Deerenberg EB, Harlaar JJ, Steyerberg EW, et al. Small bites versus large bites for closure of abdominal midline incisions (STITCH): a double-blind, multicentre, randomised controlled trial. Lancet 2015;386(10000):1254–60.

112. Simon J, Bartsch G Jr, Kufer R, et al. Neobladder emptying failure in males: incidence, etiology and therapeutic options. J Urol 2006;176(4 Pt 1): 1468–72 [discussion: 1472].

113. Anderson CB, Cookson MC, Chang SS, et al. Voiding function in women with orthotopic neobladder urinary diversion. J Urol 2012;188(1):200–4.

114. Anderson CB. Voiding function in women with orthotopic neobladders. Curr Bladder Dysfunct Rep 2015;10(4):411–8.

115. Holmes DG, Thrasher JB, Park GY, et al. Long-term complications related to the modified Indiana pouch. Urology 2002;60(4):603–6.

116. Ardelt PU, Woodhouse CR, Riedmiller H, et al. The efferent segment in continent cutaneous urinary diversion: a comprehensive review of the literature. BJU Int 2012;109(2):288–97.

117. McAndrew HF, Malone PS. Continent catheterizable conduits: which stoma, which conduit and which reservoir? BJU Int 2002;89(1):86–9.

118. Wiesner C, Stein R, Pahernik S, et al. Long-term followup of the intussuscepted ileal nipple and the in situ, submucosally embedded appendix as continence mechanisms of continent urinary diversion with the cutaneous ileocecal pouch (Mainz pouch I). J Urol 2006;176(1):155–9 [discussion: 159–60].

119. Watson HS, Bauer SB, Peters CA, et al. Comparative urodynamics of appendiceal and ureteral Mitrofanoff conduits in children. J Urol 1995;154(2 Pt 2):878–82.

120. Marien T, Robles J, Kammann TM, et al. Characterization of urolithiasis in patients following lower urinary tract reconstruction with intestinal segments. J Endourol 2017;31(3):217–22.

121. Okhunov Z, Duty B, Smith AD, et al. Management of urolithiasis in patients after urinary diversions. BJU Int 2011;108(3):330–6.

122. van Hemelrijck M, Thorstenson A, Smith P, et al. Risk of in-hospital complications after radical cystectomy for urinary bladder carcinoma: population-based follow-up study of 7608 patients. BJU Int 2013;112(8):1113–20.

123. Ferriero M, Guaglianone S, Papalia R, et al. Risk assessment of stone formation in stapled orthotopic ileal neobladder. J Urol 2015;193(3):891–6.

124. Terai A, Ueda T, Kakehi Y, et al. Urinary calculi as a late complication of the Indiana continent urinary diversion: comparison with the Kock pouch procedure. J Urol 1996;155(1):66–8.

125. Hensle TW, Bingham J, Lam J, et al. Preventing reservoir calculi after augmentation cystoplasty and continent urinary diversion: the influence of an irrigation protocol. BJU Int 2004;93(4):585–7.

126. Mansson W, Bakke A, Bergman B, et al. Perforation of continent urinary reservoirs. Scandinavian experience. Scand J Urol Nephrol 1997;31(6):529–32.

127. Carmel ME, Goldman HB, Moore CK, et al. Transvaginal neobladder vaginal fistula repair after radical cystectomy with orthotopic urinary diversion in women. Neurourol Urodyn 2016;35(1):90–4.

Secondary Tumors After Urinary Diversion

Roger Li, MD, Janet E. Baack Kukreja, MD, MPH, Ashish M. Kamat, MD, MBBS*

KEYWORDS

- Urinary diversion • Secondary malignancy • Ureterosigmoidostomy • Cystoplasty • Neobladder
- Urinary conduit

KEY POINTS

- Secondary malignancies are estimated to arise in 0.18% to 15.00% of patients undergoing various urinary diversions.
- Secondary malignancies occur most frequently after ureterosigmoidostomies and cystoplasties.
- Long-term vigilance is essential because reported latency period ranges from 2 to more than 30 years, with most lesions detected a decade after urinary diversion.
- Current surveillance protocols include patient history, imaging, urinalysis, and endoscopic evaluation, with biopsies reserved for suspicious lesions.

INTRODUCTION

The development of secondary malignancies after interposition of urinary and bowel mucosa has been recognized since its first description by Hammer in 1929.[1] Altogether, more than 300 secondary tumors have been reported within various urinary diversion constructs.[2] The risk for cancer arising from the intestinal segments used for urinary diversion has been estimated to be between 8- and 477-fold higher.[3,4] Preclinical and clinical studies have been conducted to define the mechanism of carcinogenesis in this unique microenvironment with several interesting hypotheses. In this review, we summarize the current knowledge on the developmental patterns and carcinogenic mechanisms of secondary malignancy after urinary diversions. The pressing need for consensus guidelines pertaining to cancer screening after urinary diversion is also highlighted.

URETEROSIGMOIDOSTOMY

Historically, ureterosigmoidostomy (**Table 1**) was the urinary diversion of choice in patients with nonfunctional bladders.[5] However, the propensity for neoplastic changes at the ureterosigmoid junction has been recognized since the early 1960s.[6] Although the development of junctional adenocarcinoma has been described as early as 2 years after ureterosigmoidostomy creation, the mean latency period ranges between 20 and 26 years.[7]

The incidence of adenocarcinoma has been found to be cumulative over the duration of the diversion.[8] Compared with other exstrophy patients, those having undergone ureterosigmoidostomy were 7000 times as likely to develop malignancies.[9] Described incidences range from 2% to 15%.[7] The majority of tumors follow the typical course of transforming from polyps to adenoma, and eventually to adenocarcinoma.[7,10]

The unacceptably high incidence of secondary malignancies has spelled the end to the routine use of ureterosigmoidostomies. In the unlikely event that diversion using the sigmoid colon is necessary, every effort must be made for its use as an isolated segment to prevent mixing urine with stool.[11–14] Owing to its limited usage, whether this alternative sigmoid diversion leads to reduced

Disclosure Statement: The authors have nothing they wish to disclose.
Department of Urology, The University of Texas MD Anderson Cancer Center, 1515 Holcombe Boulevard, Unit 1373, Houston, TX 77030, USA
* Corresponding author.
E-mail address: akamat@mdanderson.org

Table 1
Ureterosigmoidostomy series

	Number of Patients	Incidence (%)	Latency Period (y)	Histology
Azimuddin et al,[7] 1999	—	2–15	20–26	Adenocarcinoma
Tollefson et al,[65]	51	0	10–45	—
Gobert et al,	42	2.30	—	Adenocarcinoma
Hurlstone et al,	42	24	1–26	Adenocarcinoma

tumorigenesis remains relatively unknown. Instead, urologists have mainly used segments from elsewhere in the intestinal tract for the purpose of urinary diversion.

URINARY DIVERSION USING ISOLATED GUT
Early Findings

Owing to its rarity, early attempts to study the patterns of secondary malignancy after urinary diversion using isolated gut were limited to small single-center case reports and series. From a cohort of 645 patients after urinary reconstruction, Ali-El-Dein and colleagues[15] found 6 patients developing secondary malignancy at the uroinstestinal junction. Specifically, cancer was discovered in 3 of 54 patients (5.5%) after ileocystoplasty, 2 of 258 patients (0.8%) after ileal ureter, and 1 of 348 patients (0.3%) after ileal conduit. Unlike the prevalence of adenoma and adenocarcinoma subsequent to ureterosigmoidostomy, a wide range of pathologies including urothelial carcinoma, squamous cell carcinoma, mucinous adenoma and adenocarcinoma were found. Another pattern that emerged was the increased incidence subsequent to cystoplasties compared with other forms of intestinal diversion. However, the small sample size made it impossible to draw conclusions regarding secondary tumor incidence relative to the primary indication for urinary diversion, histologic makeup of the secondary tumors, origin of the diverting intestinal segment, or whether diversion was fashioned for urinary continence.

The analysis of an exhaustive list of 81 secondary tumors helped to shed light on some of these questions.[16] With regard to the primary indication for urinary diversion, secondary malignant tumors occurred much quicker after diversion for malignant disease at a median of 8 years versus 21.5 years for benign disease. In contrast, the latency period before developing benign and malignant secondary tumors were comparable in patients diverted for benign indications (median of 22.0 years vs 21.5 years, respectively). This is in contrast with the adenoma–adenocarcinoma sequence spanning 6 years observed after ureterosigmoidostomies.[4]

With regard to the origin of the diverting intestinal segment, 41.8% of the evaluable malignant tumors developed in isolated colonic segments, whereas 58.2% developed in ileal segments.[16] However, because the number of urinary diversions using each segment was unknown, no conclusions could be drawn regarding the relative incidence in the different intestinal segments. Nevertheless, it is clear that secondary malignancies can arise from diversion using either ileum or colon.

Of the evaluable tumors, 80.8% arose in continent urinary reservoirs versus 19.2% in conduits.[16] This finding corroborated with the observation made by Ali-El-Dein and associates that more secondary malignancies occurred in cystoplasties than conduits. Compounded with the lower usage rate of cystoplasties, the incidence of secondary malignancy seemed higher in this setting. However, the fact that conduits are frequently used for malignant indications has to be considered. These patients have a poor prognosis and may not outlive the latency period before developing secondary malignancies.

Focus on Cystoplasty

Even with limited data, a trend toward a higher incidence of secondary cancer was evident after cystoplasty. Interestingly, cystoplasties from early studies were mostly performed in adults for contractile bladders secondary to genitourinary infections, most commonly tuberculosis and schistosomiasis.[15,16] Thus, in these patients, carcinogenesis may not be solely due to the urinary reconstruction, because it was suspected that the infections themselves could lead to cancer.[17,18] Furthermore, the patients' age and history of exposure to environmental carcinogens, such as tobacco smoke, can also confound the described incidences.

Beginning in the 1980s, augmentation cystoplasty was increasingly adopted for pediatric patients with nonfunctioning bladders owing to exstrophy, posterior urethral valves, or neuropathic etiologies. As these patients reached latency period for developing malignancies, they provided important insight into the patterns of carcinogenesis subsequent to urinary diversions. A flurry of case series emerged documenting malignancies found in augmented bladders constructed using segments from the entire length of the gastrointestinal tract.

Initially, malignancies were reported predominantly in cystoplasties incorporating ileum and colon.[19,20] Single-center experiences revealed incidence rates ranging from 1.2% to 4.6%, with a median latency interval of between 19 and 32 years. Histologic findings were varied, consisting of transitional cell carcinoma and adenocarcinoma. An important finding was the increased incidence in immunosuppressed patients after renal transplantation. Husmann and Rathbun[19] reported an alarming 20% rate of tumor formation in 15 transplant recipients. The authors further noted positive reactivity to cytomegalovirus and Epstein-Barr virus in these patients and postulated that virally induced oncogenic pathways may be in play. In contrast, the prevalence of asymptomatic bacteriuria was not found to correlate with tumor incidence.[19]

The lack of association between infection and tumorigenesis contradicted the prevailing thought that oncogenesis stemmed from chronic irritation owing to infections and mucus.[21–23] In fact, the proposition to use gastrocystoplasty was partly predicated on the lower rates of subsequent infection, mucus production, and stone formation.[24] The superiority of gastrocystoplasties was seemingly validated by a small histologic study examining endoscopic biopsies taken from the bladder, augment and anastomosis at 2- to 4-year intervals postoperatively.[24] Compared with colocystoplasty, gastrocystoplasty patients exhibited no bladder calculi, fewer urinary infections, and mild histologic changes with no incipient malignancy. Vajda and colleagues[24] went as far as suggesting that gastric mucosa was more recalcitrant to the formation of malignant lesions owing to their acidic microenvironment and lower rate of bacterial colonization.

Thereafter, several case reports/series of carcinoma in gastrocystoplasties began to appear.[25–27] Castellan and colleagues[26] and Vemulakonda and colleagues[27] reported rates of 2.8% and 3.4%, and median latency periods of 13 years and 16.5 years, respectively. Adenocarcinoma was the most common histology, along with anaplastic signet ring cell and transitional carcinomas also being described.[25,26] In addition, accompanying premalignant lesions such as atrophy, urothelial and intestinal metaplasia, and carcinoma in situ were frequently found in the surgical specimens.[25,26] Of concern, no discrete lesions were seen on cystoscopy in any of the patients, and the majority had locally advanced or metastatic disease at presentation. Again, an increased risk was observed in the immunosuppressed population: of the 7 cases reported, 2 occurred in transplant recipients.

A recent metaanalysis summed up the findings for 64 malignant transformations after cystoplasties reported in the literature.[28] Estimated rates ranged from 0 to 272 per 100,000 patients per year, with no difference between gastroplasties, ileoplasties, and colocystoplasties. The median latency period, however, was shorter after gastroplasties versus ileoplasties and colocystoplasties (14 years vs 21 years and 20 years, respectively). Just 10% of the tumors occurred within 10 years of surgery. With respect to pathology, adenocarcinoma was the most common histologic type, making up 50% of the tumors. Of those staged, 35.3% were locally advanced ($\geq$pT3) and 31.2% were lymph node positive.

In considering malignancies after cystoplasties, several points are worthy of mention. The rate of carcinogenesis needs to be placed in the context of incidence of bladder cancer in the general population at large, estimated to be between 2.5 and 10.1 per 100,000 patients per year by Husmann[3]; cystoplasties using various gastrointestinal segments increased bladder cancer rates by 7- to 15-fold. However, this comparison underestimates the oncogenic potential of the dysfunctional bladder owing to exstrophy, neuropathy, or posterior urethral valves.[29] In a thoughtful case control study, Higuchi and colleagues[30] demonstrated no difference in cancer incidence in dysfunctional bladder patients managed with ileal or colonic bladder augment versus intermittent catheterization (4.6% vs 2.6%; P = .54).

Additionally, as discussed, whether the use of gastrocystoplasty increases cancer risk is debated. Husmann[3] cites the malignant transformation at the junction of gastric–small bowel anastomosis in Billroth II procedures as evidence for the increased malignant potential associated with gastric patches. The prevalence of premalignant lesion in gastrocystoplasties was also used to support the increased risk of malignancy.[3] However, similar rates of malignancies have been reported in single center case series for gastroplasties versus ileoplasties and colocystoplasties.[19,20,26,27] Moreover, in the metaanalysis encompassing all 3 types of augments, no difference in incidence was found.[28] Nevertheless, the failure of cystoscopic screening and the advanced staging on presentation are of concern.

The German Perspective

In the most comprehensive effort to date, the records of 17,758 urinary diversion patients from 44 German clinics were reviewed, yielding 32 secondary tumors for an incidence of 0.18%.[2] For the first time, the secondary malignancy patterns after ureterosigmoidostomies, cystoplasties, and diversions using isolated intestinal segments could be directly compared. Incidence of ureterosigmoidostomies (22-fold) and cystoplasties (13-fold) were found to be much higher than all other continent urinary diversions. The median latency periods for the development of benign and malignant secondary lesions were 6 and 12 years for diversions using isolated intestinal segments, 18 and 21.5 years for cystoplasties, and 22.5 and 29 years for ureterosigmoidostomies (**Table 2**). The vast majority (94%) of tumors developing after ureterosigmoidostomy occurred at the ureteroenteric junction. In contrast, 44% of the tumors arose exclusively from the intestinal portion of the reconstructed reservoir after diversion using isolated intestinal segments. Histologically, all but one of the tumors arising after ureterosigmoidostomies were adenoma or adenocarcinoma, whereas those found after diversion using isolated intestinal segments consisted of adenocarcinoma, squamous cell carcinoma, and desmoid and carcinoid tumors.

In addition, the risk for a secondary malignancy was different depending on whether the diversion was fashioned for urinary continence, as well as the origin of the diversional segment. Continent diversions (0.13%) were found to have higher tumor risk than their incontinent counterparts (0.03%; $P = .009$). Of the continent diversions, those incorporating colon (1.29%) were at higher risk for developing secondary tumors than ileoneobladders (0.05%; $P = .0001$). Of the incontinent diversions, a trend for higher malignant potential was found in colonic conduits (0.23%) than ileoconduits (0.02%; $P = .2$). Overall, diversions incorporating colon (0.27%) were found to have a higher risk than those incorporating ileum (0.03%; $P = .00001$). Furthermore, it was noted that all tumors within colonic diversions arose from the intestinal component, whereas those in ileal diversions originated from the uroenteric anastomosis. From this, it can be speculated that the higher incidence of secondary malignancies in colonic diversions can at least be partly due to the general higher tumor risk in colon versus the ileum.

MECHANISM OF CARCINOGENESIS

Studies have been conducted using preclinical murine models to better understand carcinogenesis

Table 2
Isolated intestinal series

	Diversion Type	No. of Patients	Incidence (%)	Latency Period (y)	Histology
Ali-El-Dein et al,[15] 2002	Cystoplasty, ileal conduit, ileoureter	645	0.9	4–32	Adenocarcinoma, urothelial carcinoma, squamous cell carcinoma
Husmann and Rathbun,[19] 2008	Cystoplasty	153	4.6	32	Urothelial carcinoma, adenocarcinoma
Soergel et al,[20] 2004	Cystoplasty	260	1.2	19	Urothelial carcinoma
Castellan et al,[26] 2007	Gastrocystoplasty	119	3.4	12.75	Adenocarcinoma, urothelial carcinoma
Vermulakonda et al,[27] 2008	Gastrocystoplasty	72	2.8	14	Adenocarcinoma
Kalble et al,[2] 2011	Ureterosigmoidostomy, cystoplasty, orthotopic colonic neobladder, ileal neobladder, ileocecal pouch, ileal conduit, colon conduit	17,758	0.2	6–29	Adenoma, adenocarcinoma, squamous cell carcinoma, desmoid tumor, carcinoid tumor

after urinary diversions that expose bowel segments to urine. Several factors lead to the increased incidence of malignancies in urinary diversions. Because malignant neoplasms were frequently found in ureterosigmoidostomies, the mixing of urine and stool was first implicated in the onset of carcinogenesis. Crissey and colleagues[31] devised a rat model in which tumors were found after vesicosigmoidostomies. More important, tumorigenesis was prevented using colostomies constructed proximal to the anastomosis, thereby eliminating the admixture of urine and stool. The authors hypothesized that urinary hydrolytic enzymes activated carcinogenic precursors present in the stool, leading to tumorigenesis at the junction of ureterosigmoidostomies.

Further studies pinpointed nitrosamine (N,N-dimethylnitrosamine) as the mutagenic agent.[11] These compounds not only had malignant potential, but also were found to gradually increase in the rectal slurry with complete penetrance in female Sprague-Dawley rats undergoing ureterosigmoidostomies by week 14.[32] Similarly, increased levels were detected in the rectal slurry and urine collected from patients with bladder augments or enteric conduits.[33,34]

The mechanism of nitrosamine activation was thought to be due to bacterial nitrate reductase, the essential catalytic enzyme for N-nitrosation.[35] Studies in Sprague-Dawley rats indicated an increased rate of tumorigenesis with concurrent urinary tract infections and exposure to the carcinogen 5-nitrofuran, N-[4-(5-nitro-2furyl)-2-thiazolyl] formamide (FANFT).[36] Furthermore, bacteriuria was frequently observed in patients after urinary diversions using enteric segments.[19] As such, some believed that the use of stomach patch for diversion can reduce the incidence of bacteriuria and, in turn, the rate of secondary malignancies. However, the perceived advantage of gastrocystoplasties as a result of less frequent bacteriuria was debunked by the emergence of multiple case series documenting secondary malignancies,[20,26,27,37,38] as well as multiple histologic studies using rat gastrocystoplasty models that consistently demonstrated proliferative lesions appearing at the urogastric anastomosis.[39–41] Additionally, later studies showed similar rates of bacteriuria between patients with and without secondary malignancies after cystoplasties,[30] raising the question whether bacteriuria truly played a role in carcinogenesis.

Notwithstanding its unclear mechanism of activation, nitrosamines are thought to promote secondary malignancies by inducing ornithine decarboxylase (ODC), an enzyme essential for polyamine biosynthesis.[42] Increased levels of ODC and polyamine have been found in colorectal carcinomas compared with normal rectal mucosa.[43] In vitro and in vivo experiments have linked mutant APC (the most commonly mutated tumor suppressor gene in colon cancer) to elevation in c-MYC and ODC activity, leading to increased polyamine production.[44,45] Germane to the development of secondary malignancies after urinary diversion, increased ODC levels have also been found at the vesicosigmoidostomy anastomotic sites compared with normal colonic mucosa in Wistar rats.[46]

However, the theory of nitrosamine-induced carcinogenesis has been challenged by more recent experimental and clinical data demonstrating a lack of association between high nitrosamine levels and the onset of carcinoma.[4,47] In addition, inhibition of nitrosamine by ascorbic acid failed to reduce the rate of cancer occurrence.[48] Furthermore, several reports described malignancies at the remnant ureterosigmoidostomy junction found years after additional diversion procedures rendered the junction free of urine.[49,50] These findings impugned the notion that the carcinogen was derived from the mixture of urine and stool.

Postoperative inflammatory changes may play a large role in the neoplastic changes occurring at the urointestinal junction.[51] Histologic studies in postdiversion intestinal segments revealed lymphoplasmocytic infiltration.[52] Substances released by the infiltrating immune cells may promote carcinogenesis in the uniquely juxtaposed uroenteric epithelium.[16] For example, DNA damage brought on by the increased production of reactive oxygen species from activated macrophages[53] may be precipitated by the antioxidant deficiency in the postenterocystoplasty microenvironment.[54] Additionally, increased levels of growth factors, cytokines, and cyclooxygenase-2 activity found at the urointestinal junction may also promote tissue proliferation, leading to eventual carcinogenesis.[16]

The juxtaposition of urinary and intestinal tissues within the heterotypic uroenteric chimera may also lead to aberrant stromal–epithelial cell signaling. Tissue recombinant experiments revealed plasticity of the urothelium to change into intestinal-like epithelium under the influence of adjacent rectal mesenchyme.[55] This transformational potential demonstrates the possibility for adenocarcinoma to arise from the urothelium. Whether the stromal–epithelial interaction is capable of promoting carcinogenesis warrants further investigation.

Finally, the increased risk for secondary malignancies in immunocompromised patients after renal transplant has been noted.[3] Moreover, these malignancies were found in patients testing positive for oncogenic viruses, suggesting a potential causal mechanism. In contrast, the possibility of oncogenesis as a result of failed immune surveillance also needs to be considered.

Despite the extensive efforts with preclinical animal studies and histologic evaluations, the mechanism of carcinogenesis in urinary diversion constructs has yet to be defined clearly. Far from being a singular entity, secondary malignancies are immensely heterogeneous with respect to latency period, tissue origin, histology, and perhaps mechanism of onset. Their rarity and the long latency periods make secondary malignancies especially difficult to study. However, the chimeric nature of urinary diversions offers a unique model to study potential mechanisms of carcinogenesis owing to the juxtaposition of tissues of different embryologic origins.

SURVEILLANCE

Owing to the prevalence of secondary malignancies after ureterosigmoidostomies, clear guidelines have been established mandating annual flexible sigmoidoscopy starting a decade after surgery.[56] Unfortunately, no consensus guideline exists for cancer screening after other forms of urinary diversion. There is clearly the need for a well-defined, evidence-based guidelines for cancer surveillance, especially with the use of cystoplasties in the pediatric urology realm.

Most experts suggest annual screenings with history and physical, endoscopy, and urine cytology to start 3 to 10 years after urinary diversion and cystoplasty,[16,20,57] with the caveat of decreasing the frequency in patients with cancer and conduits.[57] However, all of the proposed screening procedures are fraught with shortcomings. From the history and physical examination, the clinician may elicit critical symptoms such as hematuria. However, as many as 46% of patients after urinary diversion will have hematuria on urinalysis,[58] reducing the specificity to unacceptably low levels. Urine cytology is less reliable, because the enteric epithelium had been found to give rise to exfoliated ileal or colonic epithelial cell clusters resembling urothelial carcinoma.[59] In addition, chronic pyuria and intermittent catheterization by patients after urinary diversion can also lead to cellular artifacts used to identify atypia.[59] Even endoscopy, the benchmark of cancer surveillance in the urinary and enteric tracts, had been found to be inconsistent in the postdiversion cancer screening.[27] As a result, some authors have recommended interval biopsies to be incorporated into the surveillance regimen.[27,60]

As with all other screening protocols, the cost-to-benefit ratio needs to be assessed carefully. To that end, Husmann[3] estimated that more than 980 annual cystoscopies are required to find 1 secondary cancer in cystoplasty patients. In another study, Hamid and colleagues[60] found no secondary malignancies in 92 asymptomatic patients undergoing routine annual surveillance cystoscopy and biopsy 10 years after cystoplasty. Using a Markov model, Kokorowski and colleagues[61] estimated an incremental cost of $273,718 per life-year gained.

In an attempt to improve detection, additional screening methods had been explored. Although some have shown efficacy, none has yet been adopted into clinical practice. Ivil and colleagues[62] demonstrated the ability of fluorescence in situ hybridization to detect chromosomal losses and gains suggestive of genetic instability. In this study, fluorescence in situ hybridization was also found to have greater sensitivity than conventional urine cytology. A similar study examining the use of fluorescence in situ hybridization for surveillance after radical cystectomy for bladder cancer demonstrated high false-positive rates, but an impressive 99.5% negative predictive value.[63] Urinary microsatellite analysis has also been shown to be capable of identifying secondary adenocarcinoma arising several years after bladder augmentation.[64]

TREATMENT

No clear guideline exists for the management of secondary malignancies arising after urinary diversion. However, principles in the treatment of urothelial cancer are followed. In addition, therapeutic strategies are guided by the pathologic composition of the tumor. Although endoscopic resection followed by vigilant surveillance may suffice for benign or superficial lesions, radical extirpative surgery may be required for invasive tumors. As discussed, added caution is necessary during the surveillance of gastrocystoplasties, because no discrete lesions may be detected on endoscopic screening, leading to the development of locally invasive or metastatic disease. Owing to the rarity of the disease, no meaningful cancer-specific outcomes have been compiled subsequent to surgical intervention.

SUMMARY

Much has been learned about the development of secondary malignancies after urinary diversion. Described incidence rates range between 0.18%

to 15.00%, with ureterosigmoidostomies and cystoplasties at much greater risk. The latency period ranges between 2 years to more than 30 years, thus making long-term surveillance critical in this population. Current surveillance protocols include patient history, imaging, urinalysis, and endoscopic evaluation, with biopsies reserved for suspicious lesions.

Some knowledge gaps do, however, remain. First, the mechanism of onset remains elusive. Because cystoplasties are increasingly used for children with dysfunctional bladders, and the survival of patients undergoing urinary diversions improve, effective screening protocols are direly needed to prevent the dreaded consequence of cancer metastasis. Equally important, a better grasp of the oncogenic mechanism leading to secondary malignancies after urinary diversion may help to further the understanding of cancers of the urinary and intestinal tracts.

REFERENCES

1. Hammer E. Cancer du colon sigmoide dix ans après implantation des uretères d'une vessie exstrophiée. J Urol (Paris) 1929;28:260–3.
2. Kalble T, Hofmann I, Riedmiller H, et al. Tumor growth in urinary diversion: a multicenter analysis. Eur Urol 2011;60(5):1081–6.
3. Husmann DA. Malignancy after gastrointestinal augmentation in childhood. Ther Adv Urol 2009; 1(1):5–11.
4. Kalble T, Tricker AR, Friedl P, et al. Ureterosigmoidostomy: long-term results, risk of carcinoma and etiological factors for carcinogenesis. J Urol 1990; 144(5):1110–4.
5. Corbett CR, Lloyd-Davies RW. Long-term survival after urinary diversion. A reappraisal of ureterosigmoidostomy. Eur Urol 1976;2(5):221–5.
6. Amar AD. Neoplastic obstruction of the ureterosigmoid anastomosis. J Urol 1961;86:334–5.
7. Azimuddin K, Khubchandani IT, Stasik JJ, et al. Neoplasia after ureterosigmoidostomy. Dis Colon Rectum 1999;42(12):1632–8.
8. Arakawa K, Ishihara S, Kawai K, et al. Asynchronous bilateral anastomosis site sigmoid colon cancer after ureterosigmoidostomy: a case report. World J Surg Oncol 2016;14(1):180.
9. Eraklis AJ, Folkman MJ. Adenocarcinoma at the site of ureterosigmoidostomies for exstrophy of the bladder. J Pediatr Surg 1978;13(6d):730–4.
10. Dunn M, Roberts JB, Smith PJ. Benign tumours developing at the site of ureterosigmoidostomy. Br J Urol 1979;51(4):260–3.
11. Malone MJ, Khauli RB, Lowell J. Use of small and large bowel in renal transplantation. Urol Clin North Am 1997;24(4):837–43.
12. Boyce WH, Kroovand RL. The Boyce-Vest operation for exstrophy of the bladder. 35 years later. Urol Clin North Am 1986;13(2):307–20.
13. Carswell JJ 3rd, Skeel DA, Witherington R, et al. Neoplasia at the site of ureterosigmoidostomy. J Urol 1976;115(6):750–2.
14. Kroovand RL. Isolated ureterosigmoidostomy and isolated vesicorectal anastomosis. The rectal bladder. Urol Clin North Am 1991;18(4):603–8.
15. Ali-El-Dein B, El-Tabey N, Abdel-Latif M, et al. Late uro-ileal cancer after incorporation of ileum into the urinary tract. J Urol 2002;167(1):84–8.
16. Austen M, Kalble T. Secondary malignancies in different forms of urinary diversion using isolated gut. J Urol 2004;172(3):831–8.
17. Khalaf I, Shokeir A, Shalaby M. Urologic complications of genitourinary schistosomiasis. World J Urol 2012;30(1):31–8.
18. Takayama K, Kumazawa J, Minoda K. Bladder tumor occurring in the contracted bladder following urinary tract tuberculosis. Eur Urol 1986;12(6):448–50.
19. Husmann DA, Rathbun SR. Long-term follow up of enteric bladder augmentations: the risk for malignancy. J Pediatr Urol 2008;4(5):381–5 [discussion: 386].
20. Soergel TM, Cain MP, Misseri R, et al. Transitional cell carcinoma of the bladder following augmentation cystoplasty for the neuropathic bladder. J Urol 2004;172(4 Pt 2):1649–51 [discussion: 1651–2].
21. Adams MC, Mitchell ME, Rink RC. Gastrocystoplasty: an alternative solution to the problem of urological reconstruction in the severely compromised patient. J Urol 1988;140(5 Pt 2):1152–6.
22. DeFoor W, Minevich E, Reeves D, et al. Gastrocystoplasty: long-term followup. J Urol 2003;170(4 Pt 2): 1647–9 [discussion: 1649–50].
23. Sheldon CA, Gilbert A, Wacksman J, et al. Gastrocystoplasty: technical and metabolic characteristics of the most versatile childhood bladder augmentation modality. J Pediatr Surg 1995;30(2):283–7 [discussion: 287–8].
24. Vajda P, Kaiser L, Magyarlaki T, et al. Histological findings after colocystoplasty and gastrocystoplasty. J Urol 2002;168(2):698–701 [discussion: 701].
25. Baydar DE, Allan RW, Castellan M, et al. Anaplastic signet ring cell carcinoma arising in gastrocystoplasty. Urology 2005;65(6):1226.
26. Castellan M, Gosalbez R, Perez-Brayfield M, et al. Tumor in bladder reservoir after gastrocystoplasty. J Urol 2007;178(4 Pt 2):1771–4 [discussion: 1774].
27. Vemulakonda VM, Lendvay TS, Shnorhavorian M, et al. Metastatic adenocarcinoma after augmentation gastrocystoplasty. J Urol 2008;179(3):1094–7.
28. Biardeau X, Chartier-Kastler E, Rouprêt M, et al. Risk of malignancy after augmentation cystoplasty: a systematic review. Neurourol Urodyn 2016;35(6):675–82.
29. Austin JC, Elliott S, Cooper CS. Patients with spina bifida and bladder cancer: atypical presentation,

advanced stage and poor survival. J Urol 2007; 178(3 Pt 1):798–801.

30. Higuchi TT, Granberg CF, Fox JA, et al. Augmentation cystoplasty and risk of neoplasia: fact, fiction and controversy. J Urol 2010;184(6):2492–6.

31. Crissey MM, Steele GD, Gittes RF. Rat model for carcinogenesis in ureterosigmoidostomy. Science 1980;207(4435):1079–80.

32. Cohen MS, Hilz ME, Davis CP, et al. Urinary carcinogen [nitrosamine] production in a rat animal model for ureterosigmoidostomy. J Urol 1987; 138(2):449–52.

33. Nurse DE, Mundy AR. Assessment of the malignant potential of cystoplasty. Br J Urol 1989;64(5): 489–92.

34. Stewart M, Hill MJ, Pugh RC, et al. The role of N-nitrosamine in carcinogenesis at the ureterocolic anastomosis. Br J Urol 1981;53(2):115–8.

35. Calmels S, Ohshima H, Bartsch H. Nitrosamine formation by denitrifying and non-denitrifying bacteria: implication of nitrite reductase and nitrate reductase in nitrosation catalysis. J Gen Microbiol 1988;134(1): 221–6.

36. Johansson SL, Anderstrom C, von Schultz L, et al. Enhancement of N-[4-(5-nitro-2-furyl)-2-thiazolyl] formamide-induced carcinogenesis by urinary tract infection in rats. Cancer Res 1987;47(2):559–62.

37. Qiu H, Kordunskaya S, Yantiss RK. Transitional cell carcinoma arising in the gastric remnant following gastrocystoplasty: a case report and review of the literature. Int J Surg Pathol 2003;11(2):143–7.

38. Zhang X, Gupta R, Nicastri AD. Bladder adenocarcinoma following gastrocystoplasty. J Pediatr Urol 2010;6(5):525–7.

39. Buson H, Diaz DC, Manivel JC, et al. The development of tumors in experimental gastroenterocystoplasty. J Urol 1993;150(2 Pt 2):730–3.

40. Little JS Jr, Klee LW, Hoover DM, et al. Long-term histopathological changes observed in rats subjected to augmentation cystoplasty. J Urol 1994; 152(2 Pt 2):720–4.

41. Close CE, Tekgul S, Ganesan GS, et al. Flow cytometry analysis of proliferative lesions at the gastrocystoplasty anastomosis. J Urol 2003;169(1):365–8.

42. Rial NS, Meyskens FL, Gerner EW. Polyamines as mediators of APC-dependent intestinal carcinogenesis and cancer chemoprevention. Essays Biochem 2009;46:111–24.

43. Hixson LJ, Garewal HS, McGee DL, et al. Ornithine decarboxylase and polyamines in colorectal neoplasia and mucosa. Cancer Epidemiol Biomarkers Prev 1993;2(4):369–74.

44. Erdman SH, Ignatenko NA, Powell MB, et al. APC-dependent changes in expression of genes influencing polyamine metabolism, and consequences for gastrointestinal carcinogenesis, in the Min mouse. Carcinogenesis 1999;20(9):1709–13.

45. Fultz KE, Gerner EW. APC-dependent regulation of ornithine decarboxylase in human colon tumor cells. Mol Carcinog 2002;34(1):10–8.

46. Weber TR, Westfall SH, Steinhardt GF, et al. Malignancy associated with ureterosigmoidostomy: detection by mucosa ornithine decarboxylase. J Pediatr Surg 1988;23(12):1091–4.

47. Kalble T, Tricker AR, Mohring K, et al. The role of nitrate, nitrite and N-nitrosamines in carcinogenesis of colon tumours following ureterosigmoidostomy. Urol Res 1990;18(2):123–9.

48. Stribling M, Cohen MS, Fagan JD, et al. The effect of ascorbic acid on urinary nitrosamines and tumor development in a rat animal model for ureterosigmoidostomy. Dallas (TX): AUA; 1989 [abstract: 540].

49. Schipper H, Decter A. Carcinoma of the colon arising at ureteral implant sites despite early external diversion: pathogenetic and clinical implications. Cancer 1981;47(8):2062–5.

50. Weinstein T, Zevin D, Kyzer S, et al. Adenocarcinoma at ureterosigmoidostomy junction in a renal transplant recipient 15 years after conversion to ileal conduit. Clin Nephrol 1995;44(2):125–7.

51. Gittes RF. Carcinogenesis in ureterosigmoidostomy. Urol Clin North Am 1986;13(2):201–5.

52. Parenti A, Aragona F, Bortuzzo G, et al. Abnormal patterns of mucin secretion in ileal neobladder mucosa: evidence of preneoplastic lesion? Eur Urol 1999;35(2):98–101.

53. Weitzman SA, Weitberg AB, Clark EP, et al. Phagocytes as carcinogens: malignant transformation produced by human neutrophils. Science 1985;227(4691):1231–3.

54. Barrington JW, Jones A, James D, et al. Antioxidant deficiency following clam enterocystoplasty. Br J Urol 1997;80(2):238–42.

55. Li Y, Liu W, Hayward SW, et al. Plasticity of the urothelial phenotype: effects of gastro-intestinal mesenchyme/stroma and implications for urinary tract reconstruction. Differentiation 2000;66(2–3):126–35.

56. Woodhouse CR. Guidelines for monitoring of patients with ureterosigmoidostomy. Gut 2002; 51(Suppl 5):V15–6.

57. Filmer RB, Spencer JR. Malignancies in bladder augmentations and intestinal conduits. J Urol 1990; 143(4):671–8.

58. Husmann DA, Fox JA, Higuchi TT. Malignancy following bladder augmentation: recommendations for long-term follow-up and cancer screening. AUA Update Ser 2011;30(24):221–8.

59. Watarai Y, Satoh H, Matubara M, et al. Comparison of urine cytology between the ileal conduit and Indiana pouch. Acta Cytol 2000;44(5):748–51.

60. Hamid R, Greenwell TJ, Nethercliffe JM, et al. Routine surveillance cystoscopy for patients with augmentation and substitution cystoplasty for benign urological conditions: is it necessary? BJU Int 2009;104(3):392–5.

61. Kokorowski PJ, Routh JC, Borer JG, et al. Screening for malignancy after augmentation cystoplasty in children with spina bifida: a decision analysis. J Urol 2011;186(4):1437–43.

62. Ivil KD, Doak SH, Jenkins SA, et al. Fluorescence in-situ hybridisation on biopsies from clam ileocysto-plasties and on a clam cancer. Br J Cancer 2006; 94(6):891–5.

63. Fernandez MI, Parikh S, Grossman HB, et al. The role of FISH and cytology in upper urinary tract surveillance after radical cystectomy for bladder cancer. Urol Oncol 2012;30(6):821–4.

64. Docimo SG, Chow NH, Steiner G, et al. Detection of adenocarcinoma by urinary microsatellite analysis after augmentation cystoplasty. Urology 1999; 54(3):561.

65. Tollefson MK, Elliott DS, Zincke H, et al. Long-term outcome of ureterosigmoidostomy: an analysis of patients with >10 years of follow-up. BJU Int 2010; 105(6):860–3.

Quality of Life and Urinary Diversion

Scott M. Gilbert, MD, MS[a,b,*]

KEYWORDS

- Urinary diversion • Health-related quality of life • Improving quality of life

KEY POINTS

- Health-related quality-of-life outcomes after urinary diversion vary significantly.
- Preserving and even improving health-related quality of life are highly relevant to urinary diversion.
- Life after urinary diversion is fundamentally different than before.

INTRODUCTION

Urinary diversion, performed either as a stand-alone reconstructive procedure or in conjunction with radical cystectomy, is associated with a host of functional, metabolic, and physical changes that combined affect quality of life.[1,2] Health-related quality-of-life (HRQOL) outcomes after urinary diversion, however, vary significantly depending on the extent and burden of patient symptoms, problems and health status before and after surgery, and the reason for and objective of the diversion surgery itself. Performed to palliate symptoms or manage severe bladder dysfunction, for example, urinary diversion can alleviate burdensome symptoms, reduce patient suffering, and significantly improve overall quality of life.[3,4] In contrast, when performed as part of a radical cystectomy in cases of bladder cancer, urinary diversion may lead to quality-of-life deficits, principally as a result of the loss of normal body function, unanticipated physical and functional challenges that persist after surgery, or unavoidable permanent consequences, such as altered body image associated with some forms of urinary diversion.[5–8]

Whether positive or negative, several facets of HRQOL are affected by urinary diversion. Often referred to as domains, these areas reach beyond physical concerns and involve self-image, emotional well-being, and even social function. Consider an example of a healthy and fully functional man treated with cystectomy and urinary diversion who experiences erectile dysfunction, incontinence, and bowel dysfunction after surgery. Life after urinary diversion is fundamentally different than before. His sexual dysfunction may strain his relationship with his spouse. Problems with urine leakage and lack of control may limit his interest in social outings and change his self-perception. If his symptoms are severe enough and his coping skills and social support network are marginal, he may experience distress, anxiety, or even depression. Although perhaps an outlier example, most surgeons who perform a large number of cystectomy and urinary diversion surgeries will recognize this story. Urinary diversion can give a person their life back, or it can change life in profound and deleterious ways.

Given these potential changes, there is considerable interest in how urinary diversion impacts

Disclosure: The author has nothing to disclose.
[a] Department of Genitourinary Oncology, H. Lee Moffitt Cancer Center and Research Institute, 12902 Magnolia Drive, Tampa, FL, USA; [b] Department of Health Outcomes and Behavior, H. Lee Moffitt Cancer Center and Research Institute, 12902 Magnolia Drive, Tampa, FL, USA
* Department of Genitourinary Oncology, H. Lee Moffitt Cancer Center and Research Institute, 12902 Magnolia Drive, Tampa, FL.
E-mail address: scott.gilbert@moffitt.org

quality of life, both among cystectomy patients and patients managed with diversion for purely reconstructive purposes.[9,10] Indeed, development of continent urinary diversion was driven primarily to avoid the need for an external stoma and urostomy appliance and restore anatomic and volitional voiding with the objective of preserving quality of life in patients who require urinary diversion.[11,12] This presumption was in part supported by several early studies comparing ileal conduit to continent urinary diversions that reported better physical, social and functional outcomes in patients who received continent diversion.[13,14] Clearly, preserving and even improving HRQOL are highly relevant to urinary diversion. This review is structured to examine how and in what areas urinary diversion may impact patient quality of life and selectively reviews research findings from recent HRQOL studies performed in the urinary diversion patient population.

HEALTH-RELATED QUALITY-OF-LIFE DEFINITIONS, FRAMEWORK, AND DOMAINS

Several definitions of HRQOL have been proposed, but most focus on several common themes. For example, both the World Health Organization and Centers for Disease Control and Prevention definitions include language linking HRQOL to perceived physical and emotional function and health within the context of a person's goals, standards, and concerns for their health.[15,16] Stated more explicitly by Health People 2020, HRQOL "is a multi-dimensional concept that includes domains related to physical, mental, emotional and social functioning... [and] goes beyond direct measures of population health, life expectancy, and causes of death, and focuses on the impact health status has on quality of life."[17] Inherent in almost all definitions, HRQOL is perceived by the individual. It is the subjective reaction to health, wellness, and disease that positively or negatively affects physical function, emotional well-being, and an individual's ability to maintain social interactions and connections.[18–20]

Wilson and Cleary[21] proposed a framework for HRQOL that encapsulates many of the concepts mentioned in the above definitions.[22] In the Wilson-Cleary model, biology, physiology, patient symptoms, physical functioning, health perception, and HRQOL interconnect and interact across a causal pathway. This model suggests that individuals' personal perception of their health, coping skills, and support they receive from their social network interact with the severity of their health problem, symptoms, and resulting functional status to mediate how they experience and perceive their quality of life.[21] Consider the following example: Metabolic changes associated with urinary diversion, such as metabolic acidosis and electrolyte abnormalities (biology/physiology), may result in fatigue and lethargy (symptoms) that limit an individual's energy and impair day-to-day activities (physical and social functioning), ultimately resulting in a negative self-perception of health. In this example, as in others, the overall affect of health problems and symptoms on HRQOL varies according to the extent of the problem, how an individual experiences and copes with the problem, and external supporting factors and resources that assist them in managing the problem. Consider bowel dysfunction associated with urinary diversion as another example. One individual may have a more exaggerated response to minor changes in bowel function, such as bloating, more frequent bowel movements, and occasional diarrhea, whereas another may adapt to even moderate bowel dysfunction because they have an adaptive coping style, have greater access to resources to manage their symptoms, and are less bothered by the change in physical function and its associated consequences. The first individual is more bothered by the symptoms, experiences a greater degree of stress that may negatively impact social function, and perceives a decline in their quality of life. The experience and perception are different for the second individual even though their symptoms could be considered more severe, and as a result, their quality of life is not deflected as significantly.

As noted in the above examples, urinary diversion is associated with a range of experiences, symptoms, functional changes, and health problems that combined make up HRQOL after diversion surgery. Concerns and problem areas, also referred to as domains, that are specific to urinary diversion include bowel, sexual, and urinary function, body image, and psychosocial function, including anxiety, depression, and strain in social situations, function, or interactions. General problems and concerns experienced after surgery, such as pain, fatigue, and sleep disturbances, may also influence HRQOL among urinary diversion patients.[23]

URINARY DIVERSION-SPECIFIC HEALTH-RELATED QUALITY-OF-LIFE MEASURES

Several measures, or questionnaires, can be used to assess HRQOL after urinary diversion. In general, HRQOL measures can be divided into generic questionnaires that assess general symptoms, concerns, and problems, and condition-specific questionnaires that focus on more specific symptoms, problems, and functional states that are associated with a particular condition or apply to a specific patient population. Examples of general, or generic, HRQOL questionnaires include the Medical Outcomes Study Short Forms (SF-36 and SF-12) and EuroQol 5 dimensions questionnaire.[24–26] Questions that gauge HRQOL domains relevant to urinary diversion tend to bundle with bladder cancer HRQOL measures, such as the Functional Assessment of Cancer Therapy Bladder Cancer subscale (FACT-BL), the Vanderbilt Cystectomy Index (VCI), the Bladder Cancer Index (BCI), and the European Organization for Research and Treatment of Cancer Quality of Life Bladder Module (EORTC QLQ-BLM30).[27–30] Each of these questionnaires contains questions that are specific to symptoms, functional consequences, and health problems associated with urinary diversion. As discussed later, although most of the initial work done on HRQOL after urinary diversion was based on non–condition-specific HRQOL questionnaires, more recent research has adopted condition-specific quality-of-life measures.

Existing condition-specific questionnaires contain questions and subsections that are pertinent to the symptoms, complications, and health impairments that patients may experience after bladder removal and urinary diversion, and as a result, cover many of the health domains mentioned above. Although an in-depth review of each of the measures is beyond the scope of this review, key similarities and differences are discussed briefly. In terms of development and organization, urinary diversion–relevant HRQOL measures can be divided into 2 groups for practical purposes: (1) those developed as a module of or supplement to an existing parent questionnaire (eg, FACT-BL and FACT-VCI, EORTC-QLQ-BM30), and (2) those developed de novo without reference or connection to an existing HRQOL measure (eg, BCI). For example, both the FACT-BL and the VCI consist of supplemental questions that are specific to concerns and problems experienced by patients with bladder cancer and urinary diversion added to the general FACT core questionnaire. In the case of the FACT-BL, 12 of the 39 questions are specific to urinary diversion issues, such as stoma care, body image, and sexual function. The EORTC-QLQ-BM30 uses a modular approach by adding 30 additional questions to the base QLQ questionnaire. In contrast, the BCI consists of 36 questions that are independent of any other general HRQOL questionnaire but cover a range of health domains, including bowel, sexual, and urinary function.

Several other measures are currently in development or have been recently developed, including the Bladder Utility Symptom Scale and the Ileal Orthotopic Neobladder–Patient-Reported Outcome (IONB-PRO) questionnaire.[31,32] The Bladder Utility Symptom Scale (BUSS) is a 10-question survey designed to measure quality of life across all stages of bladder cancer that has undergone validity and reliability testing. It consists of 2 urinary questions, one bowel question, and one question on sexual function.[31] The IONB-PRO is a 23-item questionnaire that is specific to concerns and problems associated with neobladder.[32] It has been used in a multicenter Italian study that found that longer follow-up was a predictor of better emotional and social health, but urinary incontinence was associated with poorer quality-of-life outcomes among patients managed with cystectomy and neobladder.[33] The IONB-PRO cannot be used in comparative studies given that it is specific for neobladder and therefore would not provide reliable or useful information in individuals who have an ileal conduit. A summary of available condition-specific HRQOL measures is shown in **Table 1**.

REVIEW OF HEALTH-RELATED QUALITY-OF-LIFE LITERATURE

In one of the first systematic reviews targeting HRQOL among patients treated with cystectomy and urinary diversion, Porter and Penson[34] noted that of 15 studies published between 1966 and 2004 few consisted of HRQOL assessment with either a condition-specific or a validated instrument, and most omitted baseline or serial longitudinal data.[34] These findings underscore several limitations in the area of HRQOL research after urinary diversion of which the reader should be mindful. First, most of the initial studies researching HRQOL in cystectomy and urinary diversion patients relied on either general quality-of-life instruments or informal, unvalidated questionnaires (questions that did not undergo iterative development or psychometric testing). General HRQOL measures may be insensitive or unresponsive to some of the symptoms, health problems, and concerns experienced by patients who live with a urinary diversion, whereas unvalidated measures may not record reliable estimates or reflect accurate outcomes. In other words, they may be inaccurate thermometers. Second, cross-sectional HRQOL evaluations after diversion provide a limited view of HRQOL outcomes associated with urinary diversion and may misguide conclusions and inferences. A more complete and accurate picture of how diversion patients fare over

Table 1
Available condition-specific health-related quality-of-life instruments relevant to urinary diversion

Instrument	Items	Domains/Attributes	Validity Testing
FACT-BL[27]	39 (FACT-G + 12 additional questions)	Single items covering urinary, sexual, and bowel questions, ostomy care, body image, and appetite	Additional questions not formally validated
VCI-15[28]	15 (total of 42 coadministered with FACT-G)	General cancer-related domains plus urinary, bowel, ostomy, and sexual questions	Reliability and validity testing done
BCI[29]	36	Bowel, sexual, and urinary domains with function and bother subdomains	Reliability and validity testing done
EORTC-QLQ-BLM30[30]	30	Single items covering urinary symptoms, sexual function, urostomy issues, body image	Final reliability and validity evaluation underway
BUSS[31]	10	Single item covering urinary, bowel, and sexual issues, as well as body image, psychological problems, pain, and medical care	Reliability and validity testing done
IONB-PRO[32]	23	Neobladder diversion-specific questions covering symptoms, self-management, activities of daily living, emotional and social issues, and sleep fatigue	Reliability and validity testing done

time would ideally be sketched with longitudinal assessments starting before surgery. Third, there are implicit, often immeasurable factors that influence the choice or receipt of a specific type of urinary diversion that may not be appreciable, accounted for, or considered in comparative studies, but confound outcomes. Combined, these shortcomings can make results difficult to interpret and synthesis of a unified message about how patients do after urinary diversion somewhat blurry. Nevertheless, this article reviews the HRQOL literature in the context of cystectomy and urinary diversion.

To date, most HRQOL research among urinary diversion patients has focused on comparing HRQOL outcomes between different urinary diversion types (eg, ileal conduit vs neobladder vs catheterizable colon pouch).[35–44] This is not surprising given the clinical relevance and importance of HRQOL outcomes in the cystectomy and urinary diversion patient population, the constant question and debate among surgeons regarding which diversion is better, and the need for better information to help patients decide which diversion is best for them. General assessment tools, such as EQ-5D, Sickness Impact Profile, SF-12 and SF-36, and FACT, have been used to measure quality of life in urinary diversion patients, but most studies using these measures have reported similar outcomes, on average, between neobladder and ileal conduit patients.[45] More and more reports comparing HRQOL among urinary diversion patients using validated, condition-specific HRQOL measures, such as BCI, VCI, FACT-BL, QLQ-BLM30, and IONB-PRO, have been published in recent years,[46] but although improved in study design and approach, the majority have been retrospective and cross-sectional, indicating that their results should still be viewed fairly critically given the likelihood of important limitations and unavoidable biases related to choice and receipt of diversion types.[47]

For every study that suggests a HRQOL benefit for neobladder diversions there seems to be a counterpart contradicting that finding and assertion. For example, Singh and colleagues[44] reported higher physical and social functioning among neobladder patients compared with patients who received an ileal conduit in a prospective study, with scores diverging between 6 and 18 months after surgery, despite similar baseline assessment. In contrast, Anderson and colleagues[28] reported higher quality of life 1 year after ileal conduit compared with patients managed with a neobladder urinary diversion. A more recent study also reported higher

quality-of-life scores among ileal conduit patients compared with neobladder patients more than 10 years after urinary diversion, but the reasons for this finding were unclear.[48] A 2016 systematic review suggests that HRQOL outcomes reported in contemporary series favor neobladder, and a relatively large meta-analysis of observational HRQOL studies using validated questionnaires reported modestly higher HRQOL scores after neobladder diversion compared with ileal conduit, although HRQOL differences did not reach statistical significance.[49,50]

Specific health problems and functional deficits may cause patient concern without causing a large shift in overall HRQOL. Examples include sexual or urinary function and serve as a reminder of why relevant questions and domains are so important in evaluating HRQOL after urinary diversion. Several studies have examined patient distress after diversion. A study by Henningsohn and colleagues[51] suggests that patients who receive an orthotopic neobladder have similar distress levels as individuals from matched control populations 1 year following surgery. However, a study by Palapattu and colleagues[52] reported that nearly half of cystectomy patients report general distress, and Benner and colleagues[53] highlighted persistently elevated pain and fatigue scores up to 6 months after urinary diversion in their study of 33 patients treated with radical cystectomy and urinary diversion. Another study suggested that patient distress improves to baseline approximately 12 months after surgery.[54] Distress, fatigue, and disturbance of normal sleep patterns may negatively affect patient-reported HRQOL. For example, Thulin and colleagues[55] studied sleep disturbance following urinary diversion and reported that negative sleep changes (lost sleep time and quality) were notable in 37% of orthotopic neobladder patients, 14% of patients with continent reservoir, and 22% of patients who had a urostomy. The higher rate of sleep disturbance noted among patients with a neobladder most likely derives from either nighttime incontinence events or habitual reliance on a voiding alarm to manage and avoid urine leaking accidents.

Fundamental changes in urinary function after urinary diversion surgery can also affect an individual's perception of their health, vitality, and subsequently quality of life. Not surprisingly, urinary incontinence and leakage are the most commonly investigated HRQOL domain in diversion patients.[56] Leakage with conduit diversions is most commonly due to poor external appliance adherence or suboptimal stoma placement. Among ileal conduit patients, urinary leakage rates during daytime and nighttime have been reported as high as

40%, and patient anxiety related to leakage may be even higher.[57,58] Improvements in stomal creation and care, particularly with dedicated enterostomal nurse education, have largely mitigated many of these problems,[59] and most patients get to a state of good functional control with minimum urinary leaks after a few months of directed education and gaining hands-on experience changing the urostomy appliance themselves. Although continent urinary diversions are used to preserve normal anatomic urinary function and volitional voiding, urinary incontinence rates and urine leakage are still relatively high. Although most patients regain control during awake hours, nighttime incontinence can affect 40% to 50% of neobladder patients.[36,60] Leakage and lack of control of urinary function can negatively affect HRQOL. For example, incontinence and leakage accidents can lead to depressed self-esteem related to body odor, altered perception of body image, and anxiety related to fear of an accident.[61]

Changes in sexual health and function are a second important domain of urinary diversion-specific HRQOL, in terms of both physiologic dysfunction associated with the surgery itself and psychogenic sexual dysfunction related to anxiety, changes in body image, and concerns regarding other health or functional problems such as urinary dysfunction, which might interfere with sexuality. In men, erectile dysfunction has been reported in up to 80% of patients after cystectomy and ileal conduit.[62] Although condition-specific questionnaires interrogate both physical and psychosocial aspects of sexual dysfunction, other factors such as quality of erections, penile length decrease, impaired sexual function even before surgery, partner response to changes in function and appearance, and overall psychological issues may go underassessed.[63] Hekal and colleagues[64] reported that most men achieved adequate erections after nerve-sparing cystectomy and urinary diversion without needing other sexual dysfunction treatments, whereas other studies suggest that prostate-sparing cystectomy and urinary diversion may preserve sexual function postoperatively.[65–67] However, results from a large cohort of patients treated with both ileal conduit and neobladder urinary diversions reported universally low sexual function scores as measured by the BCI.[36] Several other studies are consistent with such low scores and have not shown a difference in recovery of sexual function between continent and conduit urinary diversions.[9,35–37]

In women, sexual dysfunction after urinary diversion is primarily related to changes in vaginal anatomy that impact capacity, compliance, and natural lubrication.[68] Vaginal-sparing surgical approaches used during bladder removal appear to limit dysfunction; 80% of women treated with vaginal sparing cystectomy remained sexually active in one study.[69] Other studies, however, have reported higher rates of dysfunction. For instance, Zippe and colleagues[70] reported that less than 50% of patients were sexually active and identified the most common complaints as inability to achieve orgasm (45%), decreased lubrication (41%), decreased sexual desire (37%), and dyspareunia (22%). A more recent study reported that greater than 65% of patients were sexually active after vaginal-sparing cystectomy and urinary diversion.[71]

The spectrum of bowel function and dysfunction is a third area of urinary diversion-specific HRQOL, and accordingly, most condition-specific HRQOL measures contain questions or entire domains dedicated to it. Urinary diversion affects both short-term and long-term bowel function. Although several research studies report normal bowel function after urinary diversion,[72,73] a recent report studying bowel changes up to 1 year after cystectomy found that approximately 30% of urinary diversion patients experienced frequent diarrhea, had more frequent bowel movements, suffered from episodes of fecal incontinence, and reported restrictions in their normal day-to-day lives because of bowel dysfunction.[74] These findings are further supported by those reported by Frees and colleagues[75] in which researchers found that patients managed with continent reconstructions were more likely to report frequent bowel movements, diarrhea, and lower bowel–associated quality of life than those who received an ileal conduit. These recent reports suggest that bowel dysfunction may be an underappreciated functional and quality-of-life deficit.

In the last few years, several additional comparative studies have added to the research base of HRQOL after urinary diversion, but clear winners in terms of better or worse HRQOL have not revealed themselves. Gellhaus and colleagues[76] recently surveyed more than 128 cystectomy and urinary diversion patients using the BCI and reported somewhat similar results as those reported from the original BCI cohort. Patients who received ileal conduit or a right colon pouch had higher urinary BCI scores than neobladder patients, likely because of urine leakage and incontinence associated with neobladders. Interestingly, right colon pouches were also associated with lower bowel scores among women older than age 65 years. In a 100-patient study of conduit and neobladder patients followed for 12 months after surgery with the QLQ-C30, Kretschmer and colleagues[77] reported that neobladder patients showed higher functioning and quality-of-life scores both before and

Table 2
Summary of health-related quality-of-life after urinary diversion (select studies over last 10 y)

References	Instrument	No. Pts.	Population	Findings
Gilbert et al,[36] 2007	BCI	315	US	Decreased urinary function among neobladder (NB) group
Saika et al,[80] 2007	EORTC-QLQ-C30	78	Japan	No significant difference between ileal conduit (IC) and NB
Autorino et al,[81] 2009	SF-36	79	Italy	No difference between IC and NB, but physical, emotional and social QOL scores below population norm
Sogni et al,[41] 2008	EORTC-QLQ-C30 + EORTC-QLQ-BLM30	34	Italy	Global health status higher in NB group but not significant
Philip et al,[58] 2009	SF-36, informally developed questionnaire	52	England	NB group had significantly better physical functioning
Somani et al,[10] 2009	EORTC-QLQ-C30 + SWLS	32	England	No HRQOL difference before or after cystectomy
Hedgepeth et al,[35] 2010	BCI	224	United States	No difference between IC and NB groups
Erber et al,[42] 2012	EORTC-QLQ-C30 + EORTC-QLQ-BLM30	58	Germany	Higher HRQOL scores among NB vs IC patients
Gacci et al,[82] 2013	EORTC-QLQ-C30 + EORTC-QLQ-BLM30, FACT-BL	25	Italy	No HRQOL differences among female patients
Metcalfe et al,[83] 2013	FACT-VCI	84	Canada	No HRQOL differences between IC and NB groups
Singh et al,[44] 2014	EORTC-QLQ-C30	164	India	General HRQOL better in NB group compared with IC group
Huang et al,[61] 2015	BCI	294	China	No difference in long-term HRQOL between IC and NB
Kretschmer et al,[77] 2017	EORTC-QLQ-C30	100	Germany	Higher QOL among NB patients before UD and at 3 mo, but no difference after 12 mo
Goldberg et al,[79] 2016	BCI		Israel	Lower urinary function and higher sexual function in NB patients compared with IC patients
Gelhaus et al,[76] 2017	BCI	128	United States	Lower urinary function among NB group, lower bowel scores among women with colon pouches

shortly after surgery, but scores were not significantly different between groups at 12 months. The same group also explored predictive factors associated with quality-of-life deficits after cystectomy and diversion, finding that gender, patient performance status, surgeon experience, and use of nerve-sparing were all significant predictors of general quality of life.[78] Another BCI-based comparison of long-term HRQOL outcomes between conduit and neobladder diversions reported lower urinary scores but no differences in bother scores, in addition to higher sexual function scores, but greater levels of sexual bother among patients treated with neobladder.[79]

A summary of a select group of contemporary HRQOL studies comparing outcomes between urinary diversion types is shown in **Table 2**.

FUTURE DIRECTIONS

Quality-of-life assessment after urinary diversion is a critical part of fully evaluating patient outcomes and evaluating the impact of urinary diversion on patients' lives. Although results of previous HRQOL research studies have been mixed, it should not be entirely surprising that a clear evidence-based signal differentiating ileal conduit from continent diversion has not emerged. Prior studies have predominantly used general HRQOL instruments or informally developed, unvalidated diversion questionnaires, and even in cases where condition-specific measures have been used, direct comparisons have been fundamentally limited by patient preferences and selection biases associated with choice and receipt of a conduit or continent urinary diversion. Stated more bluntly, the question of which diversion is better may be less important than many believe, and the evidence to date suggests that each diversion is associated with HRQOL deficits and that patients need to choose between tradeoffs associated with either type. Future directions in the area of patient-reported outcome and HRQOL assessments should move toward clinical translation and application, meaning that HRQOL outcomes should become part of clinical evaluation and care over the next several years. This transition from research to clinical application will enable clinicians to identify deficits and problem areas after urinary diversion, raise overall awareness of the challenges that urinary diversion patients face, and allow aggregated outcomes to be used to develop decision aids that could be used to guide patient counseling and choice before surgery. These developing areas will move HRQOL forward to a practical and clinically applicable realm and may allow us to move on from the question, "which is better?"

REFERENCES

1. Lee RK, Abol-Enein H, Artibani W, et al. Urinary diversion after radical cystectomy for bladder cancer: options, patient selection, and outcomes. BJU Int 2014;113(1):11–23.
2. Cody JD, Nabi G, Dublin N, et al. Urinary diversion and bladder reconstruction/replacement using intestinal segments for intractable incontinence or following cystectomy. Cochrane Database Syst Rev 2012;(2):CD003306.
3. Al Hussein Al Awamlh B, Lee DJ, Nguyen DP, et al. Assessment of the quality-of-life and function outcomes in patients undergoing cystectomy and urinary diversion for the management of radiation-induced refractory benign disease. Urology 2015; 85(2):394–400.
4. Kamat AM, Haung SF, Bermejo CE, et al. Total pelvic exenteration: effective palliation of perineal pain in patients with locally recurrent prostate cancer. J Urol 2003;170(5):1868–71.
5. Gandaglia G, Popa I, Abdollah F, et al. The effect of neoadjuvant chemotherapy on perioperative outcomes in patients who have bladder cancer treated with radical cystectomy: a population-based study. Eur Urol 2014;66:561.
6. Shansigh A, Korets R, Vora KC, et al. Defining early morbidity or radical cystectomy for patient with bladder cancer using a standardized reporting methodology. Eur Urol 2009;55(1):164–74.
7. Gilbert SM, Lai J, Saigal CS, et al. Urologic diseases in America project. J Urol 2013;190(3):916–22.
8. Hautmann RE, de Petriconi RC, Volkmer BG. 25 years of experience with 1,000 neobladders: long-term complications. J Urol 2011;185(6): 2207–12.
9. Månsson A, Johnson G, Månsson W. Quality of life after cystectomy: comparison between patients with conduit and those with continent caecal reservoir urinary diversion. Br J Urol 1988;62:240–5.
10. Somani BK, Gimlin D, Fayers P, et al. Quality of life and body image for bladder cancer patients undergoing radical cystectomy and urinary diversion–a prospective cohort study with a systematic review. Urology 2009;74:1138.
11. Kock NG, Nilson AE, Nilsson LO, et al. Urinary diversion via a continent ileal reservoir: clinical results in 12 patients. J Urol 1982;128(3):469–75.
12. Hautmann RE, Egghart G, Frohneberg D, et al. The ileal neobladder. J Urol 1988;139(1):39–42.
13. Hobisch A, Tosun K, Kinzl J, et al. Life after cystectomy and orthotopic neobladder versus ileal conduit urinary diversion. Semin Urol Oncol 2001;19(1):18–23.
14. Dutta SC, Chang SC, Coffey CS, et al. Health related quality of life after radical cystectomy: comparison of ileal conduit with continent orthotopic neobladder. J Urol 2002;168(1):164–7.

15. World Health Organization. Mental health program. Available at: http://www.who.int/mental_health/publications/whoqol/en/. Accessed May 1, 2017.
16. Centers for Disease Control and Prevention, definition of Health-Related Quality of Life. Available at: https://www.cdc.gov/hrqol/. Accessed May 1, 2017.
17. Healthy People 2020, Health-related quality of life and well-being. Available at: https://www.healthypeople.gov/2020/topics-objectives/topic/health-related-quality-of-life-well-being. Accessed 5/12/2017.
18. International Society of Quality of life, health-related quality of life research. Available at: http://www.who.int/mental_health/publications/whoqol/en/. Accessed May 1, 2017.
19. Schipper J, Clinch JJ, Olweny CLM. Quality of life studies: definitions and conceptual issues. In: Spilker B, editor. Quality of life and pharmacoeconomics in clinical trials. Philadelphia: Lippincott-Raven Publishers; 1996. p. 11–23.
20. Cella D. Measuring quality of life in palliative care. Semin Oncol 1995;22:73–81.
21. Wilson IB, Cleary PD. Linking clinical variables with health-related quality of life: a conceptual model of patient outcomes. JAMA 1995;273(1):59–65.
22. Ferrans CE, Zerwic JJ, Wilbur JE, et al. Conceptual model of health-related quality of life. J Nurs Scholarsh 2005;37(4):336–42.
23. Dumitrache M, Badescu DL, Rascu S, et al. Considerations on the psychological status of the patients undergoing radical cystectomy. Journal of Mind and Medical Sciences 2015;2(2):193–8. Available at: http://scholar.valpo.edu/jmms/vol2/iss2/11. Accessed October 28,2017.
24. Ware JE Jr, Sherbourne CD. The MOS 36-item short-form health survey (SF-36): I. Conceptual framework and item selection. Med Care 1992;30:473–83.
25. Ware JE Jr, Kosinski M, Keller SD. A 12-Item Short-Form Health Survey: construction of scales and preliminary tests of reliability and validity. Med Care 1996;34(3):220–33.
26. Rabin R, de Charro F. EQ-5D: a measure of health status from the EuroQol group. Ann Med 2001;33:337–43.
27. Functional assessment of cancer therapy, bladder cancer module. Available at: http://www.facit.org/FACITOrg/Questionnaires. Accessed October 9, 2016.
28. Anderson CB, Feurer ID, Large MC, et al. Psychometric characteristics of a condition-specific, health-related quality-of-life survey: the FACT-Vanderbilt cystectomy index. Urology 2012;80(1):77–83.
29. Gilbert SM, Dunn RL, Hollenbeck BK, et al. Development and validation of the bladder cancer index: a comprehensive, disease-specific measure of health related quality of life in patients with localized bladder cancer. J Urol 2010;183(5):1764–9.
30. European Organization for Research and Treatment of Cancer. Quality of life, EORTC-QLQ-BLM30 module. Available at: http://groups.eortc.be/qol/bladder-cancer-eortc-qlq-nmibc24-eortc-qlq-blm30. Accessed October 9, 2016.
31. Perlis N, Boehme K, Jamal M, et al. MP31-17 validating the Bladder Utility Symptom Scale (BUSS): a novel patient reported outcome quality of life measure for all patients with bladder cancer. J Urol 2016;195(4):e426.
32. Siracusano S, Niero M, Lonardi C, et al. Development of a questionnaire specifically for patients with ileal orthotopic neobladder (IONB). Health Qual Life Outcomes 2014;12:135.
33. Imbimbo C, Mirone V, Siracusano S, et al. Quality of life assessment with orthotopic ileal neobladder reconstruction after radical cystectomy: results from a prospective Italian multicenter observational study. Urology 2015;86(5):974–9.
34. Porter MP, Penson DF. Health related quality of life after radical cystectomy and urinary diversion for bladder cancer: a systematic review and critical analysis of the literature. J Urol 2005;173(4):1318–22.
35. Hedgepeth RC, Gilbert SM, He C, et al. Body image and bladder cancer specific quality of life in patients with ileal conduit and neobladder urinary diversions. Urology 2010;76(3):671–5.
36. Gilbert SM, Wood DP, Dunn RL, et al. Measuring health-related quality of life outcomes in bladder cancer patients using the Bladder Cancer Index (BCI). Cancer 2007;109(9):1756–62.
37. Allareddy V, Kennedy J, West MM, et al. Quality of life in long-term survivors of bladder cancer. Cancer 2006;106(11):2355–62.
38. Kikuchi E, Horiguchi Y, Nakashima J, et al. Assessment of long-term quality of life using the FACT-BL questionnaire in patients with an ileal conduit, continent reservoir, or orthotopic neobladder. Jpn J Clin Oncol 2006;36(11):712–6.
39. Mansson A, Davidsson T, Hunt S, et al. The quality of life in men after radical cystectomy with a continent cutaneous diversion or orthotopic bladder substitution: is there a difference? BJU Int 2002;90(4):386–90.
40. Yoneda T, Adachi H, Urakami S, et al. Health related quality of life after orthotopic neobladder construction and its comparison with normative values in the Japanese population. J Urol 2005;174(5):1944–7.
41. Sogni F, Brausi M, Free B, et al. Morbidity and quality of life in elderly patients receiving ileal conduit or orthotopic neobladder after radical cystectomy for invasive bladder cancer. Urology 2008;71(5):919–23.
42. Erber B, Schrader M, Miller K, et al. Morbidity and quality of life in bladder cancer patients following cystectomy and urinary diversion: a single-institution comparison of ileal conduit versus orthotopic neobladder. ISRN Urol 2012;2012:342796.

43. Large MC, Malik R, Cohn JA, et al. Prospective health-related quality of life analysis for patients undergoing radical cystectomy and urinary diversion. Urology 2014;84(4):808–13.

44. Singh V, Yadav R, Sinha RJ, et al. Prospective comparison of quality-of-life outcomes between ileal conduit urinary diversion and orthotopic neobladder reconstruction after radical cystectomy: a statistical model. BJU Int 2014;113(5):726–32.

45. Ali AS, Hayes MC, Birch B, et al. Health related quality of life (HRQoL) after cystectomy: comparison between orthotopic neobladder and ileal conduit diversion. Eur J Surg Oncol 2015;41(3):295–9.

46. Ahmadi H, Lee CT. Health-related quality of life with urinary diversion. Curr Opin Urol 2015;25(6): 562–9.

47. Evans B, Montie JE, Gilbert SM. Incontinent or continent urinary diversion: how to make the right choice. Curr Opin Urol 2010;20(5):421–5.

48. Gellhaus P, Cary KC, Johnson C, et al. MP38-13 long-term 10-year health-related quality of life outcomes following radical cystectomy. J Urol 2016; 195(4):e537–8.

49. Ghosh A, Somani BK. Recent trends in postcystectomy health-related quality of life (QoL) favors neobladder diversion: systematic review of the literature. Urology 2016;93:22–6.

50. Cerruto MA, Elia CD, Siracusano S, et al. Systematic review and meta-analysis of non RTCs on health related quality of life after radical cystectomy using validated questionnaires: better results with orthotopic neobladder versus ileal conduit. Eur J Surg Oncol 2016;42(3):343–60.

51. Henningsohn L, Steven K, Kallestrup EB, et al. Distressful symptoms and well-being after radical cystectomy and orthotopic bladder substitution compared with a matched control population. J Urol 2002;168(1):168–74 [discussion: 174–5].

52. Palapattu GS, Haisfield-Wolfe ME, Walker JM, et al. Assessment of perioperative psychological distress in patients undergoing radical cystectomy for bladder cancer. J Urol 2004;172(5 Pt 1):1814–7.

53. Benner C, Greenberg M, Shepard N, et al. The natural history of symptoms and distress in patients and families following cystectomy for treatment of muscle invasive bladder cancer. J Urol 2014;191(4): 937–42.

54. Gerharz EW, Mansson A, Hunt S, et al. Quality of life after cystectomy and urinary diversion: an evidence based analysis. J Urol 2005;174(5):1729–36.

55. Thulin H, Kreicbergs U, Wijkstrom H, et al. Sleep disturbances decrease self-assessed quality of life in individuals who have undergone cystectomy. J Urol 2010;184(1):198–202.

56. Perlis N, Krahn M, Alibhai S, et al. Conceptualizing global health-related quality of life in bladder cancer. Qual Life Res 2014;23(8):2153–67.

57. Protogerou V, Moschou M, Antoniou N, et al. Modified S-pouch neobladder vs ileal conduit and a matched control population: a quality-of-life survey. BJU Int 2004;94(3):350–4.

58. Philip J, Manikandan R, Venugopal S, et al. Orthotopic neobladder versus ilea conduit urinary diversion after cystectomy–a quality-of-life based comparison. Ann R Coll Surg Engl 2009;91(7): 565–9.

59. Li X, Fang Q, Ji H, et al. Use of urostomy bags in the management of perioperative urine leakage after radical cystectomy. Cancer Nurs 2014;37(3):170–4.

60. El Bahnasawy MS, Osman Y, Gomha MA, et al. Nocturnal enuresis in men with an orthotopic ileal reservoir: urodynamic evaluation. J Urol 2000; 164(1):10–3.

61. Huang Y, Pan X, Zhou Q, et al. Quality-of-life outcomes and unmet needs between ileal conduit and orthotopic ileal neobladder after radical cystectomy in a Chinese population: a 2-to-1 matched-pair analysis. BMC Urol 2015;15:117.

62. Matsuda T, Aptel I, Exbrayat C, et al. Determinants of quality of life of bladder cancer survivors five years after treatment in France. Int J Urol 2003; 10(8):423–9.

63. Mulhall JP. Defining and reporting erectile function outcomes after radical prostatectomy: challenges and misconceptions. J Urol 2009;181(2):462–71.

64. Hekal IA, El-Bahnasawy MS, Mosbah A, et al. Recoverability of erectile function in post-radical cystectomy patients: subjective and objective evaluations. Eur Urol 2009;55(2):275–83.

65. Nieuwenhuijzen JA, Meinhardt W, Horenblas S. Clinical outcomes after sexuality preserving cystectomy and neobladder (prostate sparing cystectomy) in 44 patients. J Urol 2008;179(5 Suppl):S35–8.

66. Ong CH, Schmitt M, Thalmann GN, et al. Individualized seminal vesicle sparing cystoprostatectomy combined with ileal orthotopic bladder substitution achieves good functional results. J Urol 2010; 183(4):1337–41.

67. Basiri A, Pakmanesh H, Tabibi A, et al. Overall survival and functional results of prostate-sparing cystectomy: a matched case-control study. Urol J 2012;9(4):678–84.

68. Modh RA, Mulhall JP, Gilbert SM. Sexual dysfunction after cystectomy and urinary diversion. Nat Rev Urol 2014;11(8):445–53.

69. Game X, Mallet R, Guillotreau J, et al. Uterus, fallopian tube, ovary and vagina-sparing laparoscopic cystectomy: technical description and results. Eur Urol 2007;51(2):441–6.

70. Zippe C, Nandipati K, Agarwal A, et al. Sexual dysfunction after pelvic surgery. Int J Impot Res 2006;18(1):1–18.

71. Wishahi M, Elganozoury H. Survival up to 5-15 years in young women following genital sparing radical

cystectomy and neobladder: oncological outcome and quality of life. Single-surgeon and single-institution experience. Cent European J Urol 2015; 68(2):141–5.

72. Hautmann RE, Volkmer BG, Schumacher MC, et al. Long-term results of standard procedures in urology: the ileal neobladder. World J Urol 2006;24(3): 305–14.

73. Fung B, Kessler TM, Haeni K, et al. Bowel function remains subjectively unchanged after ileal resection for construction of continent ileal reservoirs. Eur Urol 2011;60(3):585–90.

74. Kramer MW, von Klot CA, Kabbani M, et al. Long-term bowel disorders following radial cystectomy: an underestimated issue? World J Urol 2015; 33(10):1373–80.

75. Frees S, Schenk AC, Rubenwolf P, et al. Bowel function in patients with urinary diversion: a gender-matched comparison of continent urinary diversion with the ileocecal pouch and ileal conduit. World J Urol 2017;35(6):913–9.

76. Gellhaus PR, Cary C, Kaimakliotis HZ, et al. Long-term health related quality of life outcomes following radical cystectomy. Urology 2017;106: 82–6.

77. Kretschmer A, Grimm T, Buchner A, et al. Prospective evaluation of health-related quality of life after radical cystectomy: focus on peri- and postoperative complications. World J Urol 2017; 35(8):1223–31.

78. Kretschmer A, Grimm T, Buchner A, et al. Prognostic features for quality of life after radical cystectomy and orthotropic neobladder. Int Braz J Urol 2016; 42(6):1109–20.

79. Goldberg H, Baniel J, Mano R, et al. Orthotropic neobladder vs. ileal conduit urinary diversion: a long-term quality-of-life comparison. Urol Oncol 2016;34(3):121e1-7.

80. Saika T, Arata R, Tsushima T, et al, Okayama Urological Research Group. Health-related quality of life after radical cystectomy for bladder cancer in elderly patients with an ileal conduit, ureterocutaneostomy, or orthotopic urinary reservoir: a comparative questionnaire survey. Acta Med Okayama 2007;61(4): 199–203.

81. Autorino R, Quarto G, Di Lorenzo G, et al. Health related quality of life after radical cystectomy: comparison of ileal conduit to continent orthotopic neobladder. Eur J Surg Oncol 2009;35(8):858–64.

82. Gacci M, Saleh O, Cai T, et al. Quality of life in women undergoing urinary diversion for bladder cancer: results of a multicenter study among long-term disease-free survivors. Health Qual Life Outcomes 2013;11:43.

83. Metcalfe M, Estey E, Jacobsen NE, et al. Association between urinary diversion and quality of life after radical cystectomy. Can J Urol 2013;20(1):6626–31.

Urinary Diversion in Renal Transplantation

Mohamed Eltemamy, MD, Alice Crane, MD, PhD, David A. Goldfarb, MD*

KEYWORDS

- Renal transplantation • Urinary diversion • Bladder augmentation

KEY POINTS

- Renal transplantation in patients with urinary diversion is feasible with comparable long-term graft function despite higher overall rates of infectious complications.
- Careful preoperative assessment of patients should be done before proceeding with transplant.
- Knowledge of the unique surgical challenges of this specific cohort of patients is mandatory to achieve favorable outcomes.

INTRODUCTION

Patients with anatomically and/or functionally abnormal lower urinary tracts present a unique challenge for the renal transplant surgeon. In a subset of these patients, the native bladder may be suitable for transplantation. In others, intestinal reconstruction or diversion may have been already performed or be required at the time of presentation. For the latter group, questions of timing of surgery and type of diversion must be addressed (**Box 1**).

Kelly and colleagues[1] were the first to report the feasibility of transplantation in patients with an ileal diversion in 1966, providing hope for a desperate group of patients. At that time, an intact natural or reconstructed lower urinary tract was considered mandatory to be eligible for transplantation because of fear of recurrent infection and urosepsis in immunocompromised patients. Reports followed over the years describing renal transplantation after other types of urinary diversion. Tunner and colleagues[2] reported the first transplantation in patients with a colon conduit in 1971, and more recently, renal transplantation has been described in patients with more complex continent diversions.[1,3,4]

Approximately 6% of patients receiving a kidney transplant in the United States have end-stage renal disease (ESRD) attributable to lower urinary tract abnormalities.[5] Among pediatric patients, 24.1% of ESRD cases are attributed to congenital abnormalities of the kidney and urinary tract (CAKUT) as of 2016.[6] The most common causes of CAKUT are posterior urethral valves, vesicoureteral reflux, and neurogenic bladder, including spina bifida. Bladder exstrophy complex, prune-belly syndrome, and other rare syndromes comprise the rest. In transplant patients with hostile bladders, possible nonnative urinary systems include bladder augmentation with gastric, intestinal, or ureteric segments, continent cutaneous diversions, and ileal and colonic conduits. Orthotopic continent reservoirs are more likely to be performed well after transplantation in older patients with development of bladder cancer after transplant.[7] Rates of renal transplantation into patients with supravesical diversion range from 0.4% to 2.3%.[8,9] Rates of transplantation into a prior bladder augmentation is similarly rare with overall rates of ~1%.[10]

The original fear of uroseptic complications in those with intestinal diversion and reconstruction has not been entirely alleviated. In 1997, Alfrey and colleagues[11] cautioned against bladder augmentation before renal transplantation citing

Disclosure: The authors have nothing to disclose.
Glickman Urological and Kidney Institute, Department of Urology, Cleveland Clinic, 9500 Euclid Avenue, Cleveland, OH 44195, USA
* Corresponding author.
E-mail address: goldfad@ccf.org

Box 1
Options for urinary anastomosis in kidney transplantation with abnormal lower urinary tract

- Intestinal conduits
  - Uretero intestinal
  - Uretero ureteral
- Augmentation
  - Uretero intestinal
  - Uretero vesical
  - Uretero ureteral
- Cutaneous ureterostomies
  - Uretero ureteral
- Donor cutaneous ureterostomy

increased risk of recurrent urinary tract infection (UTI), sepsis, graft loss, and death. Most recent reports, however, are at odds with this view, and there is a strong body of evidence to support transplantation in these individuals and those with diversions.[1–5,8–10,12] Although there does seem to be a high incidence of infection in these patients after transplant, with complication rates of UTI and pyelonephritis of 24% and 13%, respectively, this has not been proven to translate into poorer patient or graft survival.[5,13–15]

WORKUP FOR PATIENTS WITH URINARY DIVERSION

It is critical to determine which patients will need staged or simultaneous surgical urinary reconstruction to achieve a mechanism for unobstructed low-pressure elimination. It is critical to determine which patients will need staged or simultaneous surgical urinary reconstruction to achieve a mechanism for unobstructed low-pressure elimination. This distinction is particularly important in patients who developed ESRD secondary to a lower urinary tract abnormality, which is more common in the pediatric population.[16]

A thorough history is paramount to establish a clear timeline of lower urinary tract dysfunction in relation to development of ESRD. Low urine outputs in ERSD patients can lead to a defunctionalized bladder due to the absence of bladder cycling. Errando and colleagues[17] thought that bladders that cycle less than 300 mL daily are defunctionalized. The ability of these bladders to recover was first shown by Tanagho[18] and MacGregor and colleagues,[19] who went on to demonstrate gradual improvement in these bladders. They were even

able to reverse the diversion in some patients with overall good long-term outcomes. They emphasized the importance of distinguishing defunctionalized bladder (usable bladders) and those with pathologic contracture owing to extensive mural fibrosis or multiple bladder surgeries (nonusable bladders). This important distinction has been corroborated by other researchers.[19,20] Serrano and colleagues[21] reported using the native bladders of 5 male patients who had prior ileal conduit diversion for small bladder capacities and uninhibited detrusor contractions. After bladder rehabilitation and renal transplantation, the mean bladder capacity was increased 10 times with resolution of the uninhibited detrusor contractions.

Imaging

Some investigators recommended voiding cystourethrogram (VCUG) as a part of the standard workup[22,23] for adult transplant candidates; however, the necessity of routine VCUG is debatable. Glazier and colleagues[24] questioned the cost-effectiveness of routine VCUG in transplant candidates when they retrospectively reviewed 517 VCUGs in pretransplant patients. Only 13 (2.5%) patients were found to have abnormal imaging, and of those, only 3 (0.6%) required pretransplant surgical intervention. A positive urologic history was common in all the 13 patients. Performing VCUG and urodynamic study (UDS) only in patients with LUTS, defunctionalized bladder, and extensive urologic history demonstrated abnormal findings in 45% of the patients, significantly improving the yield of those studies.[17]

Routine VCUG has been described in the pediatric pretransplant population[25] owing to their previously mentioned higher rate of lower urinary tract abnormalities. These patients usually have had a VCUG study during workup for their original disease. Careful review of those images is required. Requesting repeat studies on patients with images more than 1 year old is reasonable because the underlying abnormality is usually dynamic.[26]

The authors suggest that a reasonable strategy would be to obtain a VCUG in only those adult patients with a compelling urologic history while maintaining a lower threshold for pediatric patients, especially when their cause of ESRD is poorly characterized.

Imaging with a loopogram may also be warranted in patients with a preexisting ileal conduit, especially in those with low or no urine output. A loopogram is prudent in this scenario in order to exclude conduit abnormality, such as stomal stenosis or contracture. In their limited series of 6 patients transplanted to their ileal conduits, a loopogram was routinely performed for all patients at 6-month intervals to assess the length of the conduit and the patency of the uretero-ileal anastomoses.[13] Similarly, requesting a cystogram/pouchogram is reasonable in patients with bladder augmentation or orthotopic urinary diversion. The authors find that endoscopic evaluation of these reservoirs can sometimes obviate a dedicated contrast study.

Urinary Tract Infection

The incorporation of intestinal segments in the urinary tract is associated with an increased prevalence of bacteriuria.[27] One of the reasons that has been postulated is that unlike the urothelium, the intestinal epithelium lacks the inhibitory actions against bacterial adherence.[28] This hospitable environment allows the bacteria to proliferate in urinary reservoirs with integrated intestinal segments. Most of those reconstructed reservoirs also lack the complete emptying mechanism provided by the normal bladder, which encourages bacterial growth.[29]

Obtaining a urine culture in patients with urinary diversion or augmentation should be done cautiously because the interpretation is challenging. Most of these patients will have a positive urine culture even in the absence of symptoms (asymptomatic bacteriuria). The distinction between asymptomatic bacteriuria and true urinary infection is of utmost importance. The general consensus is to avoid using antibiotics in the scenario of asymptomatic positive urine cultures.[30] In renal transplant patients with urinary diversion, immunosuppression increases the complexity of decision making regarding treatment of positive cultures.

In a report of 24 patients with renal transplantation following urinary diversion and augmentation, Rigamonti and colleagues[12] reported using routine prophylactic antibiotics. In a report on 59 patients with staged renal transplantation and ileal conduit urinary diversion, Surange and colleagues[9] emphasized the importance of diligent eradication of all sources of infection during the creation of the conduit. This included unilateral or bilateral nephroureterectomies, excision of old conduits, and supratrigonal cystectomies.

Regardless of the chosen prophylactic antibiotic protocol, the utilization of therapeutic antibiotics should be culture specific and symptom driven.

Urodynamic Studies

Urodynamic studies should be used selectively based on history and particularly in patients with multiple prior bladder surgeries or other abnormality that could lead to bladder fibrosis.[31,32] It is well documented that a detrusor leak point pressure >40 cm H_2O is associated with upper tract deterioration and may lead to ESRD.[33] In a review of 300 cadaveric pediatric renal transplants, Churchill and colleagues[34] reported that graft survival was markedly decreased in patients with uncorrected lower urinary tract dysfunction. Urodynamic evaluation is less useful in patients with a defunctionalized bladder, which will commonly exhibit uninhibited detrusor contractions. These contractions usually resolve following transplantation and bladder cycling.[21]

Preoperative Compliance Assessment

Many patients with continent urinary diversion and bladder augmentation rely on clean intermittent catheterization (CIC) to empty their urinary reservoir. Assessing and improving the compliance of those patients with CIC is critical for improvement of graft survival. Determination of manual dexterity is a key component of the history because some patients may lack the manual dexterity to perform CIC and are better served with a noncontinent urinary diversion.[35]

SURGICAL TECHNIQUE
Timing

In patients without preexisting diversion or augmentation, the perfect timing of lower urinary tract reconstruction is debatable. Patients requiring bladder augmentation or complete urinary diversion may have this procedure before, during, or after transplantation. Proponents of pretransplant augmentation or urinary diversion contend that this approach will allow proper healing of the urinary tract in the absence of immunosuppressive drugs and corticosteroids.[36–40] In anuric and oliguric patients, some investigators proposed that periodic irrigation of those reservoirs is mandatory to avoid mucus accumulation and reservoir contracture,[41,42] whereas others argued against these maneuvers.[43] Most investigators recommended having this separate procedure at least 6 weeks before transplant.[8,12,44]

Advocates of posttransplant augmentation or urinary diversion think that the optimal timing is when renal function is stabilized and immunosuppressive drugs are reduced.[37] This approach carries the advantage of avoiding the scenario of a dry diversion or augmentation, which is associated with increased mucus production and pyocystitis.[15,37,42] These investigators also claim that cystoplasty necrosis secondary to surgical mishaps at the time of the transplantation is obviated.

McInerney and colleagues[45] reported one case of cystoplasty necrosis due to injury of the vascular pedicle and 2 cases of persistent mucus production that necessitated suprapubic placement and repeated bladder lavage in their series of 8 transplants into augmented bladders. Rigamonti and colleagues[12] reported one case of contraction of the augmented bladder. The development of a cycling regimen (300 mL twice daily) eliminated further complications with pretransplant augmentation and urinary diversion in their review of 24 patients. Performing the augmentation or diversion concurrently with the transplant surgery is discouraged by most investigators because this approach carries a higher surgical and infectious risk.[1,8]

Kidney Position

The transplant kidney orientation in patients with cystoplasty is similar to regular transplants. However, in patients with urinary diversion, placing the kidney in an upside-down position is usually preferred to reduce the journey of the transplanted ureter and allow a smooth-running course with no ureteral kinking.[13] Antegrade urinary flow is dependent on active ureteral peristalsis, not gravity. The site of the kidney placement in relation to the urinary reservoir is a debatable matter. Some investigators recommended ipsilateral placement of graft, claiming that this would allow a shorter linear distance of the graft ureter.[46] Others advised contralateral graft placement.[13] The authors think that surgeons should have a flexible mindset with these patients. The authors usually make the final decision after simulation of the kidney lie in the surgical field and find that the upside-down position is often more favorable. The laterality issue is usually dependent on the length of ureter provided, the expected amount of tension following anastomosis, and the space left for the kidney.

Urinary Anastomosis

In a patient with normal anatomy, the donor ureter is usually anastomosed to the native bladder. Any refluxing or nonrefluxing, intravesical or extravesical surgical technique is acceptable.[47–49] Primary ureteroureteral anastomosis between the donor ureter and the recipient ureter is favored by some surgeons for preserving the natural antireflux mechanism.[50] It is also useful for short or poorly vascularized donor ureters.[51,52]

Intestinal conduits

Although any segment of the intestine can be used for the construction of intestinal conduits, the ileum is the most commonly used segment.[53] In this scenario, end-to-side single-layer anastomosis of the graft ureter to the intestinal loop is preferred.[8,54] In donor kidneys with a short ureter or in patients with a planned left-side transplantation and a contralateral conduit, anastomosis to the native ureter may provide a tension-free anastomosis.[13] Chaykovska and colleagues[13] reported using this technique in 6 patients with renal transplantation with preexisting conduits and used ureteral stents in all cases. An end- (transplant ureter) to-side (native ureter) technique was used to prevent devascularizing the previously reimplanted ureter. In pouches created from large intestine segments, as in Indiana and Bricker pouches, the anastomosis can be fashioned end to side to the terminal ileum or the taenia.[55]

Augmentation

Cystoplasty is usually a last resort option for patients with neurogenic bladder after failure of more conservative treatment options. Various segments of the gastrointestinal tract have been used to augment the bladder (stomach, ileum, colon). Ileocystoplasty is the most common form of bladder augmentation.[56] Ureterocystoplasty is also a potential option in some patients.[57] Some investigators recommend anastomosis of the donor ureter to the native bladder whenever possible to avoid disruption of the augmenting-patch blood supply.[10,55] However, most reports on transplantation into an augmented bladder reported anastomosis to the bowel segment and to the ipsilateral ureter.[10,39] An ipsilateral native nephrectomy might be indicated in transplant candidates with a high urinary output then using a ureteroureteral approach. Others thought that anastomosis to the native bladder should preferably be avoided, because in many cases, those hostile bladders are the primary ESRD cause.[35] Anastomosis to the ureteric portion of the ureterocystoplasty has also been described.[12,39] The authors cannot overemphasize the importance of having a high degree of flexibility in these circumstances. In patients with thick pathologic bladders, the authors try to avoid the native bladder by anastomosing the ureter to the intestinal pouch as long as the vascular supply of the pouch is not compromised. Otherwise, the anastomosis locates at the most favorable portion of the augmented bladder.

Cutaneous ureterostomy

Cutaneous ureterostomy has for the most part fallen out of favor in both children and adults. The advantage was thought to lie in avoiding an intestinal anastomosis, which is considered the most morbid part of urinary diversion. However, because of the high stricture rate and infectious complications, it was mostly abandoned.[58–62] Older reports of anastomosis of the donor ureter to the native ureter implicated in ureterocutaneous anastomosis has been described with good overall outcome. In most cases, a native nephrectomy is performed to avoid ascending pyelonephritis. It is imperative to perform preoperative ureterography to exclude the presence of strictures. Obviously, this option should be completely discarded if this diversion is thought to play a role in the development of ESRD in those patients.[19,63,64]

Prieto and colleagues[65] reported donor cutaneous ureterostomy in 6 patients. They reported unacceptable bacteriuria rates with a high incidence of symptomatic UTI. Most patients suffered from stomal stenosis that required repeated dilatation. These discouraging results should dissuade surgeons from considering this option.

OUTCOMES

It is difficult to compare outcomes because of the small number of transplants into patients with diversions and the numerous different types of diversions and transplant techniques involved. Many reports pool adult and pediatric recipients and all types of urinary diversion. However, 5-year graft survival in the literature for any type of diversion is between 63% and 78% considering both pediatric and adult literature.[9,12,36,66,67] The few studies with long-term follow-up out to 15 years report graft survival rates of 69%.[9,12]

In one of the largest populations studied, Surange and colleagues[9] looked at 59 transplants in 54 adult and pediatric patients with a prior ileal conduit. Patient and graft survival at 5 years was 83% and 63%, respectively. Importantly, although UTI was noted in 65% of these patients, no graft loss was due to infection and survival was comparable to grafts transplanted into patients without diversions during the same timeframe. In a smaller study of 6 patients with intestinal urinary conduits (5 ileal, 1 colon) and ureteroureterostomy to the native ureter as opposed to the conduit itself, the overall 5-year functional outcome was good with a patient and graft survival rate of 100% and 83.3%, respectively.[13] Although proving this anastomotic approach technically feasible when necessary, there was a high rate of complications requiring secondary interventions. Two patients required management of subsequent ureteral obstruction and 4 of the 6 patients required native nephrectomy for recurrent pyelonephritis.

In one of the few case control studies, Warholm and colleagues[36] had similar outcomes with a mixed patient group of ileal conduits and continent reservoirs (27 grafts in 22 patients) with graft survival of 70% at 5 years and comparable to controls. Chronic bacteriuria was almost universally encountered in diverted patients, and no effect on survival was seen despite relaxation of treatment of asymptomatic bacteriuria over the time course studied. Consistent with studies in adult or mixed-age populations, Hatch and colleagues[67] found increased rates of infection without effect on graft survival in a purely pediatric population with mostly bladder augmentation or incontinent urinary conduits. Graft survival in this population was 78% at 5 years and 60% at 10 years in 30 patients with no losses due to infection.

Regarding patients with prior augmentation only, a small study of 6 adult patients with mostly remote prior bladder augments experienced loss of 3 (50%) of their grafts with a mean follow-up of 56 months, due to frequent infection, but no graft loss due to infectious cause.[35] There is a general trend toward worse outcomes with enterocystoplasty as opposed to intestinal urinary diversion.[11,45]

Chronic and acute rejection are consistently found to be the most frequent cause of allograft loss, implying that the limiting factor of graft survival is the same regardless of the anatomy of the patient's lower urinary tract. However, this is not without some controversy. There have been recent reports of renewed concern over infection and graft survival in these reconstructed patients.[68] A 2016 study retrospectively comparing 21 recipients with urinary diversion or augment to patients labeled with "bladder dysfunction" without reconstruction and patients with normal bladder function reported a 3.57 risk of graft failure and a trend toward increased risk of patient death. Five-year graft survival in the reconstructed group was 66.6%. Interestingly, 14 of the 21 patients had an orthotopic neobladder, accounting for 4 of the graft losses with the other 3 in patients with augmentation cystoplasty. Two of their 5 graft losses were due to infection, suggesting perhaps a higher burden of infection or even graft loss depending on predominant type of reconstruction, although a small number of patients and variations across time and institutions make direct comparisons difficult.

COMPLICATIONS
Infectious Complication

Chronic bacteriuria and UTI are extremely common with intestinal reconstruction. As previously discussed, although this does significantly increase the morbidity of transplant patients, it does not have an effect on graft survival.

The overall incidence of UTI has been reported at 50% to 67% in the literature. Technique and timing of both urinary reconstruction and renal transplantation may affect infectious complications. McInerney and colleagues[45] reported recurrent pyocystitis as a complication of cystoplasties performed before transplant in anuric patients. Native nephrectomies for recurrent pyelonephritis, reported as a frequent complication with ureteroureterostomy in conduit patients, were rare in other series with direct implantation or unspecified ureteral anastomosis.[13] One rare but feared complication reported is perforated augmented bladder and peritonitis.[14] Signs of this occurring may be subtle in the immunocompromised reconstructed patient.

The general consensus for urinary diversion is that performing diversion before transplantation leads to lower infectious risk compared with the greater burden of immunosuppression if conducted during transplantation[15] despite the risk of performing surgery on a dry system. A recent large cohort of 46 pediatric patients with mixed urinary reconstruction was reported to have no significant difference in UTI between the 80.4% that underwent pretransplant intervention and the 19.6% that underwent posttransplant intervention.[68]

Metabolic Complications

Metabolic derangement, usually in the form of metabolic acidosis given the common use of ileum and colon, is a well-known complication of intestinal diversion. The longer the contact between urine and bowel mucosa, the more profound the metabolic change. This translates into a less profound effect in incontinent diversions with short dwell times. Hatch[5] reported 2 of 7 children with significant acidosis with continent diversion and reported 5 of 30 children requiring alkali therapy in their later series.[67] Another study by Koo and colleagues[69] experienced metabolic acidosis requiring alkali therapy in 8 of 9 pediatric patients with a bowel-containing reservoir.

Most studies in reconstructed and transplanted patients do not mention metabolic acidosis, choosing to focus on graft and infectious outcomes. The ESRD patient population also has an extremely high incidence of metabolic acidosis due to renal failure going into surgery, suggesting more of a failure to correct than a complication.

Stones

Calculi are cited to occur in up to 52% of patients with bladder augmentation.[70,71] The increased rate compared with those with native lower urinary tract is attributable to increased urinary stasis, metabolic acidosis, increased rates of bacteriuria, and mucus production, which can serve as a nidus for stone formation. In Hatch's 2001 series, only one patient experienced a stone, and they hypothesized the lower rate was due to the inherent aggressive follow-up and management of urinary drainage in a transplant cohort.[67] Rigamonti and colleagues[12] experienced 3 out of 16 patients (18.7%) with continent diversions developing bladder or upper tract stones and 1 out of 7 (14.3%) with an incontinent diversion. Other reports confirm relatively low incidence of stone formation in diverted transplant patients,[36] although one series had a rate approaching 30% in patients with ileal conduits.[72] Dedicated care, including adequate oral hydration, pouch irrigation, prophylactic antibiotics, and management of metabolic derangements, can decrease the risk for not only infection but also stone formation, which can be surgically challenging to manage in reconstructed systems.[70,73,74]

Other Surgical Complications

Complication rates of transplantation into a reconstructed lower urinary tract are higher than transplant recipients with a functional bladder.[15] Complications include stomal stenosis, conduit prolapse, intestinal and urinary fistula, wound dehiscence, and urine leak. One complication unique to transplantation after enterocystoplasty is damage to the vascular pedicle of the previously mobilized bowel, causing necrosis of the enteric segment.[45]

Surange and colleagues[9] noted a role for the conduit itself in 60% of their total surgical complications and significantly higher rates of urinary leakage or obstruction (15%) in transplant patients (N = 52) with an ileal conduit than in their nondiverted patients (6%). They recommended close follow-up and low threshold for intervention for the first 3 years and, as in past 3 years, only stomal complications arose. They did not lose any grafts to urologic complications. Smaller studies have also reported a significant rate of complications involving the ileal conduit and ureteroenteric anastomosis without leading to graft loss.[8,36,55] Two out of 6 patients with prior conduit that underwent ureteroureterostomy in the literature developed ureteral complications, hinting at a possible increased rate of obstruction with this technique, although the sample size is very small.[13]

A recent report of 17 patients in Ireland did not report any mechanical complications stemming from the conduit itself in patients with an ileal conduit created in 16/17 patients, although they did have a high rate of stone formation (29.4%), as previously noted.[72] Similarly, Srinivasan and colleagues[66] interestingly had a higher overall rate of complications in patients with bladder reconstruction (majority neobladder) but had no urologic complications in that group. Al-Khudairi and colleagues[68] reported only 3 urine leaks in their population of 46 pediatric reconstructed patients, most of whom had augmentations and/or the Mitrofanoff procedure. They had 6 wound dehiscences in the same population.

Although the studies are uniformly small, there appears to be a general trend over time in the decline of urinary complications as surgical comfort with these patients increases. One area that remains uncertain is the incidence of secondary malignancy of intestinal segments in the transplanted population. In 2004, there were 81 known case reports of secondary malignancy in all types of intestinal urinary tract diversion and augmentation in nontransplant series.[75] Unlike the well-known complication of adenocarcinoma after ureterosigmoidostomy, tumors arising in urinary diversions are of varied histology with ~75% being adenocarcinoma and the remainder transitional cell, squamous cell, and others. The investigators at that time recommended yearly endoscopic investigation starting at year 3. It is logical that transplant patients would be at higher risk for the development of malignancy given their immunosuppressed state, but there is no consensus on appropriate surveillance. There has been one report of adenocarcinoma of the urachal remnant in a woman with bladder exstrophy 16 years after transplant with ureterosigmoidostomy converted to ileal conduit.[75] To the authors' knowledge, there has not yet been a report of secondary malignancy in the intestinal segment itself after transplantation, although a high suspicion should be held because long-term outcomes remain unclear.

REFERENCES

1. Kelly W, Merkel F, Markland C. Ileal urinary diversion in conjunction with renal homotransplantation. Lancet 1966;287:222–7.
2. Tunner WS, Whitsell JC 2nd, Rubin AL, et al. Renal transplantation in children with corrected abnormalities of the lower urinary tract. J Urol 1971;106:133–9.
3. Djakovic N, Wagener N, Adams J, et al. Intestinal reconstruction of the lower urinary tract as a prerequisite for renal transplantation. BJU Int 2009;103: 1555–60.
4. Kocot A, Spahn M, Loeser A, et al. Long-term results of a staged approach: continent urinary diversion in preparation for renal transplantation. J Urol 2010; 184:2038–42.
5. Hatch DA. Kidney transplantation in patients with an abnormal lower urinary tract. Urol Clin North Am 1994;21:311–20.
6. United States Renal Data System. 2015 USRDS annual data report: epidemiology of kidney disease in the United States. National Institutes of Health, National Institute of Diabetes and Digestive and Kidney Diseases. Bethesda (MD): USRDS; 2015. Available at: https://www.usrds.org/2015/view/. Accessed March 19, 2017.
7. Manassero F, Di Paola G, Mogorovich A, et al. Orthotopic bladder substitute in renal transplant recipients: experience with Studer technique and literature review. Transpl Int 2011;24:943–8.
8. Coosemans W, Baert L, Kuypers D, et al. Renal transplantation onto abnormal urinary tract: ileal conduit urinary diversion. Transplant Proc 2001; 33(4):2493–4.
9. Surange RS, Johnson RW, Tavakoli A, et al. Kidney transplantation into an ileal conduit: a single center experience of 59 cases. J Urol 2003;170(5):1727–30.
10. Power RE, O'Malley KJ, Khan MS, et al. Renal transplantation in patients with an augmentation cystoplasty. BJU Int 2007;86:28–31.
11. Alfrey E, Conley SB, Tanney DC, et al. Use of an augmented urinary bladder can be catastrophic in renal transplantation. Transplant Proc 1997; 29(1–2):154–5.
12. Rigamonti W, Capizzi A, Zacchello G, et al. Kidney transplantation into bladder augmentation or urinary diversion: long-term results. Transplantation 2005; 80:1435–40.
13. Chaykovska L, Deger S, Wille A, et al. Surgical techniques in urology kidney transplantation into urinary conduits with ureteroureterostomy between transplant and native ureter: single-center experience. URL 2008;73:380–5.
14. Parada B, Figueiredo A, Mota A, et al. Renal transplantation in patients with lower urinary tract dysfunction. Transplantation 2010;89(11):1299–307.
15. Sullivan ME, Reynard JM, Cranston DW. Renal transplantation into the abnormal lower urinary tract. BJU Int 2003;92:510–5.
16. DeFoor W, Minevich E, McEnery P, et al. Lower urinary tract reconstruction is safe and effective in children with end stage renal disease. J Urol 2003;170: 1497–500.
17. Errando C, Batista JE, Caparros J, et al. Urodynamic evaluation and management prior to renal transplantation. Eur Urol 2000;38:415–8.
18. Tanagho EA. Congenitally obstructed bladders: fate after prolonged defunctionalization. J Urol 1974;111: 102–9.
19. MacGregor P, Novick AC, Cunningham R, et al. Renal transplantation in end stage renal disease patients with existing urinary diversion. J Urol 1986; 135:686–8.

20. Cerilli J, Anderson GW, Evans WE, et al. Renal transplantation in patients with urinary tract abnormalities. Surgery 1976;79:248–52.

21. Serrano DP, Flechner SM, Modlin CS, et al. Transplantation into the long-term defunctionalized bladder. J Urol 1996;156:885–8.

22. Reinberg Y, Bumgardner GL, Aliabadi H. Urological aspects of renal transplantation. J Urol 1990;143: 1087–92.

23. Jefferson R, Burns JR. Urological evaluation of adult renal transplant recipients. J Urol 1995;153:615–8.

24. Glazier DB, Whang MI, Geffner SR, et al. Evaluation of voiding cystourethrography prior to renal transplantation. Transplantation 1996;62:1762–5.

25. Najarian JS, Matas AJ. The present and future of kidney transplantation. Transplant Proc 1991;23: 2075–82.

26. Bauer SB. Neurogenic bladder: etiology and assessment. Pediatr Nephrol 2008;23:541–51.

27. Wood DP, Bianco FJ, Pontes JE, et al. Incidence and significance of positive urine cultures in patients with an orthotopic neobladder. J Urol 2003; 169:2196–9.

28. Bruce AW, Reid G, Chan RC, et al. Bacterial adherence in the human ileal conduit: a morphological and bacteriological study. J Urol 1984;132:184–8.

29. Wullt B, Agace W, Mansson W. Bladder, bowel and bugs–bacteriuria in patients with intestinal urinary diversion. World J Urol 2004;22:186–95.

30. Suriano F, Gallucci M, Flammia GP, et al. Bacteriuria in patients with an orthotopic ileal neobladder: urinary tract infection or asymptomatic bacteriuria? BJU Int 2008;101:1576–9.

31. Crowe A, Cairns HS, Wood S, et al. Renal transplantation following renal failure due to urological disorders. Nephrol Dial Transplant 1998;13:2065–9.

32. Cairns HS, Leaker B, Woodhouse CR, et al. Renal transplantation into abnormal lower urinary tract. Lancet 1991;338:1376–9.

33. McGuire EJ, Woodside JR, Borden TA, et al. Prognostic value of urodynamic testing in myelodysplastic patients. J Urol 1981;126:205–9.

34. Churchill BM, Sheldon CA, McLorie GA, et al. Factors influencing patient and graft survival in 300 cadaveric pediatric renal transplants. J Urol 1988; 140:1129–33.

35. Blanco M, Medina J, Pamplona M, et al. Outcome of renal transplantation in adult patients with augmented bladders. Transplant Proc 2009;41: 2382–4.

36. Warholm C, Berglund J, Andersson J, et al. Renal transplantation in patients with urinary diversion: a case-control study. Nephrol Dial Transplant 1999; 14:2937–40.

37. Fontaine E, Gagnadoux MF, Niaudet P, et al. Renal transplantation in children with augmentation cystoplasty: long-term results. J Urol 1998;159:2110–3.

38. Thomalla JV, Mitchell ME, Leapman SB, et al. Renal transplantation into the reconstructed bladder. J Urol 1989;141:265–8.

39. Hatch DA. A review of renal transplantation into bowel segments for conduit and continent urinary diversions: techniques and complications. Semin Urol 1994;12:108–13.

40. Zaragoza MR, Ritchey ML, Bloom DA, et al. Enterocystoplasty in renal transplantation candidates: urodynamic evaluation and outcome. J Urol 1993;150: 1463–6.

41. Heritier P, Perraud Y, Relave MH, et al. Renal transplantation and Kock pouch: a case report. J Urol 1989;141:595–6.

42. Martín MG, Castro SN, Castelo LA, et al. Enterocystoplasty and renal transplantation. J Urol 2001;165: 393–6.

43. Wegner HE, Meier T, Schwarz A, et al. Ileal conduit urinary diversion 16 months before renal transplantation in a case of non-functioning lower urinary tract. Int Urol Nephrol 1994;26:661–4.

44. Hatch DA, Belitsky P, Barry JM, et al. Fate of renal allografts transplanted in patients with urinary diversion. Transplantation 1993;56:838–42.

45. McInerney PD, Picramenos D, Koffman CG, et al. Is cystoplasty a safe alternative to urinary diversion in patients requiring renal transplantation? Eur Urol 1995;27:117–20.

46. Malone MJ, Khauli RB, Lowell J. Use of small and large bowel in renal transplantation. Urol Clin North Am 1997;24:837–43.

47. Hakim NS, Benedetti E, Pirenne J, et al. Complications of ureterovesical anastomosis in kidney transplant patients: the Minnesota experience. Clin Transplant 1994;8:504–7.

48. Pleass HC, Clark KR, Rigg KM, et al. Urologic complications after renal transplantation: a prospective randomized trial comparing different techniques of ureteric anastomosis and the use of prophylactic ureteric stents. Transplant Proc 1995;27:1091–2.

49. Shokeir AA, Sobh MA, Bakr MA, et al. Vesico-ureteral reimplantation in kidney transplantation from living relative donor: extravesical or transvesical? Urologic complications and long-term results evaluation. Prog Urol 1992;2:241–8 [in French].

50. Gurkan A, Yakupoglu YK, Dinckan A, et al. Comparing two ureter reimplantation techniques in kidney transplant recipients. Transpl Int 2006;19: 802–6.

51. Chava SP, Singh B, Stangou A, et al. Simultaneous combined liver and kidney transplantation: a single center experience. Clin Transplant 2009;24:E62–8.

52. Fong TL, Khemichian S, Shah T, et al. Combined liver-kidney transplantation is preferable to liver transplant alone for cirrhotic patients with renal failure. Transplantation 2012;94:411–6.

53. Lee RK, Abol-Enein H, Artibani W, et al. Urinary diversion after radical cystectomy for bladder cancer: options, patient selection, and outcomes. BJU Int 2014;113:11–23.

54. Sheldon CA, Gonzalez R, Burns MW, et al. Renal transplantation into the dysfunctional bladder: the role of adjunctive bladder reconstruction. J Urol 1994;152:972–5.

55. Slagt IK, Ijzermans JN, Alamyar M, et al. Long-term outcome of kidney transplantation in patients with a urinary conduit: a case–control study. Int Urol Nephrol 2013;45(2):405–11.

56. Biers SM, Venn SN, Greenwell TJ. The past, present and future of augmentation cystoplasty. BJU Int 2012;109:1280–93.

57. Taghizadeh A, Mahdavi R, Mirsadraee S, et al. Ureterocystoplasty is safe and effective in patients awaiting renal transplantation. Urology 2007;70:861–3.

58. Feminella JG, Lattimer JK. A retrospective analysis of 70 cases of cutaneous ureterostomy. J Urol 1971;106:538–40.

59. Kogan BA, Gohary MA. Cutaneous ureterostomy as a permanent external urinary diversion in children. J Urol 1984;132:729–31.

60. MacGregor PS, Kay R, Straffon RA. Cutaneous ureterostomy in children–long-term followup. J Urol 1985;134:518–20.

61. MacGregor PS, Montie JE, Straffon RA. Cutaneous ureterostomy as palliative diversion in adults with malignancy. Urology 1987;30:31–4.

62. Kearney GP, Docimo SG, Doyle CJ, et al. Cutaneous ureterostomy in adults. Urology 1992;40:1–6.

63. McDonald MW, Zincke H, Engen DE, et al. Adaptation of existing cutaneous ureterostomy for urinary drainage after renal transplantation. J Urol 1985;133:1026–8.

64. Purohit RS, Bretan PN. Successful long-term outcome using existing native cutaneous ureterostomy for renal transplant drainage. J Urol 2000;163:446–9.

65. Prieto M, Sierra M, de Francisco AL, et al. Long-term outcome in renal transplantation with terminal cutaneous ureterostomy. Br J Urol 1993;72:844–7.

66. Srinivasan D, Stoffel JT, Mathur AK, et al. Long-term outcomes of kidney transplant recipients with bladder dysfunction: a single-center study. Ann Transplant 2016;21:222–34.

67. Hatch DA, Koyle MA, Baskin LS, et al. Kidney transplantation in children with urinary diversion or bladder augmentation. J Urol 2001;165:2265–8.

68. Al-Khudairi N, Riley P, Desai DY, et al. Interventions for impaired bladders in paediatric renal transplant recipients with lower urinary tract dysfunction. Transpl Int 2013;26:428–34.

69. Koo HP, Bunchman TE, Flynn JT, et al. Renal transplantation in children with severe lower urinary tract dysfunction. J Urol 1999;161:240–5.

70. Okhunov Z, Duty B, Smith AD, et al. Management of urolithiasis in patients after urinary diversions. BJU Int 2011;108:330–6.

71. Palmer LS, Franco I, Kogan SJ, et al. Urolithiasis in children following augmentation cystoplasty. J Urol 1993;150:726–9.

72. McLoughlin LC, Davis NF, Dowling CM, et al. Outcome of deceased donor renal transplantation in patients with an ileal conduit. Clin Transplant 2014;28:307–13.

73. Seth JH, Promponas J, Hadjipavlou M, et al. Urolithiasis following urinary diversion. Urolithiasis 2016;44:383–8.

74. Austen M, Kälble T. Secondary malignancies in different forms of urinary diversion using isolated gut. J Urol 2004;172:831–8.

75. Fanning DM, Sabah M, Conlon PJ, et al. An unusual case of cancer of the urachal remnant following repair of bladder exstrophy. Ir J Med Sci 2011;180:913–5.

Advances in Pediatric Urinary Diversion

Jeffrey D. Browning, MD[a], Heidi A. Stephany, MD[b],*

KEYWORDS

- Pediatric • Diversion • Techniques • Urinary • Bladder

KEY POINTS

- Urinary diversion in pediatric patients is used for unique indications and utilizes distinct techniques.
- Pediatric patients who require or may require urinary diversion should be followed closely by a pediatric urologist with a wide breath of knowledge of the various techniques for urinary diversion.
- Optimal management of pediatric patients requiring diversion should be tailored to individual patients.

INTRODUCTION

Urinary diversion in pediatric patients is used for a distinct set of indications to address the unique surgical and technical challenges of this patient population. The management of spina bifida has evolved over the past century with the advent of clean intermittent catheterization and the judicious use of anticholinergic medicines; however, urinary diversion remains an important treatment modality for a certain subset of patients. The indications for and the various types of diversions as well as the relevant and emerging techniques are reviewed.

The primary indication for surgical invention and urinary diversion in pediatric patients is the preservation of renal function and prevention of upper tract deterioration secondary to a hostile lower urinary tract. In addition, reconstruction of the urinary tract to allow for urinary continence is particularly important with a significant effect on quality of life in these patients. A majority of patients requiring such techniques have a neurogenic bladder as a result of myelodysplasia.[1] Although there is an increased emphasis on optimizing bladder function via medical management and pharmacotherapy, several patients still require a form of urinary diversion, whether temporary or permanent. In 1981, McGuire and colleagues[2] reported his findings linking detrusor leak point pressures greater than 40 cm H_2O with increased risk of upper tract damage. Passive filling pressures greater than 40 cm H_2O become clinically pathologic, leading to impaired ureteral drainage.[3] Elevated bladder pressure can produce hydroureteronephrosis, which can result in an associated decrease in glomerular filtration rate (GFR). Moreover, elevated bladder pressures can cause secondary vesicoureteral reflux (VUR).[1]

Other indications for urinary diversion include temporizing newborns with severe VUR and febrile urinary tract infections (UTIs) as well as outlet obstruction secondary to conditions, including posterior urethral valves and bilateral ectopic ureters. Bladder exstrophy and other cloacal malformations require more complex urinary reconstruction.

TYPES OF URINARY DIVERSION

Urinary diversion can be subdivided into 2 categories: continent and incontinent (**Table 1**). Continent urinary diversion seeks to maintain the continence mechanism using a continent catheterizable channel. Although intermittent catheterization and anticholinergic medications can obviate

Disclosure Statement: The authors have nothing to disclose.
[a] Department of Urology, University of Pittsburgh Medical Center, 3471 Fifth Avenue, Suite 700, Pittsburgh, PA 15213, USA; [b] Department of Urology, University of California, Irvine and Children's Hospital of Orange County, 505 S. Main Street, Orange, CA 92868, USA
* Corresponding author.
E-mail address: hstepha1@uci.edu

Table 1
Pediatric urinary diversion

Continent	Incontinent
Mitrofanoff APV	Cutaneous vesicostomy
Monti procedure	
Continent catheterizable vesicostomy	Cutaneous ureterostomy
Button vesicostomy	Ileovesicostomy
Indiana pouch	Ileal conduit
Augmentation cystoplasty	
Ureterosigmoidostomy	

surgical repair in some cases, long-term urethral catheterization may be difficult for many patients. Orthopedic contractures, diminished manual dexterity, and other comorbidities can impede ease of routine catheterization and incontinent diversion may be the best alternative in these patients. Continent catheterizable channels allow an alternative route to drain the bladder with or without bladder augmentation or reconstruction of the bladder neck. Bladder augmentation and bladder neck reconstruction are important methods used in patients to improve not only continence but concerning urodynamic parameters that can subsequently affect the upper urinary tract.[1] Social circumstances precluding strict compliance to a catheterization regimen is a critical factor in selecting the best treatment option and urologists must take this into consideration.

INCONTINENT URINARY DIVERSION
Cutaneous Vesicostomy

Background and indications
Lapides and colleagues[4] first proposed the use of a cutaneous vesicostomy in the 1960s. Many infants with myelodysplasia and resultant neurogenic bladder were treated with a cutaneous vesicostomy as a temporizing measure to protect the upper urinary tracts from a hostile bladder. With the introduction of clean intermittent catheterization, the use of vesicostomies as a form of diversion has decreased significantly, yet there remains a subset of patients with specific indications requiring a urinary diversion.[5] Various indications include recurrent febrile UTIs, progressively worsening hydronephrosis with decreasing renal function, and outlet obstruction, such as posterior urethral valves when cystoscopy is not possible.[6]

Technique
The Blocksom technique of vesicostomy creation begins with a 2-cm midline transverse incision made approximately midway between the pubic

symphysis and the umbilicus.[7] The rectus muscles are separated and the bladder is exposed and secured with traction sutures. The peritoneum is mobilized cephalad to free the dome and posterior wall of the bladder and the urachus is ligated. The bladder is opened in the longitudinal axis and secured circumferentially to the skin. The posterior wall should be kept taut to prevent prolapse of the bladder through the incision.[4] **Fig. 1** shows a vesicostomy performed at the time of bladder closure in an infant with cloacal exstrophy.

Complications
Complications related to cutaneous vesicostomy include stenosis, contact dermatitis, and mucosal prolapse (**Fig. 2**). Prudente and colleagues[6] evaluated 21 patients with a vesicostomy to determine long-term complications. Indications for the vesicostomy included posterior urethral valves and myelomeningocele. Renal function remained stable or improved in 95.2% and there was a decrease in the number of UTIs by 38.1% and VUR in 71.4%. As for complications, they reported stomal stenosis (38%), dermatitis (24%), and mucosal prolapse (29%). **Fig. 2** demonstrates mucosal prolapse.

Cutaneous Ureterostomy

Background and indications
Definitive surgical treatment of VUR and megaureter is indicated in the setting of recurrent febrile UTIs or upper tract deterioration. Failure of expectant management is particularly challenging in infants less than 1 year because surgical repair can be difficult. Ureteral reimplantation prior to 1 year of age has an increased rate of reoperation and revision.[8] For those patients less than 1 year of age, an end cutaneous ureterostomy can be used as a temporizing measure to allow the patient time to grow prior to definitive reimplantation.

Technique
Extraperitoneal exposure of the ureter can be carried out through an ipsilateral modified Gibson incision. The ureter is exposed and transected

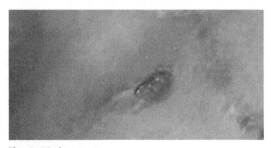

Fig. 1. Vesicostomy.

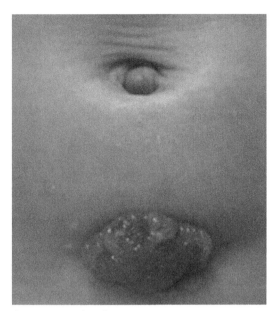

Fig. 2. Mucosal prolapse.

near its insertion into the bladder with the ureteral stump oversewn with absorbable suture.[9] The ureterostomy can also be created in a loop fashion without complete transection of the ureter and may prevent disruption of the ureteral blood supply.[10] The ureteral stoma is created in the lateral aspect of the incision. The ureteral adventitia is anchored to the underlying fascia and skin. If bilateral diversion is required, a Pfannenstiel incision can be used.

Complications
Postoperative complications related to creation of end cutaneous ureterostomy include stomal stenosis and febrile UTI/pyelonephritis. One series demonstrated a rate of stomal stenosis of 3% and pyelonephritis of 31%.[9] Some investigators advocate creating a temporary refluxing ureteral reimplant as an alternative to a ureterostomy, thus negating the risk of stomal stenosis.[11] The frequency of pyelonephritis is similar, however, with rates of 18% in the most recent series.[12]

Ileovesicostomy

Background and indications
Ileovesicostomy was first described in the 1950s and its use in the pediatric population has previously been somewhat limited.[13] An ileovesicostomy serves as a low-pressure diversion without the need for intermittent catheterization. This can be particularly useful in patients with significant emotional, social, cognitive, and physical barriers to intermittent catheterization. It boasts an additional advantage in that it is reversible if circumstances change allowing for a continent diversion.[14]

Technique
A segment of at least 15 cm to 20 cm of ileum proximal to the ileocecal valve with adequate mesentery to reach the bladder is used. The proximal end of the segment is anastomosed to the bladder whereas the distal end is matured as a stoma to the lower abdominal wall. The ureters are left in their native location. The length of the segment is tailored to the patient ensuring no significant redundancy to allow adequate drainage.[13] The same procedure has also been performed robotically in an entirely intracorporeal approach in adults.[15]

Complications
Complications include ileus, wound infection, UTI, stomal stenosis, and temporary urethral leakage. One series evaluated 9 patients who had an ileovesicostomy performed for various reasons and reported 2 immediate postoperative complications, including an ileus requiring total parental nutrition and a wound infection. Long-term complications included urinary tract infection in 2 patients, temporary urinary leakage in 1, and stomal issues in 2.[14] Long-term follow-up is vital to these patients and should be stressed to the patients and families. As they transition to adulthood, rates of obesity and associated complications, such as stomal stenosis and/or mechanical loop obstruction, increase. These later complications have been found associated with upper tract deterioration in as many as 60% of patients.[16]

Ileal Conduit

Background and indications
Urinary diversion through use of an ileal conduit is common for adult patients undergoing radical cystectomy. Ileal conduit had been applied to pediatric patients too young to undergo continent urinary diversion, those lacking family support, and those with poor manual dexterity. Several studies, however, have shown high complication rates and renal deterioration with its use in pediatric populations; thus, ileal conduit use in the pediatric population is typically reserved for those with no other options for urinary diversion.[17]

Technique
Similar to an ileovesicostomy and augmentation cystoplasty, a segment of at least 15 cm to 20 cm of ileum proximal to the ileocecal valve with adequate mesentery is used. The proximal end of the segment is used as a landing site for the bilateral native ureters and the distal end is

matured as a stoma to the lateral abdominal wall. The bladder may be left in situ or removed depending on the clinical indication for diversion.[17]

Complications

Like any procedure using a segment of bowel, complications include ileus, adhesions, and bowel obstruction. Addition complications include stomal stenosis, ureteral stricture, pyelonephritis, and progression of renal deterioration. A review of 29 children (mean age 10 years) who underwent creation of an ileal conduit for neurogenic bladder in most cases were followed for a mean of 91 months.[18] Although there was no statistically significant difference between baseline and last follow-up GFR, stage of chronic kidney disease had worsened in 44.8% of patients and end-stage kidney disease developed in 11 patients and 9 had died.[18]

CONTINENT URINARY DIVERSION
Mitrofanoff Appendicovesicostomy

Background and indications

First described in 1980, the Mitrofanoff appendicovesicostomy (APV) is a continent catheterizable channel that used the appendix to create a flap valve.[19] The appendix is an ideal structure for diversion because it can be safely removed from the gastrointestinal tract without significant morbidity. Continence can be achieved with an appendiceal tunnel of only 2 cm.[20] The appendix can be implanted into the native bladder or into bowel segments used for augmentation cystoplasty during more complex repairs. The procedure is ideal in pediatric patients with a relatively long appendiceal segments and generally thinner abdominal walls. The procedure overall has a lower morbidity than other surgeries requiring bowel resection.

In recent years, minimally invasive techniques, in particular robotic-assisted laparoscopy, have been used to create APVs. Reviews have demonstrated no significant differences in effectiveness, morbidity, and immediate postoperative and long-term complications when compared with the open procedure.[21] There is, however, significantly increased mean operative time when comparing the 2 techniques, with 623 minutes for a robotic-assisted procedure versus 267 minutes in the open procedure ($P<.01$).[22] Operative times can improve with accumulated experience.

Indications for a Mitrofanoff APV are well documented. **Fig. 3** lists indications for a continent catheterizable channel in a retrospective review of cases over a 20-year period by Faure and colleagues,[23] with neurogenic bladder the most common.

Technique

Exposure to the appendix and bladder can be achieved through a low midline or transverse incision. The ascending colon may need to be mobilized along the line of Toldt to gain better access and length to the appendix and its mesentery.[24] Colonic mobilization is especially important in

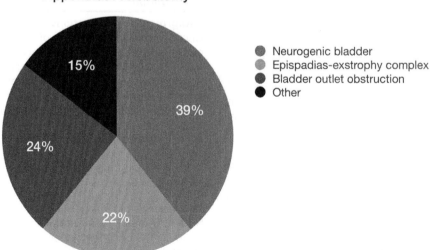

Fig. 3. Indications for a continent catheterizable channel in a retrospective review of cases over a 20-year period. (*From* Faure A, Cooksey R, Bouty A, et al. Bladder continent catheterizable conduit (the Mitrofanoff procedure): long-term issues that should not be underestimated. J Pediatr Surg 2016;52(3):470; with permission.)

spina bifida patients with prior abdominal surgeries or those with a ventriculoperitoneal shunt. Special care should be taken in these patients, particularly if the procedure is performed robotically to avoid bowel injury during trocar placement. The appendix and a small portion of the cecum are amputated and cecal cuff closed. A larger portion of cecum can be taken if there is concern for insufficient length of the appendix. The distal appendix is tunneled into the bladder to provide continence after the end is amputated. The conduit should be maintained as short as possible to prevent difficulty with catheterization caused by kinking. For all procedures involving catheterizable channels, the channel should be catheterized at each step of the procedure to ensure ease of passage.[1]

Complications

The most common complication after an APV is stomal stenosis, with rates ranging from 6% to 10% of patients.[25] Some retrospective studies have demonstrated much higher complication rates, however. In a retrospective review by Faure and colleagues,[23] the revision rate was as high as 60%, of which most occurred within the first 2 years. Patients with posterior urethral valves seemed to have higher rate of revisions. Additional complications include leakage, conduit stricture, angulation of the conduit, difficulty with catheterization, and prolapse. The timing of complications has also been evaluated. A single institution review by Thomas and colleagues[25] demonstrated a 23% complication rate in continent catheterizable stomas at a mean of 28.4 months of follow-up. The majority developed in the first 12 months and none was observed after 24 months. This study also included Malone Antegrade Continence Enema (MACE) channels. In a more recent review from the same institution, extending the period of follow-up to an average of 80.1 months, the investigators found complications related to a catheterizable channel were more common in the first 2 years after surgery and then significantly decreased.[26]

Mitrofanoff Modifications—Monti Procedure

Background and indications

There are many circumstances where the appendix is not available or appropriate for use in urinary diversion and other options must be explored. The appendix may not be ideal if it has a precarious blood supply, insufficient length, or a short mesentery. There can be histopathologic changes, such as chronic inflammation or a fibrous lumen obstruction, precluding its use as well.[27] In some, the appendix may have already been removed for use in other surgical procedures,

such as a MACE procedure. A wide range of structures have been utilized in these circumstances, including ureter, ileum, stomach, cecal flaps, fallopian tube, colon, and bladder flaps.[27] The quality of the resulting channel, however, was often believed inferior.

In 1993, Yang[28] was the first to describe transverse tubularization of 2 small detubularized ileal segments to be implanted into an ileal reservoir in a patient undergoing radical cystectomy. This alternative technique, however, remained relatively unknown until 1997, when Monti and colleageus[29] independently detailed construction of single and double ileal tubes in dogs. This review focuses on the Monti procedure using a tubularized ileal segment because this is the most commonly performed technique in pediatric urology when the appendix is not a viable option.

Technique

In general, a segment of ileum measuring 2 cm to 2.5 cm is sufficient to allow construction of a tube, which accommodates passage of a 16F to 18F catheter. Preservation of the vascular pedicle is key and ideally the tube is kept as short as possible, with a single tube usually preferred to avoid kinking.[1] The determining factor as to whether or not a single or double tube is required is the thickness of the abdominal wall. Two stay sutures are placed at both ends of the bowel patch and tubularization is performed with absorbable 3-0 or 4-0 running sutures over a 12F catheter. The new tube is implanted into the bladder using the Le Duc technique in which an intramural tunnel is created in an antirefluxing fashion.[30] The reservoir is fixed to the anterior abdominal wall at a site immediately adjacent to the site of implantation to prevent kinking of the tube. The stoma can be positioned in any quadrant but the umbilicus allows for use of a single tube with a good cosmetic result.[1]

Modifications of the Monti procedure include the Casale procedure, also known as the spiral Monti. The advantage of the spiral Monti is that it provides a channel with double the length without a circular anastomosis, which is a theoretic disadvantage of the classic double Monti tube.[31]

Complications

Complications are similar to that of the APV; however, there are higher rates of early postoperative complications associated with bowel resection, including ileus and small bowel obstruction. Cain and colleagues[32] reported on approximately 200 patients who underwent Monti and Casale procedures with an overall success rate of

97.5% at a mean follow-up of 28 months. Early complications generally occurred in patients who had simultaneous bladder augmentations. Stomal revision was required in 8% (n = 16) for stomal stenosis, prolapse, or superficial stomal problems. Primary channel revisions were required in 9.5% of patients for indications, including channel elongation/angulation, insufficient tunnel length, and stenosis.[32] Overall, channel incontinence was rare and only occurred in 4 patients. Complication rates are similar between the Monte and Casale techniques, with the exception of stomas placed in the umbilicus using the Casale technique found to have twice the complications.[33] A recent study retrospectively evaluated 510 consecutive catheterizable channels and found that Monti channels were 2.09 times more likely to require surgical revision than APVs.[34] It was thought the difference between the 2 channels was a result of a naturally occurring appendiceal lumen as well as the greater surface area of the appendiceal mesentery.

Mitrofanoff Modifications—Continent Catheterizable Vesicostomy and Button Vesicostomy

There are many variations derived from the Mitrofanoff technique, including a continent catheterization vesicostomy used in patients with a large bladder capacity. Peard and colleagues[35] described a technique using an intussuscepted bladder flap as the channel and continence mechanism. This spares the appendix or the need for a bowel resection. Early results have been encouraging; however, other investigators have reported higher stenosis rates using similar techniques in long-term follow-up compared with intestinal channels.[36]

In 2007, the button vesicostomy, which uses a short gastrostomy tube, was described as an alternative short-term or medium-term option for a catheterizable continent urinary stoma.[37] Through a 2-cm transverse skin incision in the lower abdomen, the bladder apex is accessed and the tube is secured in place with a purse string suture. The tube is brought out through a separate stab incision inferiorly. The procedure is associated with minimal morbidity and postoperative maintenance is well tolerated by patients and their families. In a review of 30 patients over 13 years, minor complications, including transient leakage, wound infection, and overgranulation, occurred in 44% of patients. Major complications included major leaks and device failure occurred in 20% of patients.[37]

Indiana Pouch

Background and indications

The Indiana pouch urinary diversion has been used since its initial description in the late 1980s.[38] In children with complex lower urinary tract abnormalities, an Indiana pouch can provide catheter-based continence.[39] In a review by Chowdhary and colleagues,[40] indications included those patients with multiple failed surgeries for exstrophy-epispadias complex, residual disease in the trigone after chemotherapy for genitourinary rhabdomyosarcoma, and nephrogenic metaplasia in patients with a neurogenic bladder.

Technique

In general, a short segment of the terminal ileum is used as an efferent limb. This limb is kept as short and straight as possible to facilitate easy catheterization. The continence mechanism is provided by the ileocecal valve rather than the length of the efferent limb.[1] Imbrication is usually secured with interrupted, permanent sutures, involving the distal ileum and ileocecal valve and is carried onto the cecum.[40]

Complications

Complications are similar to both the Monti and APV procedures, including incontinence (daytime or nocturnal), calculi, stricture, and VUR.[41,42] Changes in bowel function are rare and most are related to disruption of the ileocecal valve. Removing this is more likely to cause diarrhea, with rates reportedly ranging from 10% to 23%, and can also allow bacterial backflow into the ileum altering fat and vitamin B_{12} absorption.[43]

Augmentation Cystoplasty

Background and indications

Frequently augmentation cystoplasty is performed in patients undergoing reconstruction of a catheterizable channel. Overall, the number of bladder augmentations has decreased in the United States by 25% according to a study looking at national trends in augmentation rates in the 2000s. Although multifactorial, this likely reflects in part the evolving practice patterns in this subset of patients.[44] It remains an important consideration after failed medical management in children with evidence of persistent lower urinary tract dysfunction threatening upper tract integrity because it improves bladder compliance and capacity in such patients. In addition, it provides an option for reconstruction using the native bladder and a continent catheterizable channel to achieve continence. The importance of careful patient selection cannot be stressed enough. Patients and caregivers must comply with a strict catheterization regiment to prevent severe, life-threatening complications, such as a bladder perforation. Age and maturity level should be considered as well as their social support system. Patients requiring complete ablation of the bladder neck or significant reconstruction of the bladder neck to allow for continence are at particular risk because they no longer have any type of pop-off mechanism if unable to catheterize their channel.[1]

Technique

Bladder augmentation is classically performed via an open abdominal approach; however, with the advancement of minimally invasive techniques, some investigators have described laparoscopic techniques, which typically require much longer operative times.[45] In general, augmentation cystoplasty is performed through a low midline incision, although a lower transverse incision can be used if there has been no prior abdominal surgery. The native bladder is incised in a sagittal plane from a point several centimeters cephalad to the bladder neck to a position just above the trigone posteriorly. A variety of intestinal segments have been used, including gastric, jejunal, ileal, and colonic. The choice of segment is individualized to each patient based on numerous characteristics, such as previous surgical history, ease of mobilization of a segment, and renal function. Regardless of segment, the bowel is isolated, detubularized, and reconfigured to achieve the most spherical shape possible to maximize bladder capacity. The most commonly used technique is ileocystoplasty because the ileum has been found to be the most compliant and least contractile.[1] The segment of ileum must be at least 15 cm to 20 cm proximal to the ileocecal valve and should have adequate mesentery to reach the native bladder without tension. The ileal segment is folded into a U shape with the bowel anastomosed to itself with running absorbable sutures. The anastomosis of the bladder to the ileum may be done in 1 or 2 layers using absorbable suture. A suprapubic tube is generally placed as well as a pelvic drain.[1]

Complications

Complications are common and include intestinal, infectious, and metabolic abnormalities. Immediate perioperative complications include prolonged ileus and respiratory complications. In a large series, including 500 patients, the prevalence of complications requiring bladder level surgical intervention was 34%. Bowel obstruction occurred in approximately 3% of patients, most commonly with gastrocystoplasties, presumably

due its longer mesenteric course. A second augmentation was required in 9.4% due to incontinence or limited capacity with a mean time of 7.5 years to the second operation. Symptomatic UTI was identified in 22.7% of patients with lower rates in those patients where a gastric segment was used.[46] Data from the Pediatric Health Information System, including patients who underwent an augmentation cystoplasty from 1999 to 2010, demonstrated a 10-year cumulative incidence ranges, including pyelonephritis (16.1%–37.1%), bladder rupture (2.9%–6.4%), and small bowel obstruction (5.2%–10.3%). Urologic procedures after an augmentation included cystolithalopaxy (13.3%–35.1%), and reaugmentation (5.2%–13.4%). There was an increased hazard of bladder rupture (hazard ratio 1.9; 95% CI, 1.1–3.3) in patients undergoing simultaneous bladder neck surgery.[47]

Complications specific to the bowel segment vary based on the secretion of the segment. The acidic nature of gastric secretions can result in hematuria-dysuria syndrome.[48] Symptoms of hematuria-dysuria syndrome include bladder spasms, suprapubic pain, dysuria, and gross hematuria. The net loss of acid can result in hypokalemic, hypochloremic metabolic acidosis.[1] Mucous production, which is greatest in the colon, can impede bladder emptying and predispose patients to UTIs. Mucous and infection have been long known to be related to the high rate of bladder and renal stone formation in this patient population.[49] Recent studies, however, have demonstrated noninfectious stones in one-third of bladder stones and one-half of renal stones. There were also no clinical variables associated with infectious stones suggesting a possible metabolic component to stone formation after bladder augmentation.[50]

Complications involving loss of intestinal segment include metabolic abnormalities, such as vitamin B_{12} deficiency, anemia, and diminished bone mineral density. A recent analysis of children who underwent augmentation cystoplasty demonstrated higher rates of osteopenia and osteoporosis relative to controls on dual-energy x-ray absorpiometry scan. Decreased bone mineral density was also associated with decreased GFR.[51]

The risk of malignancy in an augmented bladder is a significant concern that was originally observed as a late complication of ureterosigmoidostomy and is now understood to be associated with any bowel segment not exposed to a fecal stream.[52] Tumors can arise from all associated tissues with reported malignancies, including transitional cell carcinoma, adenocarcinoma, and benign polyps. Pathogenesis includes effects of chronic inflammation as well as nitrosamine-producing bacteria. In a series of 153 patients who were followed for a minimum of 10 years, a total of 7 (4.5%) cases of malignancy were reported, including urothelial and adenocarcinoma.[52] The median time to tumor development after augmentation was 32 years. Currently, cystoscopy is recommended for screening starting 10 years after bladder augmentation, but some studies have shown this may not be cost effective because a majority of patients are symptomatic on presentation.[53]

Ureterosigmoidostomy

Background and indications

The use of ureterosigmoidostomy in the United States in pediatric populations is generally historic and has fallen out of favor due to many significant complications. Knowledge of this technique and its complications, however, is wise because there are certain populations of patients this may prove the most viable option.

Technique

Dating back as far as the 1800s, anastomosing the ureters to the bowel has been described in patients with exstrophy.[54] This technique uses the rectosigmoid colon as the reservoir with the anus serving as the continence mechanism for both feces and urine. It was advantageous in that the new method for ureterointestinal anastomosis decreased the risk of reflux and subsequent pyelonephritis.[55] Another modification was the Mainz II pouch in which the colon is incised along the anti-mesenteric border and reconfigured to establish a rectosigmoid reservoir with lower pressures to protect the upper tracts.[56] Prior to any surgical intervention, the anal sphincter must be tested using manometry or an oatmeal enema to ensure competence of the sphincter to avoid stool and urinary incontinence. Neurogenic patients with fecal incontinence are not candidates for this procedure.

Complications

The most significant complication of ureterosig-moidostomy is the risk of colorectal adenocarci-noma with rates reportedly as high as 15%.[57] A Swedish review of 25 patients who underwent the procedure between 1944 to 1961 demonstrated development of invasive colorectal adenocarcinoma in 7 patients and colorectal adenocarcinoma in situ in 1. Five patients died because of the malignancy. The mean time from ureterosigmoidostomy to diagnosis of invasive colorectal adenocarcinoma was 38 years (range

23–55).[55] Compared with the general population, the risk of colorectal adenocarcinoma was increased 42 times. The incidence of poorly differentiated disease was also very high. Despite conversion to other forms of diversion, Sohn and colleagues[58] found the risk persists even years later. Other significant complications include hyperchloremic metabolic acidosis, hydronephrosis, reflux, and pyelonephritis.

SUMMARY

Urinary diversion is performed for a unique set of indications in the pediatric population. Although surgical intervention has decreased in necessity overall due to advances in expectant management, it remains an important tool. These patients require long-term follow-up with a urologist to ensure preservation of renal function as well as regular monitoring for the various complications associated with urinary diversion.

REFERENCES

1. Adams MC, Joseph DB, Thomas JC. Urinary tract reconstruction in children. In: Wein AJ, Kavoussi LR, Partin AW, et al, editors. Campbell-walsh urology. 11th edition. Philadelphia: Elsevier; 2016. p. 3330–67.
2. McGuire EJ, Woodside JR, Borden TA, et al. Prognostic value of urodynamic testing in myelodysplastic patients. J Urol 1981;126(2):205–9.
3. Wang SC, McGuire EJ, Bloom DA. A bladder pressure management system for myelodysplasia–clinical outcome. J Urol 1988;140(6):1499–502.
4. Lapides J, Ajemian EP, Lichtwardt JR. Cutaneous vesicostomy. J Urol 1960;84:609–14.
5. Lee MW, Greenfield SP. Intractable high-pressure bladder in female infants with spina bifida: clinical characteristics and use of vesicostomy. Urology 2005;65(3):568–71.
6. Prudente A, Reis LO, Franca RD, et al. Vesicostomy as a protector of upper urinary tract in long-term follow-up. Urol J 2009;6:96–100.
7. Nerli RB, Patil RA, Ghagane SC. Revisited Blocksom vesicostomy: operative steps. J Sci Soc 2017;44: 58–60.
8. Peters CA, Mandell J, Lebowitz RL, et al. Congenital obstructed megaureters in early infancy: diagnosis and treatment. J Urol 1989;142(2 Pt 2):641–5.
9. Kitchens DM, DeFoor W, Minevich E, et al. End cutaneous ureterostomy for the management of severe hydronephrosis. J Urol 2007;177(4):1501–4.
10. Mor Y, Ramon J, Raviv G, et al. Low loop cutaneous ureterostomy and subsequent reconstruction: 20 years of experience. J Urol 1992;147(6):1595–7.
11. Lee SD, Akbal C, Kaefer M. Refluxing ureteral reimplant as temporary treatment of obstructive

megaureter in neonate and infant. J Urol 2005; 173(4):1357–60.

12. Kaefer M, Misseri R, Frank E, et al. Refluxing ureteral reimplantation: a logical method for managing neonatal UVJ obstruction. J Pediatr Urol 2014; 10(5):824–30.

13. Cordonnier JJ. Ileocystostomy for neurogenic bladder. J Urol 1957;78(5):605.

14. Ching CB, Stephany HA, Juliano TM, et al. Outcomes of incontinent ileovesicostomy in the pediatric patient. J Urol 2014;191(2):445–50.

15. Dolat MT, Moore BW, Grob BM, et al. Completely intracorporeal robotic-assisted laparoscopic ileovesicostomy: initial results. J Robot Surg 2014;8(2):137–40.

16. Burgess K, Lightner D, Husmann D. Management outcomes in the severely impaired patient with moribund obesity and iatrogenic intrinsic sphincteric deficiency. Neurourol Urodyn 2011;30:251.

17. Cass AS, Luxenberg M, Gleich P, et al. A 22-year followup of ileal conduits in children with a neurogenic bladder. J Urol 1984;132(3):529–31.

18. Abdelhalim A, Elshal AM, Elsawy AA, et al. Bricker conduit for pediatric urinary diversion—should we still offer it? J Urol 2015;194(5):1414–9.

19. Mitrofanoff P. Trans-appendicular continent cystostomy in the management of the neurogenic bladder. Chir Pediatr 1980;21(4):297–305.

20. Kaefer M, Retik AB. The Mitrofanoff principle in continent urinary reconstruction. Urol Clin North Am 1997;24:795–811.

21. Famakinwa OJ, Rosen AM, Gundeti MS. Robot-assisted laparoscopic Mitrofanoff appendicovesicostomy technique and outcomes of extravesical and intravesical approaches. Eur Urol 2013; 64(5):831–6.

22. Murthy P, Cohn JA, Selig RB, et al. Robot-assisted laparoscopic augmentation ileocystoplasty and Mitrofanoff appendicovesicostomy in children: updated interim results. Eur Urol 2015;68(6):1069–75.

23. Faure A, Cooksey R, Bouty A, et al. Bladder continent catheterizable conduit (the Mitrofanoff procedure): long-term issues that should not be underestimated. J Pediatr Surg 2016;52(3):469–72.

24. Cadeddu JA, Docimo SG. Laparoscopic-assisted continent stoma procedures: our new standard. Urology 1999;54:909–12.

25. Thomas JC, Dietrich MS, Trusler L, et al. Continent catheterizable channels and the timing of their complications. J Urol 2006;176(4):1816–20.

26. Jacobson DL, Thomas JC, Pope J 4th, et al. Update on continent catheterizable channels and the timing of their complications. J Urol 2017 Mar;197(3 Pt 2):871–6.

27. Monti PR, de Carvalho JR, Arap S. The Monti procedure: applications and complications. Urology 2000;55(5):616–21.

28. Yang WH. Yang needle tunneling technique in creating antireflux and continent mechanisms. J Urol 1993;150(3):830–4.

29. Monti PR, Lara RC, Dutra MA, et al. New techniques for construction of efferent conduits based on the Mitrofanoff principle. Urology 1997;49(1):112–5.

30. Le Duc A, Camey M, Teillac P. An original antireflux ureteroileal implantation technique: long-term followup. J Urol 1987;137(6):1156–8.

31. Casale AJ. A long continent ileovesicostomy using a single piece of bowel. J Urol 1999;162(5):1743–5.

32. Cain MP, Dussinger AM, Gitlin J, et al. Updated experience with the Monti catheterizable channel. Urology 2008;72(4):782–5.

33. Leslie JA, Cain MP, Kaefer M, et al. A comparison of the Monti and Casale (spiral Monti) procedures. J Urol 2007;178(4):1623–7.

34. Szymanski KM, Whittam B, Misseri R, et al. Long-term outcomes of catheterizable continent urinary channels: what do you use, where you put it, and does it matter? J Pediatr Urol 2015;11:210.e1-7.

35. Peard L, Fox PJ, Andrews WM, et al. Continent catheterizable vesicostomy: an alternative surgical modality for pediatric patients with large bladder capacity. Urology 2016;93:217–22.

36. Cain MP, Rink RC, Yerkes EB, et al. Long-term followup and outcome of continent catheterizable vesicostomy using the Rink modification. J Urol 2002; 168(6):2583–5.

37. Bradshaw CJ, Gray R, Downer A, et al. Button vesicostomy: 13 years of experience. J Pediatr Urol 2014;10(1):80–7.

38. Randall G, Rowland RG. Indiana continent urinary reservoir. J Urol 1987;137:1136.

39. Rowland RG, Kropp BP. Evolution of the Indiana continent urinary reservoir. J Urol 1994;152(6 Pt 2):2247–51.

40. Chowdhary SK, Rao KL, Kandpal DK, et al. Indiana pouch in children: a 15-year experience. J Pediatr Urol 2014;10(5):911–6.

41. Leonard MP, Gearhart JP, Jeffs RD. Continent urinary reservoirs in pediatric urological practice. J Urol 1990;144(2 Pt 1):330–3.

42. Bassiouny IE. Continent urinary reservoir in exstrophy/epispadias complex. BJU Int 1992;70(5):558–62.

43. Roth S, Semjonow A, Waldner M, et al. Risk of bowel dysfunction with diarrhea after continent urinary diversion with ileal and ileocecal segments. J Urol 1995;154(5):1696–9.

44. Schlomer BJ, Saperston K, Baskin L. National trends in augmentation cystoplasty in the 2000s and factors associated with patient outcomes. J Urol 2013; 190(4):1352–7.

45. Gundeti MS, Acharya SS, Zagaja GP, et al. Paediatric robotic-assisted laparoscopic augmentation ileocystoplasty and Mitrofanoff appendicovesicostomy (RALIMA): feasibility of and initial experience with

the University of Chicago technique. BJU Int 2014; 107(6):962–9.

46. Metcalfe PD, Rink RC. Bladder augmentation: complications in the pediatric population. Curr Urol Rep 2007;8(2):152–6.

47. Schlomer BJ, Copp HL. Cumulative incidence of outcomes and urologic procedures after augmentation cystoplasty. J Pediatr Urol 2014;10(6):1043–50.

48. Leonard MP, Dharamsi N, Williot PE. Outcome of gastrocystoplasty in tertiary pediatric urology practice. J Urol 2000;164(3):947–50.

49. Palmer LS, Franco I, Kogan SJ, et al. Urolithiasis in children following augmentation cystoplasty. J Urol 1993;150(2 Pt 2):726–9.

50. Szymanski KM, Misseri R, Whittam B, et al. Bladder stones after bladder augmentation are not what they seem. J Pediatr Urol 2016;12(2):98.e1.

51. Hensle TW, Reiley EA, Fam MM, et al. Enterocystoplasty: the long-term effects on bone mineral density. J Pediatr Urol 2016;12(4):245.e1.

52. Shokeir AA, Shamaa M, El-Mekresh MM, et al. Late malignancy in bowel segments exposed to urine without fecal stream. Urology 1995;46(5):657–61.

53. Soergel TM, Cain MP, Misseri R, et al. Transitional cell carcinoma of the bladder following augmentation cystoplasty for the neuropathic bladder. J Urol 2004;172:1649.

54. Lloyd M. Ectopia vesicae (absence of the anterior walls of the bladder), operation, and subsequent death. Lancet 1851;2:370–2.

55. Pettersson L, Tranberg J, Abrahamsson K, et al. Half century of followup after ureterosigmoidostomy performed in early childhood. J Urol 2013;189(5):1870–5.

56. Stein R, Fisch M, Beetz R, et al. Urinary diversion in children and young adults using the Mainz pouch I technique. BJU Int 1997;79(3):354–61.

57. North AC, Lakshmanan Y. Malignancy associated with the use of intestinal segments in the urinary tract. Urol Oncol 2007;25(2):165–7.

58. Sohn M, Füzesi L, Deutz F, et al. Signet ring cell carcinoma in adenomatous polyp at site of ureterosigmoidostomy 16 years after conversion to ileal conduit. J Urol 1990;143(4):805–7.

Tissue Engineering and Conduit Substitution

Scott C. Johnson, MD[a],*, Zachary L. Smith, MD[a], Bryan S. Sack, MD[b], Gary D. Steinberg, MD[a]

KEYWORDS

- Urinary diversion • Radical cystectomy • Tissue engineering • Regenerative medicine • Scaffolds

KEY POINTS

- Radical cystectomy with urinary diversion is associated with significant morbidity, which could be reduced substantially with a tissue engineered substitute for bowel.
- Efforts to develop a tissue engineered urinary conduit have involved scaffolds with or without cell seeding.
- Significant hurdles remain to the development of a clinically useful tissue engineered urinary conduit.

INTRODUCTION

For centuries, regeneration observed in organisms such as amphibians and crustaceans has fueled enthusiasm for the potential of regenerative medicine. The ability to recreate functional biological structures through tissue engineering (TE) represents a substantial goal, which would have a dramatic impact across multiple fields of medicine, including organ transplantation, reconstruction, and oncology. Although pioneering work on TE has been ongoing for decades, intense media interest was ignited in 1995, when images of the "auriculosaurus" were broadcast by the British Broadcasting Company (**Fig. 1**). The now highly recognized mouse—which appeared as if it was growing a human ear along its dorsum—immediately captured the imagination of the public and many believed rapid advancements in the field of TE were forthcoming. In reality, the synthetic ear-shaped scaffold, which was seeded with bovine cells and implanted on the back of a nude mouse by Charles Vacanti and his team, represented an important proof of concept in TE, but not the advent of xenotransplantation. Nevertheless, substantial attention and lofty expectations resulted in high enthusiasm for the promise of TE and regenerative medicine. The seemingly limitless possibilities of regenerative medicine were explored in popular culture as evidenced by major motion pictures such as *The Island* (Warner Bros. Entertainment Inc), which portrayed a dystopian world where humans were cloned for producing autografts. Headlines such as *Grow Your Own Replacement Parts* were seen on mainstream media outlets, signaling an impending medical revolution.[1] Despite the initial excitement, it has now been more than 2 decades since the auriculosaurus caught our attention, and although significant advances have been made, widespread clinical applications of TE remain very limited.

Some pioneering TE efforts have come in the field of urology. In 2006, Atala and colleagues[2] published what was viewed as significant breakthrough at the time, detailing the creation and implantation of tissue engineered bladders in 7 patients with myelomeningocele. Synthetic and composite synthetic natural bladder–shaped scaffolds were seeded with bladder cells obtained via

Disclosure: The authors have nothing they wish to disclose.
[a] Department of Surgery, Section of Urology, The University of Chicago, 5841 South Maryland Avenue, MC-6038, Chicago, IL 60637, USA; [b] Department of Urology, Boston Children's Hospital, 300 Longwood Avenue, Hunnewell 3, Boston, MA 02115, USA
* Corresponding author.
E-mail address: scott.johnson@uchospitals.edu

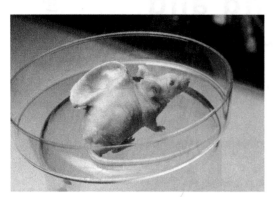

Fig. 1. Images of the "auriculosaurus," a mouse with a subcutaneously implanted ear-shaped scaffold were broadcast by the British Broadcasting Company in 1995, catapulting the prospect of tissue engineering into public consciousness. (*Courtesy of* the British Broadcasting Corporation London, United Kingdom; with permission.)

biopsy and incubated for several weeks. The engineered bladders were then used to augment the native bladder and preliminary results were encouraging—after a mean follow-up of 46 months, the bladders were functioning normally. In 2011, Raya-Rivera and coworkers[3] reported promising results in 5 boys who underwent urethral reconstruction with tissue-engineered tubular urethras. Autologous muscle and epithelial cells were seeded onto a synthetic tubular scaffold in vitro and the engineered urethras were used in posterior urethroplasty. After a median follow-up of 71 months, the urethras remained patent and biopsies confirmed normal urethral histology.

For numerous reasons, the bowel is used frequently in urinary reconstruction. Its relatively abundant supply and rich vascularization make it an attractive substitute for urothelium; however, its absorptive nature is not ideal for use in the urinary system and results in a number of metabolic disturbances. These limitations were a major motivation in efforts to design a tissue engineered bladder augment. Urinary diversion after radical cystectomy (RC) represents the most common uses of bowel in urology. RC with urinary diversion is associated with significant morbidity; nearly two-thirds of patients experience a perioperative complication, of which the majority are gastrointestinal in nature.[4] The development of a tissue-engineered substitute for urinary diversion likely would dramatically reduce the perioperative and metabolic morbidity associated with the use of bowel after RC. A fully functional, continent replacement bladder would represent a remarkable achievement in TE, but is far from clinical reality with our current technology. Recent efforts

have instead focused on developing a tubular conduit for use in incontinent urinary diversion. Although there are significant challenges in any TE application, tubular structures such as a conduit represent a lower level of complexity than hollow, distensible organs such as the bladder and far less complexity than end-organs such as kidneys. In this paper, we review the current approaches for TE, limitations of current technology as well as clinical experience with the development of tissue-engineered urinary conduits (TEUC).

TISSUE ENGINEERING APPROACHES

There are several approaches that have been explored for TE. The bulk of efforts at developing a TEUC have used scaffolds with or without cell seeding. Scaffolds are an acellular matrix that provides structural support and a backbone for cells to proliferate. Cell seeding has been attempted with several different cell types, all with particular advantages and significant hurdles. Finally, and possibly most challenging, is that a suitable host environment needs to exist to promote the expansion and organization of cells. This includes adequate vascularization, appropriate growth factors, and immune regulation. There are efforts underway to understand and harness the natural self-assembly of cells for scaffold-free approaches to TE, but the majority of clinical applications now use the scaffold and cell seeding approach.

Scaffolds

A particular challenge with many TE applications is that target tissue has not have fully developed at the time of implantation, yet it must immediately perform as a functioning organ. In the case of a TEUC, once surgically implanted, it must immediately serve its basic function, passively transporting urine to the external environment and also must act as an impenetrable barrier to urine, which can diffuse into surrounding tissue, resulting in inflammation and fibrosis. Additionally, cells need a physical structure on which to migrate and guide growth into the desired tissue architecture. Scaffolds help to solve these issues as a 3-dimensional structure that provides physical support and an organizing template for cells to proliferate. The ideal scaffold would provide adequate mechanical support, allow for rapid cell ingrowth, elicit no adverse physiologic or immunologic reaction, and completely dissolve over time. Unfortunately, a material that perfectly fulfills these requirements has yet to be identified; these qualities often juxtapose one another. For example, to enhance cellular ingrowth a TEUC scaffold needs to be sufficiently porous, however, this sacrifices its mechanical strength and function as a barrier to urine. Furthermore, scaffolds that completely degrade release byproducts, which may lead to a foreign body reaction.

Materials for use as scaffolds are generally organized into 3 categories: acellular tissue matrices such as small intestine submucosa or decellularized bladder matrix, naturally derived materials such as collagen or silk, and synthetic polymers such as polylactic acid, polyglycolic acid (PGA), and polylactic-glycolic acid (PLGA). Acellular tissue matrices have been created from a variety of sources, both allogeneic and xenogeneic. They are created by decellularization of harvested tissue and their architecture is based on the tissue from which they are derived. Once processed, what remains is a protein matrix consisting largely of collagen and elastin. These materials are attractive for use because they provide a 3-dimensional microstructure conducive to cellular ingrowth and organization. Additionally, they contain growth factors, which may aid in cellular migration and differentiation.[5] Small animal studies using these materials in urologic applications have shown some promise,[6,7] but a number of factors have limited their clinical investigation. First, the cost and availability of these materials can be prohibitive, whether they are sourced from animals or cadavers. Additionally, as a result of decellularization and heterogenic structure, they have limited, unreliable mechanical properties, which may make them unsuitable for use as a TEUC.

Naturally derived materials such as collagen, silk, and alginate have been developed for use in TE applications and offer some distinct advantages. These natural polymers are highly biocompatible and have found numerous medical applications.[8] They also biodegrade over time and allow engineered tissue to create their own extracellular matrix. Alginate is unlikely to be useful in a TEUC because it lacks mechanical the strength that would be required.[8] Silk is a naturally derived material that has been used for multiple medical uses owing to its versatility and biocompatibility. It has not been explored specifically in the context of a TEUC; however, preclinical research as a TE scaffold in the urinary system has been encouraging.[9] Collagen is a ubiquitous structural protein and has been studied extensively as a possible scaffold in urothelial TE applications. It is a versatile material that can be fabricated in a number of configurations and densities. To allow maximal cell ingrowth and nutrient diffusion, the matrix should be maximally porous[10]; however, this can result in inadequate

mechanical strength. The development of collagen hybrid materials may overcome some of these mechanical limitations while allowing adequate tissue development.[11]

Synthetic biomaterials overcome many of the structural and mechanical shortcomings of other materials. Polymers such as polylactic acid, PGA, and PLGA can be manufactured with precise, reliable mechanical properties in virtually any size or configuration desired.[12] The US Food and Drug Administration has approved the use of these materials for a variety of applications, including sutures. Although the versatility and structural properties of synthetic scaffolds make them very appealing, their main disadvantage is poor biocompatibility and the ability to invoke a foreign body reaction. This factor is partially owing to the acidic microenvironment created with hydrolytic degradation of the polymer. Further work to create a pH-neutral material[13] or the incorporation of growth factors may help to develop a synthetic scaffold that better supports the cellular development of a graft.

Cells

The use of unseeded scaffolds is limited by the presence and proximity of native cells, which only have the ability to migrate very small distances.[14] Owing to this limitation, seeding of scaffolds with cells has proved essential for most tubular applications in humans. De Filippo and colleagues[15] showed that urethroplasty with unseeded tubularized grafts invariably resulted in fibrosis and stricture, whereas seeded grafts maintained patency and developed normal urethral architecture. Similarly, Drewa and colleagues[16] demonstrated in a rat model that synthetic bladder augments seeded with fibroblasts resulted in complete epithelization, whereas unseeded grafts lacked epithelization in the central portion of the graft, highlighting the limited ingrowth ability of native cells.

Multiple cell lines and sources have been attempted and no perfect cell has been identified for cell seeding. The ideal cell would be easy to obtain, and proliferate efficiently in culture conditions without invoking a detrimental immune response. A functioning TEUC would resemble other urothelial tissue in the body, consisting of urothelial cells (UC) to form an impermeable barrier to urine and smooth muscle cells (SMC) to provide structure and contractility for urine transport. Whether the seeded cell should be fully differentiated, capable of target cell differentiation, or unrelated to the target cell line but exist to supply a suitable environment for target cell ingrowth is still being investigated. It may, in fact, be a combination of cell types that is most appropriate. With each cell type, there exists unique challenges to overcome. Ideally, an autologous cell would be used to avoid an immune response, but this introduces issues associated with cell harvest. Furthermore, the use of autologous cells raises significant concerns in the setting of malignancy, specifically with the use of differentiated UC lines. Another challenge with suitable cell identification for TE is the proliferative capacity of a cell, which is inherent to the cell itself, the cell line, and the culture conditions. This point is especially salient in the setting of bladder cancer, because delays in cystectomy can lead to poor outcomes. From harvest to implantation, an acceptable TEUC using autologous cells would need to be produced without introducing further delays in time to RC.

Urothelial Cells

Typically, cells for use in TE applications can be obtained from biopsies of autologous healthy tissue. The use of UC from the bladder may be appropriate for benign applications of a TEUC; however, it introduces the risk of malignancy in the setting of bladder cancer. The use of any autologous UC carries theoretic risk, but some investigators have suggested that UC from the upper tract may be acceptable evidenced by the relatively low risk of upper urinary tract disease in patients with bladder cancer.[17] UCs have successfully been cultured for decades[18] and have numerous applications in vitro. Liao and colleagues[7] reported that the use of grafts seeded with UCs in a rabbit model resulted in less fibrosis and obstruction. They concluded that preseeding with UCs reestablished a blood–urine barrier, which allows successful regeneration to occur in the absence of toxic metabolites present in urine. Conversely, Geutjes and colleagues[19] evaluated a TEUC in a pig model with and without seeding of UC cells obtained by bladder biopsy. In their study, the TEUC resulted in obstruction and hydronephrosis in all cases and no benefit was found for UC seeding of the scaffold. It is not clear whether seeding with UC alone provides substantial benefit, and the inherent risks associated with their use may hamper their clinical investigation.

Smooth Muscle Cells

Whereas UC form the impermeable outer layer of urothelial tissue, SMCs help to provide support and allow contractility. SMCs have been used alone and in conjunction with UCs for the purpose of seeding engineered scaffolds. Attempts at creating TE bladders for augmentation cystoplasty in neurogenic bladder patients used constructs seeded with UCs and SMCs, and resulted in the formation of normal appearing urothelial histology.[2] Similar to UCs, SMCs can be harvested from a patient's own urothelial tissue, but this too raises concerns in the setting of malignancy. Fortunately, SMCs can be harvested from a variety of tissues, including adipose, peripheral blood, cord blood, and bone marrow. In a pig model, Basu and colleagues[20] showed that SMCs derived from either adipose tissue, peripheral blood, or urothelium could be used successfully for seeding tubular scaffolds. Furthermore, they showed that this process resulted in tissue histologically similar to native urothelium regardless of the SMC source.

Stem Cells

Stem cells have been the subject of intense investigation owing to their potentially broad therapeutic application. Stem cells are characterized by their regenerative ability and their ability to produce specialized tissue from an undifferentiated state. Accordingly, they could represent an ideal source of cells for use in TE. Stem cells were classically obtained from embryonic tissue or nonembryonic "adult" tissue. More recently, induced pluripotent stem cells (iPSC) have become another source of stem cells that has received much attention.

Embryonic stem cells (ESC) are derived from the inner layer of blastocysts and can give rise to any fully differentiated adult cell type. Early work showed that ESC seeding was enhanced by co-seeding with UC or SMC, suggesting that ESC may promote migration of cells and development of urothelial tissue.[21] More recently, methods for inducing the development of urothelial tissue directly from ESC have been developed in vitro.[22] Unfortunately, the clinical use of ESCs is hampered by several issues, most notably the well-publicized ethical concerns that have been raised. Additionally, implantation of ESCs has been associated with teratoma formation in vivo.[23] Finally, differentiated cells from allogeneic ESCs express foreign major histocompatibility complex molecules and may induce a rejection response.

The iPSCs are fully differentiated adult cells that have been manipulated genetically to behave similar to ESCs. The use of iPSCs overcomes the ethical issues associated with ESCs and could represent a reliable source of autologous tissue for use in TEUCs. The iPSCs have been successfully used in the laboratory to create urothelial tissue in vitro.[24,25] A significant hurdle for the clinical use of iPSCs is their malignant potential, because the genetic modifications used to create them can introduce unwanted oncogenes. Developing safe methods of cell reprogramming and successfully harnessing the pluripotent ability to form functional tissue may one day make iPSCs the ideal cell for use in TEUCs.

Adult stem cells, or somatic stem cells (SSC), have been used most extensively in TE applications. SSC are undifferentiated cells found to exist among differentiated cells throughout the body. SSC have been preferred to ESCs and iPSCs for a number of reasons. SSC are easily obtained from several sources, and their use is not ethically objected to. Additionally, the use of SSC does not introduce an inherent risk of malignancy, and the use of autologous cell lines can avoid issues with rejection. SSC from numerous sources have been used to create engineered urothelial tissue, including bone marrow,[26] adipose tissue,[27] hair follicles,[28] amniotic fluid,[29] endometrium,[30] and even urine-derived cells.[17] Adipose-derived SSC have been shown to differentiate into urothelial tissue under the correct conditions and could be an ideal source for such cells.[27,31,32] Subcutaneous adipose tissue is abundant and easily accessible via biopsy for autologous harvesting. Additionally, SSC account for 3% of isolated cells in adipose tissue, a relative abundance compared with the 0.001% that can be expected from bone marrow. An important caveat is that urothelial tissue derived from undifferentiated stem cell lines has been identified by molecular markers only and may not necessarily be phenotypically similar to native urothelial tissue. Additionally, the lifespan and regenerative ability of SSC is variable and not well-understood, which could impact the long-term success of engineered tissue using them.

Host Environment

Choosing the appropriate scaffold and cell type is not sufficient for successfully creating a TEUC. Providing the appropriate microenvironment to promote and support appropriate tissue development is essential. Our current limited understanding in this area may represent the largest hurdle to clinically useful engineered tissue. Among the challenges are understanding and maintaining the appropriate milieu of growth factors and cytokines to promote healthy tissue and avoid fibrosis. Equally important is establishing an adequate blood supply and neural innervation, a unique challenge in the development of a heterotopic neo-organ such as a TEUC.

Several growth factors have been identified as important in the development of functional urothelial tissue. Vascular endothelial growth factor is a well-recognized promoter of angiogenesis and has been shown to be crucial in cell growth and development. Loai and colleagues[33] showed that the incorporation of vascular endothelial growth factor into an acellular bladder graft resulted in improved angiogenesis as well as increased regeneration of UCs and SMCs. Fibroblast growth factor is a mediator of paracrine signaling and important in the remodeling and maintenance of urothelial smooth muscle.[34] Insulinlike growth factor-1 is a known regulator of cell growth and proliferation, and has been shown to be important in urothelial regeneration.[35] When stem cells are used, the presence of appropriate growth factors is essential to efficient and anticipated target cell differentiation. Transforming growth factor-β1, platelet-derived growth factor-BB, and epidermal growth factor have been used to successfully differentiate stem cells from bone marrow into tissue resembling native urothelium.[36] Whether differentiation is induced in vivo or in vitro, sustaining such growth factors is likely essential for ongoing cell proliferation and phenotypic stability.[37]

As mentioned, acellular organic scaffolds are attractive because they can be a source for relevant growth factors. Collagen scaffolds, for example, can be a significant source of growth factors such as vascular endothelial growth factor, transforming growth factor-β1, and fibroblast growth factor.[5] Unfortunately, these growth factors present in naturally derived scaffolds are not sufficient to maintain urothelial regeneration.[38] Alternative strategies investigated for growth factor delivery include scaffold impregnation and endogenous production from seeded cells, which could be induced through genetic manipulation. The complex microenvironment supportive of regeneration is poorly understood, however, and approaches to synthetically create such an environment have had limited success.

Establishing an adequate vascular supply and nutrient delivery to engineered tissue has been an issue for many applications. Passive diffusion of nutrients in tissue is successful for lengths of less than 1 cm,[14] highlighting a substantial obstacle in the case of a TEUC, which would span a significantly longer distance in establishing continuity from the urinary tract to the skin. One solution for providing vascular supply involves the omentum, a versatile organ that has found innumerable uses in surgery, from reconstruction to wound healing and hemostasis. It has a rich vascular supply and is mobile enough for use throughout the abdomen, making it an ideal candidate for use in TEUC. The use of omentum as a vascular supply in other TE has produced encouraging results. Autologous bladders wrapped in omentum showed improved function compared with those not incorporating omentum.[2]

Clinical Experience

Unfortunately, despite some incremental success in the laboratory, the clinical experience with TEUC has been disappointing. The neo-urinary conduit (NUC; Tengion, Inc, Winston-Salem, NC) was a commercial attempt at developing a TEUC (**Fig. 2**). It used a synthetic PGA/PLGA scaffold seeded with adipose-derived autologous SMCs. Preclinical studies in pigs undergoing urinary diversion with the NUC showed evidence of tissue regeneration after 3 months. The lumen was covered by urothelium and the smooth muscle bundles were seen in the proximal and mid sections of the NUC as demonstrated by cytokeratin-7 and calponin-1 staining, respectively.[39]

A phase I clinical trial (NCT01087697) was designed with plans to recruit 10 patients for NUC implantation after RC.[40] The goal was to establish a safety profile and evaluate structural integrity and conduit patency. Autologous adipose-derived SMCs were obtained via abdominal wall fat biopsy and expanded in vitro for approximately 3 to 4 weeks. The cells were then seeded onto a biodegradable tubular scaffold composed of PGA and PLGA. After RC, the seeded graft was used analogous to a bowel segment in an incontinent conduit diversion. The graft was wrapped in omentum to promote vascularization, an essential step recognized in preclinical animal studies. At the distal end of the graft, a flush cutaneous stoma was created owing to the difficulty of everting the graft and establishing an adequate vascular supply. A total of 9 patients underwent NUC implantation. Although there was promising evidence of urothelial-like regeneration, issues with obstruction and stricture were significant. Stomal stenosis was an anticipated obstacle based on preclinical animal studies and was managed with silicone stomal ports; however, this measure proved insufficient to maintain long-term stomal patency. Additionally, ureteral anastomotic strictures and resultant hydronephrosis were commonly seen, despite Wallace-type anastomoses. Ultimately, all surviving patients required NUC explantation. The study showed that the NUC was not able to provide a safe, effective substitute for bowel in urinary diversion (Steinberg G and collegues, unpublished data, 2017).

Despite metabolic and gastrointestinal consequences, the use of bowel in urinary reconstruction remains the best option available. Enormous effort and resources have been expended to develop a suitable engineered substitute with no clinically applicable product on the foreseeable

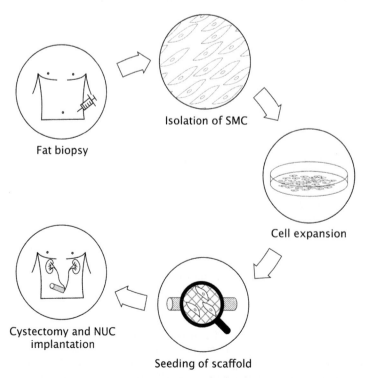

Fig. 2. Steps involved in the creation of the neourinary conduit (NUC). Autologous smooth muscle cells (SMC) are obtained by biopsy of peripheral adipose tissue, isolated, and seeded onto a synthetic polymer scaffold. The NUC is then implanted at the time of cystectomy to serve as an incontinent channel for urine to pass from the ureters to the skin level.

Fat biopsy

Isolation of SMC

Cell expansion

Seeding of scaffold

Cystectomy and NUC implantation

horizon. Unfortunately, even the more promising accomplishments have ended up leading to disappointing results. Enthusiasm surrounding the landmark report in 2006 of Dr Atala and his team creating engineered bladders for cystoplasty was tempered substantially when a subsequent phase II study showed no improvement in bladder capacity and an unacceptable safety profile.[41] On the heels of these disappointing clinical results, Tengion—the company behind development of the NUC, the TE bladder augment, and other TE ventures—declared bankruptcy in late 2014.

In the face of these clinical setbacks, investigators continue the work to develop a safe, functional substitute for urothelial tissue. A TEUC for clinical use is not likely in the short term, but further investigations are underway to identify a TE approach that translates into clinical success. Although a TEUC seems relatively simple in terms of its tubular structure, the interplay of host factors that drive the regeneration and homeostasis of a functional graft are more complex than we currently understand. Recently, Sloff and colleagues[42] described their experience with a TEUC in pigs which they preimplanted subcutaneously for 1 month before urinary diversion. This procedure resulted in improved drainage and vascularization compared with seeded or unseeded scaffolds. This strategy introduces new questions and challenges but might form the basis for overcoming issues with establishing a host environment capable of maintaining a functional TEUC. A significant amount of work has been done to identify an ideal scaffold and cell to seed it; however, the development of a successful TEUC may stem from an entirely different approach. Work in better understanding embryonic urothelial differentiation and the self-assembly of tissues is ongoing and may lead to TE approaches avoiding the use of synthetic materials.[43] Rapidly developing technology is introducing new tools that could change the way TE is approached. Notably, clustered regularly interspaced short palindromic repeats (CRISPR) technology is a new tool that allows for gene editing with unprecedented efficiency and accuracy. The potential impact and application of CRISPR technology is vast and will undoubtedly have a place in TE. It is possible that CRISPR technology may one day pave the way for the engineering of immunocompatible tissues in animals—indeed, the misconceived anticipation of the auriculosaurus more than 20 years ago.

SUMMARY

A TE alternative to the use of bowel in urinary diversion could represent a substantial reduction in the morbidity of RC. The current approach to developing a TEUC incorporates a scaffold seeded with cells; however, neither the ideal cell nor scaffold material has been identified. Supplying a suitable host environment for tissue development and support represents an additional obstacle that must be overcome before a clinically useful TEUC is attainable. Early enthusiasm for TE applications was strong, and although the rapid development of engineered tissue for clinical use has not become a reality, we have come to better understand the complex issues which must be solved for successful TE. Despite hurdles yet to be overcome, TE applications such as TEUCs have the potential to substantially reduce burden of disease for patients, fueling ongoing research in this area. Future advances in biomaterial technology and our understanding of tissue development may help overcome current hurdles in TE or lead to a new approach in TE altogether.

REFERENCES

1. Andrews W. Grow your own replacement parts. Available at: http://www.cbsnews.com/news/grow-your-own-replacement-parts/. Accessed March 1, 2017.
2. Atala A, Bauer SB, Soker S, et al. Tissue-engineered autologous bladders for patients needing cystoplasty. Lancet 2006;367:1241–6.
3. Raya-Rivera A, Esquiliano DR, Yoo JJ, et al. Tissue-engineered autologous urethras for patients who need reconstruction: an observational study. Lancet 2011;377:1175–82.
4. Shabsigh A, Korets R, Vora KC, et al. Defining early morbidity of radical cystectomy for patients with bladder cancer using a standardized reporting methodology. Eur Urol 2009;55:164–74.
5. Kanematsu A, Yamamoto S, Ozeki M, et al. Collagenous matrices as release carriers of exogenous growth factors. Biomaterials 2004;25:4513–20.
6. Drewa T. The artificial conduit for urinary diversion in rats: a preliminary study. Transplant Proc 2007;39: 1647–51.
7. Liao W, Yang S, Song C, et al. Tissue-engineered tubular graft for urinary diversion after radical cystectomy in rabbits. J Surg Res 2013;182:185–91.
8. Kim BS, Baez CE, Atala A. Biomaterials for tissue engineering. World J Urol 2000;18:2–9.
9. Sack BS, Mauney JR, Estrada CR. Silk fibroin scaffolds for urologic tissue engineering. Curr Urol Rep 2016;17:16.
10. Melchels FP, Tonnarelli B, Olivares AL, et al. The influence of the scaffold design on the distribution of adhering cells after perfusion cell seeding. Biomaterials 2011;32:2878–84.

11. Ajalloueian F, Zeiai S, Fossum M, et al. Constructs of electrospun PLGA, compressed collagen and minced urothelium for minimally manipulated autologous bladder tissue expansion. Biomaterials 2014; 35:5741–8.

12. Webb AR, Yang J, Ameer GA. Biodegradable polyester elastomers in tissue engineering. Expert Opin Biol Ther 2004;4:801–12.

13. Heffernan MJ, Murthy N. Polyketal nanoparticles: a new pH-sensitive biodegradable drug delivery vehicle. Bioconjug Chem 2005;16:1340–2.

14. Dorin RP, Pohl HG, De Filippo RE, et al. Tubularized urethral replacement with unseeded matrices: what is the maximum distance for normal tissue regeneration. World J Urol 2008;26:323–6.

15. De Filippo RE, Yoo JJ, Atala A. Urethral replacement using cell seeded tubularized collagen matrices. J Urol 2002;168:1789–92 [discussion: 1792].

16. Drewa T, Sir J, Czajkowski R, et al. Scaffold seeded with cells is essential in urothelium regeneration and tissue remodeling in vivo after bladder augmentation using in vitro engineered graft. In Transplantation proceedings 2006;38(1):133–5. Elsevier.

17. Bodin A, Bharadwaj S, Wu S, et al. Tissue-engineered conduit using urine-derived stem cells seeded bacterial cellulose polymer in urinary reconstruction and diversion. Biomaterials 2010;31: 8889–901.

18. Sutherland GR, Bain AD. Culture of cells from the urine of newborn children. Nature 1972;239:231.

19. Geutjes P, Roelofs L, Hoogenkamp H, et al. Tissue engineered tubular construct for urinary diversion in a preclinical porcine model. J Urol 2012;188: 653–60.

20. Basu J, Jayo MJ, Ilagan RM, et al. Regeneration of native-like neo-urinary tissue from nonbladder cell sources. Tissue Eng Part A 2012;18:1025–34.

21. Frimberger D, Morales N, Gearhart JD, et al. Human embryoid body-derived stem cells in tissue engineering-enhanced migration in co-culture with bladder smooth muscle and urothelium. Urology 2006;67:1298–303.

22. Osborn SL, Thangappan R, Luria A, et al. Induction of human embryonic and induced pluripotent stem cells into urothelium. Stem Cells Transl Med 2014; 3:610–9.

23. Hentze H, Soong PL, Wang ST, et al. Teratoma formation by human embryonic stem cells: evaluation of essential parameters for future safety studies. Stem Cell Res 2009;2:198–210.

24. Moad M, Pal D, Hepburn AC, et al. A novel model of urinary tract differentiation, tissue regeneration, and disease: reprogramming human prostate and bladder cells into induced pluripotent stem cells. Eur Urol 2013;64:753–61.

25. Shi L, Cui Y, Luan J, et al. Urine-derived induced pluripotent stem cells as a modeling tool to study rare human diseases. Intractable Rare Dis Res 2016;5:192–201.

26. Sharma AK, Bury MI, Marks AJ, et al. A nonhuman primate model for urinary bladder regeneration using autologous sources of bone marrow-derived mesenchymal stem cells. Stem Cells 2011;29: 241–50.

27. Shi JG, Fu WJ, Wang XX, et al. Transdifferentiation of human adipose-derived stem cells into urothelial cells: potential for urinary tract tissue engineering. Cell Tissue Res 2012;347:737–46.

28. Drewa T, Joachimiak R, Bajek A, et al. Hair follicle stem cells can be driven into a urothelial-like phenotype: an experimental study. Int J Urol 2013; 20:537–42.

29. Kang HH, Kang JJ, Kang HG, et al. Urothelial differentiation of human amniotic fluid stem cells by urothelium specific conditioned medium. Cell Biol Int 2014;38:531–7.

30. Shoae-Hassani A, Sharif S, Seifalian AM, et al. Endometrial stem cell differentiation into smooth muscle cell: a novel approach for bladder tissue engineering in women. BJU Int 2013;112:854–63.

31. Jack GS, Zhang R, Lee M, et al. Urinary bladder smooth muscle engineered from adipose stem cells and a three dimensional synthetic composite. Biomaterials 2009;30:3259–70.

32. Zhang M, Xu MX, Zhou Z, et al. The differentiation of human adipose-derived stem cells towards a urothelium-like phenotype in vitro and the dynamic temporal changes of related cytokines by both paracrine and autocrine signal regulation. PLoS One 2014;9:e95583.

33. Loai Y, Yeger H, Coz C, et al. Bladder tissue engineering: tissue regeneration and neovascularization of ha-VEGF-incorporated bladder acellular constructs in mouse and porcine animal models. J Biomed Mater Res A 2010;94:1205–15.

34. Imamura M, Kanematsu A, Yamamoto S, et al. Basic fibroblast growth factor modulates proliferation and collagen expression in urinary bladder smooth muscle cells. Am J Physiol Renal Physiol 2007;293:F1007–17.

35. Lorentz KM, Yang L, Frey P, et al. Engineered insulin-like growth factor-1 for improved smooth muscle regeneration. Biomaterials 2012;33:494–503.

36. Tian H, Bharadwaj S, Liu Y, et al. Myogenic differentiation of human bone marrow mesenchymal stem cells on a 3d nano fibrous scaffold for bladder tissue engineering. Biomaterials 2010;31:870–7.

37. Gordeladze JO, Reseland JE, Duroux-Richard I, et al. From stem cells to bone: phenotype acquisition, stabilization, and tissue engineering in animal models. ILAR J 2009;51:42–61.

38. Lam HJ, Patel S, Wang A, et al. In vitro regulation of neural differentiation and axon growth by growth factors and bioactive nanofibers. Tissue Eng Part A 2010;16:2641–8.

39. Bivalacqua T, Steinberg G, Smith N, et al. 178 Pre-clinical and clinical translation of a tissue engineered neo–urinary conduit using adipose derived smooth muscle cells for urinary reconstruction. European Urology Supplements 2014;13(1): e178.

40. Tengion. Incontinent urinary diversion using an autologous neo-urinary conduit. ClinicalTrials gov Identifier: NCT01087697. 2012. Available at: https://clinicaltrials.gov/show/NCT01087697. Accessed March 1, 2017.

41. Joseph DB, Borer JG, De Filippo RE, et al. Autologous cell seeded biodegradable scaffold for augmentation cystoplasty: phase II study in children and adolescents with spina bifida. J Urol 2014;191: 1389–95.

42. Sloff M, Simaioforidis V, Tiemessen DM, et al. Tubular constructs as artificial urinary conduits. J Urol 2016;196:1279–86.

43. Marga F, Neagu A, Kosztin I, et al. Developmental biology and tissue engineering. Birth Defects Res C Embryo Today 2007;81:320–8.

Printed and bound by CPI Group (UK) Ltd, Croydon, CR0 4YY

03/10/2024

01040302-0011